AF356657

Identification and Characterization of Genetic Components in Autism Spectrum Disorders 2020

Identification and Characterization of Genetic Components in Autism Spectrum Disorders 2020

Editor

Merlin G. Butler

MDPI • Basel • Beijing • Wuhan • Barcelona • Belgrade • Manchester • Tokyo • Cluj • Tianjin

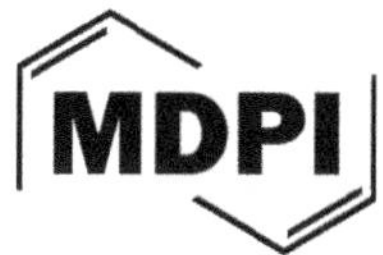

Editor
Merlin G. Butler
University of Kansas Medical
Center
USA

Editorial Office
MDPI
St. Alban-Anlage 66
4052 Basel, Switzerland

This is a reprint of articles from the Special Issue published online in the open access journal *International Journal of Molecular Sciences* (ISSN 1422-0067) (available at: https://www.mdpi.com/journal/ijms/special_issues/ASD_2020).

For citation purposes, cite each article independently as indicated on the article page online and as indicated below:

LastName, A.A.; LastName, B.B.; LastName, C.C. Article Title. *Journal Name* **Year**, *Volume Number*, Page Range.

ISBN 978-3-0365-3611-8 (Hbk)
ISBN 978-3-0365-3612-5 (PDF)

Contents

About the Editor

Merlin G. Butler MD, PhD is Professor of Psychiatry & Behavioral Sciences and Pediatrics at the University of Kansas Medical Center, Kansas City, Director of the Division of Research and Genetics and Director of the University of Kansas Health System Genetics Clinic. He received his MD degree from the University of Nebraska College of Medicine in 1978 and his PhD in Medical Genetics from Indiana University School of Medicine in Indianapolis, where he also trained and completed his postgraduate training and fellowship in medical genetics accredited by the American Board of Medical Genetics (ABMG). He received ABMG board certification in both Clinical Genetics and Clinical Cytogenetics in 1984. He is also a Founding Fellow of the American College of Medical Genetics and Genomics. He previously held faculty and academic positions at Indiana University, the University of Notre Dame, Vanderbilt University, and the University of Missouri–Kansas City prior to his arrival at the University of Kansas Medical Center in 2008.

Dr. Butler is an appointed member of local academic and state programs for genetic screening services as well as national committees engaged in the care and treatment of those with rare genetic disorders. He is also a member of federal and parent-based organizations or foundations participating in grant review study sections. He serves as a member of several editorial boards for peer-reviewed journals and is an Associate Editor of *Frontiers in Genetics* and *Frontiers in Pediatrics*. He is a recipient of local academic and national honors in recognition of his research and clinical service in genetic disorders. He is a member of advisory board organizations for rare disorders including Mowat–Wilson syndrome and is Chairperson of the Scientific Advisory Board of the Prader–Willi Syndrome Association (USA). His research interests include the genetics of developmental disorders, congenital anomalies, connective tissue disorders, autism, and mechanisms of genomic imprinting and impact on Prader–Willi, Angelman, Burnside–Butler, and fragile X syndromes. His research is focused on genotype–phenotype correlations and delineation with natural history of rare disorders as well as the use of advanced genetic technology, including high-resolution microarrays, next-generation sequencing, and pharmacogenetics testing, in clinical practice. He has published over 500 peer-reviewed articles, over 50 book chapters and authored or edited 20 books on the principles of medical genetics and clinical description, management, and care of patients with common and rare genetic disorders, specifically Prader–Willi, fragile X and Burnside–Butler syndromes, the genetics of autism and syndromic obesity, congenital anomalies, intellectual disabilities, and clinical applications of advanced genetic testing.

Preface to "Identification and Characterization of Genetic Components in Autism Spectrum Disorders 2020"

This textbook, *The Identification of the Genetic Components of Autism Spectrum Disorders 2020*, includes themes associated with autism spectrum disorders (ASD) and related conditions divided into three sections (clinical, genetics, other) covering topics discussed in 2020. These sections include: information on clinical description and phenotypic subtyping, causes, diagnosis, treatment, and characterization of ASD and biomarker development related to neurodevelopmental disorders; the overview of genetic, epigenetic, and environmental factors involved in ASD; characterization of findings in autism based on genomics advanced laboratory testing and genetics with bioinformatics and translational research and characterization of an emerging 15q11.2 BP1-BP2 deletion (Burnside–Butler) syndrome as a cause of autism and neurodevelopmental defects; and other factors contributing to our understanding of causation of ASD, including proteomics and metabolomics with approaches towards functional insights into autism.

This textbook includes nine chapters written by experts in the field of genetics, medical care with treatment approaches and diagnosis, autism research and discovery with characterization, and analysis of genetic and environmental factors. Of these, five chapters are dedicated to clinical description, treatment, and characterization with relevant reviews of ASD and related conditions or contributing factors; three chapters are dedicated to basic laboratory or translational research with genetic data analysis and reviews regarding their contribution to ASD, as 90% of individuals with autism may have a genetic component contributing to their clinical findings; and one chapter describes proteomics and metabolic approaches contributing to ASD and biomarker discovery in order to allow readers to acquire a better understanding and awareness of ASD.

This textbook should be a useful resource for scientists and clinical researchers, medical geneticists, and physicians and clinicians in caring for and managing patients with the goal to translate this information directly to the clinical setting for diagnosis, care, and treatment of patients with ASD. Other healthcare providers and paraprofessionals should be interested, particularly those engaged in teaching, research, care, and treatment, including students at all levels of training and families regarding this important neurodevelopmental disorder which is on the rise in our society and worldwide.

Ultimately, the team of healthcare professionals required to diagnose, treat and care for the growing list of problems recognized or understudied in ASD may include psychiatrists, psychologists and laboratory geneticists, clinical geneticists and genetic counselors, neurologists, special educators and paraprofessionals, child life experts, developmental specialists and pediatricians, social workers, nurses and nurse practitioners, occupational and physical therapists, as well as speech therapists and pathologists; furthermore, public health experts and community activists will find this resource helpful in recognizing features seen in autism and understanding and identifying casuses. Lastly, this book can serve as a resource for students, parents, and other family members for better awareness about the risks, features, and causes of autism as well as agencies providing care, information, resources, and services for those families with autism and/or related neurodevelopmental disorders.

Merlin G. Butler

Editor

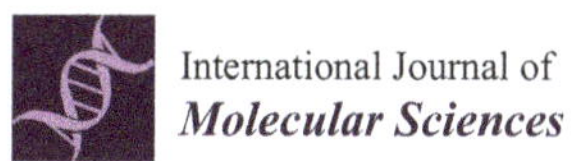

International Journal of
Molecular Sciences

MDPI

Review

Clinical Assessment, Genetics, and Treatment Approaches in Autism Spectrum Disorder (ASD)

Ann Genovese and Merlin G. Butler *

Department of Psychiatry & Behavioral Sciences, University of Kansas Medical Center, Kansas City, KS 66160, USA; agenovese@kumc.edu

* Correspondence: mbutler4@kumc.edu; Tel.: +1-913-588-1800; Fax: +1-913-588-1305

Received: 1 May 2020; Accepted: 27 June 2020; Published: 2 July 2020

Abstract: Autism spectrum disorder (ASD) consists of a genetically heterogenous group of neurobehavioral disorders characterized by impairment in three behavioral domains including communication, social interaction, and stereotypic repetitive behaviors. ASD affects more than 1% of children in Western societies, with diagnoses on the rise due to improved recognition, screening, clinical assessment, and diagnostic testing. We reviewed the role of genetic and metabolic factors which contribute to the causation of ASD with the use of new genetic technology. Up to 40 percent of individuals with ASD are now diagnosed with genetic syndromes or have chromosomal abnormalities including small DNA deletions or duplications, single gene conditions, or gene variants and metabolic disturbances with mitochondrial dysfunction. Although the heritability estimate for ASD is between 70 and 90%, there is a lower molecular diagnostic yield than anticipated. A likely explanation may relate to multifactorial causation with etiological heterogeneity and hundreds of genes involved with a complex interplay between inheritance and environmental factors influenced by epigenetics and capabilities to identify causative genes and their variants for ASD. Behavioral and psychiatric correlates, diagnosis and genetic evaluation with testing are discussed along with psychiatric treatment approaches and pharmacogenetics for selection of medication to treat challenging behaviors or comorbidities commonly seen in ASD. We emphasize prioritizing treatment based on targeted symptoms for individuals with ASD, as treatment will vary from patient to patient based on diagnosis, comorbidities, causation, and symptom severity.

Keywords: autism; ASD; genetics; heterogeneity; syndromes; assessment; medications; treatment; causes

---

1. Introduction

Leo Kanner in 1943 [1] first introduced the term autism as a diagnostic label to define a specific syndrome observed in young children manifested by early onset, characteristic symptomatology, and disrupted social and emotional relationships. Since then, autism is now recognized as Autism Spectrum Disorder (ASD), which is classified as a developmental disorder as defined in DSM-5 (Diagnostic and Statistical Manual of Mental Disorders, 5th Edition) by the American Psychiatric Association [2] and the ICD-10 (International Classification of Diseases, 10th Revision) by the World Health Organization [3]. Autism is characterized by significant impairment in social communication and atypical repetitive and/or restrictive behaviors or interests, with an onset in the early developmental period, prior to age 3 years. The American Academy of Pediatrics [4] recommends screening all infants and toddlers to identify early signs of autism at 18 months and again at 24 months of age. Rating or assessment scales that have been validated for both clinical and research purposes are helpful in establishing the diagnosis of autism. These scales include the Autism Diagnostic Interview-Revised (ADI-R) and the Autism Diagnostic Observation Schedule, Second Edition (ADOS-2) and should be administered by trained specialists in conjunction with an evaluation of the child with consideration of history and clinical presentation [5,6].

ASD affects between 1 to 2% of children in United States with a growing role for genetic factors with etiological heterogeneity. ASD can be conceptualized as a behavioral syndrome rather than a specific categorical mental disorder [7]. The concept of "syndromic autism" (ASD associated with morphological signs or symptoms helpful in the identification of specific genetic disorders) stands in contrast to "non-syndromic autism" (idiopathic ASD with no associated signs or symptoms). Multiplex autism refers to those with a positive family history of other similarly affected individuals, which highlights the heterogeneity of ASD [8,9].

Clinical and other health concerns that may be associated with ASD include intellectual disability (ID), electroencephalogram (EEG) abnormalities with or without epilepsy, dysmorphic features, and abnormal MRI findings [10,11]. About 10% of children with autism are reported to have microcephaly [12,13], which may be associated with additional findings and a poor prognosis. On the other hand, a large-appearing head size is common in children with autism along with increased brain volumes, particularly in the frontal lobes, but with smaller occipital lobes [14–19]. Mutations of the phosphatase and tensin homolog (PTEN) tumor suppressor gene were reported by Butler et al. [14] in children with autism and extreme macrocephaly. Recent studies have shown that about 20% of genes implicated in autism are also known cancer genes, thereby stimulating an interest in not only risks for cancer development in individuals with ASD but whether chemotherapeutic agents could play a role in treatment of autism [20].

Tordjman et al. [7] provided a comprehensive review of diverse genetic disorders associated with autism and considered possible common underlying mechanisms leading to a similar cognitive-behavioral phenotype of autism, while examining relevant genetics, syndromes, epigenetics, and environmental factors. Despite the recognition of nearly 800 susceptibility, clinically relevant, or known genes for autism spectrum disorder collated by Butler et al. [21] and characterized by numerous etiological studies including relevant animal models [22], it appears that no cohesive model of causation, biomarker [23], or specific mode of transmission for the development of autism has been firmly identified [24].

The cause of ASD is heterogenous involving genetics with multiple different gene variants and environmental influences triggering physiological changes in genetically sensitive individuals along with in utero and metabolic factors including mitochondria dysfunction reported in 10 to 20% of patients with ASD. Familial and heritability studies have shown that genetic factors contribute, with estimates as high as 90% with tuberous sclerosis, fragile X, and Rett syndromes as examples of single gene conditions found but accounting for less than 10% of all ASD cases [25–27]. A list of genetic syndromes and chromosomal disorders associated with ASD is illustrated as Box 1 below.

Behavioral and psychiatric comorbidities are common in individuals on the autism spectrum, and can have a substantial impact on overall health, quality of life, and long-term prognosis. Approximately 30% of individuals with ASD require psychological and psychiatric treatments including medication for behavioral problems including hyperactivity, impulsivity, inattention, aggression, property destruction, self-injury, mood disorders, and psychotic or tic disorders [28,29], a major focus of our report.

Box 1. A List of Genetic Syndromes and Chromosome Findings where Autism is a Recognized Feature.

• Adenylate succinase deficiency	• Myotonic dystrophy
• Angelman and Prader-Willi syndromes (AS–maternal or PWS–paternal 15q11-q13 deletions)	• Neurofibromatosis
• Apert syndrome	• Noonan syndrome
• 15q11.2 BP1-BP2 microdeletion (Burnside-Butler) syndrome	• Oculo-auriculo-vertebral spectrum
• CHARGE syndrome	• Phelan-McDermid syndrome (22q13 deletion)
• Chromosome 15 duplications (maternal origin)	• PTEN gene associated disorders with extreme macrocephaly (Cowden/Bannayan-Riley-Ruvalcaba syndrome)
• Chromosome 16p11.2 deletions	• Rett syndrome (MECP2 gene)
• Cohen syndrome	• Shprinzten/velo-cardio-facial/DiGeorge • (22q11 deletion)
• De Lange syndrome	• Smith-Lemli-Opitz syndrome
• Down syndrome	• Smith-Magenis syndrome (17p11.2 deletion)
• Duchenne muscular dystrophy	• Sotos syndrome
• Fragile X syndrome (FMR1 gene)	• Tuberous sclerosis
• Hypomelanosis of Ito	• Turner syndrome
• Joubert syndrome	• Untreated or poorly treated phenylketonuria (PKU)
• Mitochondrial dysfunction	• Williams syndrome
• Moebius sequence	

Modified from G.B. Schaefer and N.J. Mendelsohn, "Genetics evaluation for the etiologic diagnosis of autism spectrum disorders," Genetics in Medicine, vol. 10, pp 4–12, 2008 [25] and from M.G. Butler and others, "Assessment and treatment in autism spectrum disorders: A focus on genetics and psychiatry", Autism Research and Treatment, vol. 2012, 242537, 2012 [30].

2. Diagnosis and Genetics of ASD

ASD affects about 1 individual in 50–100 live births [31,32] and is on the increase with a higher prevalence than reported for congenital brain malformations or Down syndrome. The recurrence rate may be as high as 25–30% if a second child is also diagnosed with ASD in a family (i.e., multiplex) compared with a sporadic pattern (simplex) form of ASD. High heritability estimates have been reported in ASD, e.g., 70 to 90% concordance rate in monozygotic twins [33,34], indicating the potential importance of genetics, but studies have not identified the anticipated number of pathogenic variants to date. Those without a family history may be at a greater risk of copy number variants (CNVs) or deletions/duplications at the chromosome level using chromosomal microarray analysis and DNA probes for CNVs and comparative genomic hybridization [35]. Furthermore, 10% of the individuals with autism from simplex families had CNVs, while only 3% of individuals with autism from multiplex families with more than one family member affected showed CNVs, compared with 1% seen in normally developing children studied as controls. The majority of CNVs were of the deletion type. Single gene conditions are found in about 20% of subjects with ASD, while epigenetics impacted by environmental factors such as nutrition, infections, or toxins could alter the gene status through methylation, controlling function without changing the DNA sequence [27,36,37]. Genome-wide linkage and association studies (GWAS) have identified hundreds of ASD risk gene loci in all human chromosomes.

Autism is considered the most heritable neurodevelopmental disorder based on a large difference in concordance rates or heritability estimates between monozygotic and dizygotic twins with monozygotic twins having rates that are nearly three times higher than rates found in dizygotic twins [38]. Furthermore, a meta-analysis of twin studies on the heritability of ASD in more than 6000 twin pairs was reported by Tick et al. [39]. They found that correlations for monozygotic twins were very close to perfect at a score of 0.98 while the score for dizygotic twins was 0.53, indicating a role of shared environmental effects. Hallmayer et al. [38] concluded that susceptibility to ASD showed moderate genetic heritability and substantially shared twin environmental components, indicating a challenge to find genetic causation for autism.

Genetic investigations have identified the role of hundreds of gene variants, but risk effects are highly variable and relate to other conditions besides autism, making it difficult to find ASD-specific gene variants [40–42]. Many gene variants do impact on common biological pathways or interactions and may play a potential causative role in autism, but more research is needed to address the current challenges in translating autism genetics into clinical practice as genetic etiology and pathogenesis of ASD remain largely unclear [43–45].

Further advances made in genetic technology and testing with improved DNA sequencing and development of bioinformatics with searchable computer genetic variant databases have led to discoveries and characterization of genetic defects in the potential causation of ASD. Improvements of chromosome microarray technology with combination of probes for both copy number variants and single nucleotide polymorphisms (SNPs) have not only led to enhanced testing capabilities in identifying segmental deletions and duplications in the genome, but also the identification of pathogenic or disease-causing genes and their positions within chromosomal regions.

2.1. Genetic Factors Contributing to Autism

Advances in genetic testing and evaluation for syndromic causation of patients with ASD have identified an etiology in up to 40%, using a three-tier clinical genetic approach described by Schaefer and others in 2008 [25] and later in 2013 [34] to identify causes in children diagnosed with ASD. These include fragile X, Rett, and other genetic syndromes, such as tuberous sclerosis (10–20%), PTEN gene mutations (3%), and structural chromosomal deletions or duplications using early versions of chromosomal microarrays (3%), and an additional 10% or higher when using high-resolution microarray technology. Metabolic disorders such as mitochondrial dysfunctions are seen in 10 to 20% of patients with ASD [32,34,46]. Children with ASD reported with microdeletions or duplications involve chromosome regions 1q24.2, 2q37.3, 3p26.2, 4q34.2, 6q24.3, 7q35, 13q13.2-q22, 15q11-q13, 15q22, 16p11.2, 17p11.2, 22q11, 2q13, and Xp22 [13] and additional cytogenetic disorders associated with ASD are found with new ultra-high-resolution microarray technology (e.g., 15q11.2 BP1-BP2 deletions) [47]. Recent GWAS findings in ASD and broad autism phenotype in 28 extended pedigrees from Canada and the United States showed additional chromosome regions including 1p36.22, 2p13.1, 6q27, 8q24.22, 9p21.3, 9q31.2, 12p13.31, 16p13.2, and 18q21.1 [48].

These newer chromosomal SNP microarrays can identify abnormalities 100 times smaller than can be seen with high-resolution chromosome methods including for ASD candidate genes. A report by Shen et al. [26] on 933 patients with ASD using standard karyotype analysis, fragile X DNA testing, and chromosomal microarrays found abnormal karyotypes in 2.2%, abnormal fragile X testing in 0.5%, and microdeletions or microduplications in 18.2% of subjects. These included recurrent deletions or duplications of chromosome 16p11.2 [49] and for chromosome 15q13.2q-13.3, while new studies found chromosome 7q11, chromosome 15q11.2 BP1-BP2, and chromosome 22q11.2 [50].

Whole-exome sequencing (WES) have identified yields of up to 30% [51] but other studies show lower results (e.g., 9.3%) in individuals with ASD [52]. The vast majority of gene variants are of uncertain clinical significance due in part to the rarity found in genomic normative datasets and limitations of bioinformatics, evolutionary conservation, computational predictions, and relevance in relationship to the normal population. Likely explanations for the lack of consistency among molecular diagnostic testing results may relate to multifactorial causation of ASD influenced by a complex interplay between inheritance and environmental effects along with contributions by epigenetics on gene expression. Despite considerable interest in identifying autism-specific genes, deleterious variants have been implicated across multiple neurodevelopmental and psychiatric disorders but insufficient to date in identifying those genes that, when mutated, confer a largely ASD-specific risk [42].

An early genome-wide association study (GWAS) on 4300 affected children with ASD reported by Wang et al. [53] and 6500 controls of European ancestry found a strong association with six single nucleotide polymorphisms (SNPs) located between cadherin 10 (CDH10) and cadherin 9 (CDH9) genes located on chromosome 5 encoding neuronal cell-adhesion molecules. Since then, over 100 genetic loci have been reported to be associated with ASD [54,55], comprising genes converging on chromatin–remodeling, synaptic function in neuronal signaling, and neurodevelopment [56,57]. Furthermore, Butler et al. [21] collated about 800 genes from the literature that were implicated as clinically relevant, susceptible, or known in ASD. These multiple genes include several members of the neuroligin, neurexin, GABA receptor, cadherin, and SHANK gene families. Other genes were found to code for neurotransmitters and their receptors, transporters, oncogenes, brain-derived hormones, epigenetics, and signaling and ubiquitin pathway proteins, along with neuronal cell-adhesion molecules [21,58–61].

2.2. Metabolic Factors Contributing to Autism

Metabolic factors are now recognized as contributing to autism including the mitochondria. Next-generation DNA sequencing now allows for accurate detection of mutations or gene variants at the nuclear and mitochondrial DNA (mtDNA) level and is potentially more informative than chromosomal microarray analysis involved in structural DNA changes. This technology is now available in the clinical setting for individuals presenting with biochemical and mitochondrial disturbances and autism [21,62]. Three functional pathways to ASD are potentially involved, which include genes and pathways for chromatin remodeling, (e.g., CHD7, MECP2, DNMT3A, and PHF2), Wnt (e.g., CHD8, PAX5, and ATRX), and other signaling super-pathways (e.g., GPCR, ERK, RET, and AKT) [50,51] and mitochondrial dysfunction in ASD (e.g., [62]). High lactate levels are also reported in about one in five children with ASD, further supporting the role of the mitochondria in energy metabolism and brain development [32,46,62].

The mitochondria are intracellular organelles found in the cytoplasm which play a crucial role in adenosine 5′-triphosphate (ATP) production through oxidative phosphorylation [62–66], the latter process carried out by the electron transport chain made up of Complexes I, II, III, and IV situated in the inner membrane of the mitochondria containing about 100 proteins. Genes that encode the proteins are located in both nuclear and mitochondrial DNA [65–67] and are required for cellular energy that can impact or influence brain development and activity. There are hundreds of nuclear genes involved in mitochondrial function, while only 13 mitochondrial genes code for protein. Mitochondrial disturbances include a depletion type, or reduced number of mitochondria per cell, with a decreased quantity of mtDNA, or mtDNA mutations producing defects in biochemical reactions within the mitochondria and individual cells [32,46,65,68].

A subset of individuals with ASD can have small mitochondrial DNA deletions/duplications detectable with mitochondrial genome microarrays. Human mitochondrial DNA (mtDNA) is a circular, double-stranded DNA molecule contained within the mitochondrion and inherited solely from the mother. Each mitochondrion contains 2–10 mtDNA copies. In humans, 100–10,000 separate copies of mtDNA are usually present per cell [63–65]. Inborn errors of metabolism may contribute significantly to the causation of ASD with enzyme deficiencies leading to an accumulation of substances that can cause toxic effects on the developing brain. A common example is phenylketonuria, leading to excessive phenylalanine levels, intellectual disability, and ASD, if not diet controlled.

3. Clinical Assessment and Testing

3.1. Initial Clinical Evaluation

A healthcare professional interviews the parent or caregiver regarding presenting problems, reviews a three-generation family history, developmental milestones, and abnormal behaviors of the child, medical and surgical history, and any past or current treatments. The diagnostic evaluation is typically performed by a developmental pediatrician or a child and adolescent psychiatrist. Physical and mental status examinations are performed, and additional testing ordered, as appropriate. If a positive family history for autism is found or dysmorphic (syndromic) features, then a referral is made for clinical genetics' evaluation. Laboratory evaluations may include genetic testing, lead levels, thyroid function, lactate, pyruvate and cholesterol levels, and urine for organic acids. Referrals are made for neurological evaluations and brain imaging when clinically indicated.

3.2. High-Resolution Microarrays and ASD

Genetic testing often begins with chromosomal microarray analysis (CMA) to identify copy number variants (CNVs) to search for a cause of autism spectrum disorder and other related conditions. Microarrays employ a variety of designs and range of coverage of genomic regions, which increases the diagnostic yield as arrays have evolved over time to include better coverage and accuracy. Often the CNVs identified are unclassified or poorly understood in their role in causation of ASD.

Neurodevelopmental disorders can cumulatively affect up to 15% of children [69]. While the etiology of ASD is complex, it involves genetic factors with 800 genes recognized, accounting for 4% of all human genes that are implicated in ASD [21]. Single gene changes, large genomic structural changes (i.e., deletions or duplications), or smaller CNVs and other polygenic conditions can be influenced by the environment and epigenetic factors [70,71]. Genetic testing to pinpoint the underlying cause of ASD is critical for clinical management and counseling. Further, chromosomal microarray analysis has demonstrated the highest diagnostic yield for individuals with ASD as compared to other genetic tests as well as in individuals with ID and/ or behavioral problems, including in developing countries.

High-resolution microarrays now utilize millions of single nucleotide polymorphisms (SNPs) as probes to test the DNA from patients presenting with neurodevelopmental disorders, intellectual disabilities, and ASD. These SNP microarrays are used to identify microdeletions (or duplications) with recognition of dozens of a growing list of deletion or duplication syndromes not previously detected. For example, a study of custom-made, ultra-high-resolution microarrays reported by Ho et al. [47] in 2016 were optimized for the detection of neurodevelopmental disorders (Lineagen, Salt Lake City, Utah) on 10,351 patients presenting for genetic services for neurodevelopmental disorders, ASD, ID, behavioral problems, or with or without multiple congenital anomalies (MCA) over a period of four years. Their testing sample had a male:female ratio of 2.5:1 with a mean age of 7 years. Fifty-five percent of cases represented patients with a diagnosis of ASD with or without other features. The overall CNV detection rate of 28.1% was seen in 10,351 consecutive patients and 24.4% in those with ASD along with 33% in those with intellectual disabilities and/or MCA without autism. The rate of pathogenic findings was significantly lower (4.4%) when the diagnostic indication was ASD only compared to diagnostic indications of DD/ID/MCA without a reported diagnosis of ASD (i.e., non-ASD cohort) (12.5%).

In the ASD cohort, the overall pathogenic rate was slightly higher for individuals with ASD+ as compared to the overall pathogenic rate for individuals with ASD only. The pathogenic rate in the ASD+ cohort started at 4.1% in the youngest group and rose to 8.5% in the 5.5–10 years range. The pathogenic rate in the ASD only cohort rose gradually with age, from 3.4% in the youngest cohort (0–3.4 years) to a peak at 7.0% in adolescence. In 5694 patients classified as ASD and 4657 patients with non-ASD, the most common findings were 15q11. 2 BP1-BP2 deletions followed by proximal 16p11.2 deletions or duplications, 15q13.3 deletions, and 16p13.1 duplications (see Figure 1). The most common finding in the non-ASD cohort was the 22q11.2 deletion causing velo-cardio-facial or DiGeorge syndrome. This study illustrates the value of CMA testing and its impact on medical management is now recognized in consensus medical guidelines for the evaluation of children with ASD.

3.3. Next-Generation Sequencing (NGS)

Advances in genomics technology using next-generation sequencing (NGS) have led to discovery of many disease-causing genes using candidate gene approaches, disease-specific gene panels, or by whole-exome sequencing of patients presenting with neurodevelopmental disorders, intellectual disabilities, or ASD. Applying genomics to the study of neurodevelopment and function has identified over 5000 implicated genes using clinical exome sequencing approaches and informatics in affected individuals. In addition, disease-specific NGS gene testing panels have been developed and used in the commercial laboratory setting for testing patients presenting for genetic services, including approximately 600 genes for intellectual disabilities and over 100 genes available for testing for ASD (e.g., Fulgent Diagnostics, Irvine, California).

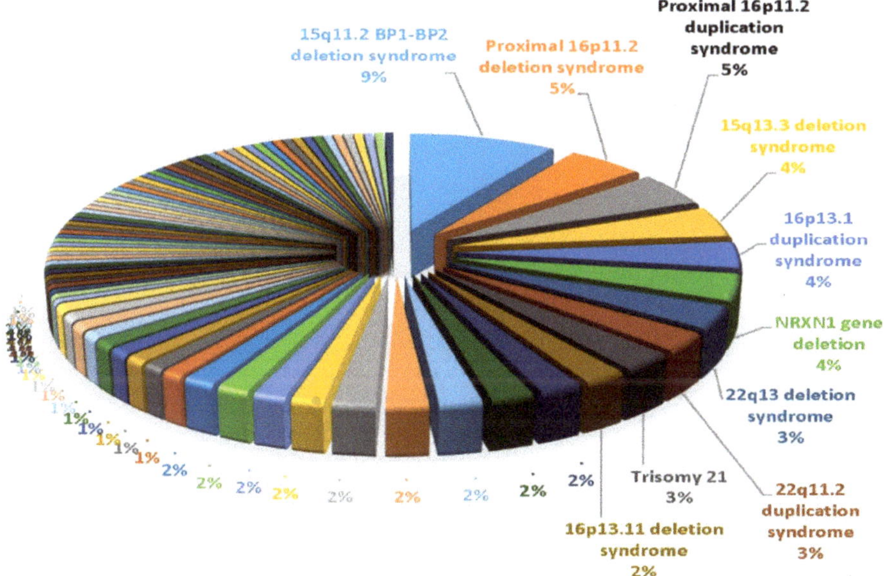

Figure 1. Pie chart showing the top 10 out of 85 genetic findings from data summarized by Ho et al. [47] using ultra-high-resolution chromosomal microarrays from over 10,000 consecutive patients presenting for genetic testing with neurodevelopmental disorders affecting brain function and/or structure of unknown cause with developmental/intellectual disabilities and/or ASD.

These types of analyses have identified pathogenic gene variants or mutations which are known to be disease-causing such as missense or nonsense, but more often variants of unknown clinical significance are found. More testing and information with better interpretations of the genomic change and impact at the protein level are needed to help determine the role, if any, of the unknown gene variants in causing the disease under study including for ASD. Hundreds of new causative genes relating to human diseases and syndromes have been identified with the use of NGS technology over the past few years, with expectations of continued success given improvements in genetic technology, bioinformatics, and expanded genomic databases to search for gene variants and in further characterizing identified genes.

Next generation DNA sequencing of the exons (referred to as exome sequencing) or whole-genome sequencing will continue to find new discoveries of disease-causing SNPs, gene regulatory sequences, or mutations of protein-coding genes for both structural and regulatory proteins. Identifying molecular signatures of novel or disturbed gene or exon expression, disease-specific profiles and patterns (i.e., expression heat maps), and recognition of interconnected gene pathways in autism and other behavioral disorders in the future by using readily available blood elements (e.g., lymphoblasts) should hold promise for treatments with pharmacological agents by regulating (either increasing or decreasing) activity of normal (or abnormal) gene function. The study of non-coding RNAs, which control the amount or quantity of gene expression coding for protein production through micro-RNAs and the quality of protein production by specific isoform development by sno-RNAs, will lead to new areas of research and medical therapies for human diseases. Therefore, this technology should be considered in the diagnostic evaluation of ASD, either sporadic or with a positive family history of others similarly affected.

Butler et al. [21] searched the literature and found approximately 800 genes implicated in autism in the literature as clinically significant, relevant, or known to contribute to the risk of ASD. Recent research revealed that ASD and cancer genes may share common genetic architecture and pathways with the first evidence of the PTEN tumor-suppressor gene playing a role in autism in 2005 [14]. Hence, approximately 800 ASD-related genes and 3500 genes in cancer were examined using the GeneAnalytics pathways and profiling software programs and found shared cell-signaling pathways, metabolic disturbances, and molecular functions in 138, or 17%, of ASD genes that overlap with cancer genes [20]. Shared mechanisms may lead to identification of common pathology and a better molecular understanding of causation as well as potential treatment options.

4. Treatment Approaches

4.1. Behavioral Interventions in ASD

4.1.1. For Children and Adolescents with ASD

Weitlauf et al. [72] reviewed 65 studies, comprising 48 randomized trials and 17 nonrandomized comparative studies, that analyzed the benefit of behavioral interventions. High-intensity applied behavior analysis (ABA) was associated with improvement in cognitive functioning and language skills relative to community controls in young children [73]. Early intensive behavioral intervention (EIBI) is a well-established treatment for young children with ASD and is based on the principles of applied behavior analysis. Delivered over a period of several years at an average of 20 to 40 hours per week, it can provide substantial benefit for core ASD symptoms, particularly in terms of communication skills [74]. Social skills' interventions including group administered training showed positive effects on social behaviors for older children [75].

4.1.2. For Adults with ASD

National Institute for Health and Care Excellence (NICE) recommended guidelines for management and support of children and young people with autism using group or individual social learning programs to improve social interaction deficits by applying behavioral therapy techniques within a social learning framework. These include using video modeling, peer feedback, imitation, and reinforcement to teach conventions of appropriate social interpersonal interaction [76]. There is evidence from observational studies in adults with ASD that social skills' groups may be effective at improving social interaction [77]. CBT can help adults with ASD across a range of domains, particularly in the context of treating anxiety and OCD, and supporting adults who have difficulties related to a history of victimization [78].

4.2. Medication Treatments in ASD

Psychopharmacological treatment of ASD is challenging due to considerable variability in the presentation of ASD and commonly occurring comorbidities. Individuals with ASD are typically more vulnerable to side effects of psychopharmacological agents than their age-matched, neuro-typically developing peers [79]. Finally, ASD impacts individuals over the course of their lifespan and most of the literature on psychotropic medications in ASD involves pediatric populations.

A psychopharmacological approach may be beneficial in the treatment of identified target symptoms in individuals with ASD. When considering the use of medications, potential benefits and risks must be weighed on a case-by-case basis. It has been reported that close to half of insured children with ASD are receiving psychopharmacological interventions, most commonly with stimulants, alpha-2 agonists, antipsychotics, anticonvulsants, and antidepressants [80].

Currently, there are no medications approved for treatment of the core symptoms of ASD including social communication deficits or repetitive behaviors. Common target symptoms for which there are effective, evidence-based medication treatment include hyperactivity, inattention, impulsivity, irritability, aggression, self-injurious behavior, repetitive behaviors (including stereotypies), and insomnia [81]. For the treatment of irritability associated with ASD, the antipsychotics risperidone and aripiprazole are licensed and approved by the US Food and Drug Administration [82].

4.2.1. For the Treatment of ADHD Symptoms in ASD

Stimulant medications are considered first line agents for attention deficit hyperactivity disorder (ADHD) in individuals with ASD, given that overall they are most often effective and generally well tolerated compared to other ADHD medications. The RUPP research team [83] and later Reichow et al. [84] demonstrated a clear superiority of methylphenidate over placebo in children with pervasive developmental disorder. However, those with ASD had a greater risk of side effects with methylphenidate including decreased appetite, insomnia, depressive symptoms, irritability, higher levels of social withdrawal, and lower treatment response rates compared to youth with ADHD alone. It should be noted that stimulant medications for ADHD in the amphetamine class are often used in children with ASD but have not been as rigorously studied.

Regarding non-stimulant medications for ADHD in ASD, both atomoxetine and alpha-2 agonists have shown benefit. Harfterkamp et al. [85], in a double-blind treatment trial of patients age 6 to 17 years with ADHD and ASD using atomoxetine 1.2 mg/kg/day or placebo for eight weeks, found that atomoxetine moderately improved ADHD symptoms, but with frequent adverse events including nausea, decreased appetite, fatigue, and early morning awakening. The alpha-2 agonist guanfacine has been shown to be effective for ADHD in children with ASD demonstrated by a double-blind, placebo-controlled trial of guanfacine extended release in which 50% of youth on active treatment improved on the Clinical Global Impression–Improvement (CGI-I) scale [86], compared to 9.4% on placebo [87], with sedation and transient lowering of blood pressure as the most common adverse effects.

4.2.2. For the Treatment of Irritability, Aggression, and Self-Injurious Behavior in ASD

Atypical antipsychotics compared to other medications have to date demonstrated the best evidence for the treatment of irritability in ASD. Risperidone in youth age 5 to 16 years with ASD [88] in three randomized, placebo-controlled trials showed an over 50% reduction in the irritability score of the Aberrant Behavior Checklist (ABC-I) irritability scale [89] and the magnitude of the response was greater when irritability was rated as moderate to severe [90].

Aripiprazole, the second antipsychotic approved by the FDA for the treatment of irritability associated with autism (in children between the age of 6 and 17 years), demonstrated significantly lower severity scores on the ABC-I and the CGI-I scales for subjects on active medication compared to placebo in two large-scale, randomized, placebo-controlled studies. Unfortunately, weight gain is a common side effect of antipsychotics, and increases in body mass index have been shown to be similar for aripiprazole and risperidone in children with ASD [91].

Anticonvulsant medications divalproex and topiramate have shown some promise for treating irritability in ASD. Divalproex was beneficial in reducing irritability in a small, randomized, placebo-controlled trial of children with ASD [92]. However, an earlier trial failed to show separation from placebo on the ABC-I [93]. Topiramate as monotherapy has no demonstrated benefit in the treatment of irritability in youth with ASD [94]; however, it reduced the ABC-I score when co-administered at an average daily dose of 200 mg with risperidone [95]. It is hypothesized that, as EEG abnormalities are common in children with ASD, symptom reduction with anticonvulsants may result from treatment of abnormal brain discharges [96].

4.2.3. For the Treatment of Repetitive Behaviors Including Stereotypies in ASD

Fluoxetine has been shown to improve repetitive behaviours in adults with ASD [97]; however, benefit has not been reliably demonstrated in pediatric populations. In fact, the Cochrane Collaboration published a systematic review [98], which concluded that for repetitive behaviors in children with ASD there is not only a lack of available evidence of benefit from treatment with selective serotonin reuptake inhibitors (SSRIs) including fluoxetine, fluvoxamine, and citalopram, but some evidence for risk of harm, given a greater incidence of adverse effects, most notably symptoms of behavioral activation.

4.2.4. For the Treatment of Persistent Insomnia in ASD

Exogenous melatonin, (available as an over-the-counter supplement) in both immediate-release and extended-release formulations, has been shown to be safe and effective in improving sleep patterns in children with ASD [99]. Some evidence suggests that children with ASD have abnormal melatonin secretion and circadian rhythm abnormalities compared to non-ASD children [100]. Clonidine (an alpha-2 agonist) has shown promise in reducing latency of sleep initiation and decreasing nighttime awakening in ASD [101].

4.3. Pharmacogenetics and Role in Medication Selection and Management

Personalized or precision medicine is emerging in clinical practice based on individual genetic patterns contributing to pharmacogenetics, particularly in the field of psychiatry and treating individuals with ASD [102–105] with behavior issues including ADHD, irritability, aggression and self-injury, repetitive behaviors, and persistent insomnia addressed above. Pharmacogenetics is a study of structural DNA variation that impacts drug metabolism [106,107] and most often based on the cytochrome P450 enzyme system, primarily active in the liver and coded by genes. Cytochrome P450 enzymes metabolize or break down drugs in the liver with most prescription drugs metabolized by this enzyme system and, thus, play a significant role in the treatment of diseases [107,108]. Variation in drug response among individuals due to metabolism differences is now recognized as a major clinical problem, especially given that the use of several medications per patient is common practice. Relevant cytochrome P450 gene polymorphisms and different racial distributions can identify sources of variability in drug response by the modulation of metabolism by the cytochrome P450 enzymes impacting treatment in ASD.

There are over 50 cytochrome P450 hepatic enzymes that are primarily found in the mitochondria [102–105]. These enzymes metabolize endogenous and xenobiotic substrates including environmental pollutants and agricultural and plant-based chemicals and are involved in biosynthesis and metabolism of steroids, vitamins, hormones, lipids, and prostaglandins. About 90% of all drugs are metabolized by seven different cytochrome enzymes including CYP1A2, CYP3A4, CYP3A5, CYPC19, CYP2D6, CYP2C9 and CYP2B6 [106,109–111]. The most commonly prescribed medications used in treating patients with psychiatric problems and ASD are broken down by CYP2D6 [102–105]. It should also be noted that many drugs are also metabolized by more than one cytochrome P450 enzyme and in addition some drugs (e.g., risperidone) require break down to generate an active metabolite or functional agent for treatment.

There is growing evidence that cytochrome P450 enzymes may be altered by the environment in the form of inhibitors or inducers as well as impacting drug–drug interactions. Known inhibitors or inducers may include common sources such as caffeine, grapefruit, broccoli, cabbage, or cauliflower by impacting the individual enzyme activity. For example, if an individual has a reduced form of a cytochrome P450 enzyme, then an inducer may increase the enzyme response in breaking down the drug to help that person in metabolizing a specific medication and, thus, impact response to treatment.

Drug–drug interactions and their concentrations and half-life along with response to inhibitors and/or inducers can all impact medication levels and treatment in the patient. It should also be noted that individuals who are either fast or slow metabolizers based on their microsomal P450 enzyme system genotype patterns may respond differently to specific medications and put them at risk for either failure of drug therapy and/or adverse side effects. Similarly, a better understanding of the metabolic differences that occur with age will further impact on drug dosage and selection of specific therapeutic agents. Therefore, personalized medicine requires the development of resources for clinicians including pharmacogenetic dosing guidelines for medications, as 25 to 50% of individuals do not respond normally to drug dosage or treatment, and this scenario also applies to those with ASD [102].

Applying this knowledge from pharmacogenomics and identifying genes and polymorphisms involved in drug metabolism will benefit patients treated for psychiatric and behavioral problems. The discovery of new classes of drugs and research on existing drugs for new purposes to treat behavioral problems in patients with ASD are under investigation including clinical trials (e.g., in fragile X syndrome), holding promise for improved therapy. In addition, the discoveries made in brain imaging such as functional MRI or PET scans in identifying regions of the brain that are affected in ASD should allow for new treatment discoveries and applications specific for the altered regions identified.

5. Future Directions

Advances and application of genomic testing technology, bioinformatic approaches, and computational predictions will strengthen genetic testing results and interpretations as more experience is gained in testing patients presenting for clinical services and diagnosis [112–114]. Increased number of next-generation sequencing (NGS) or whole-exome sequencing (WES) studies in ASD of individuals from different ethnic backgrounds will be required to gain ASD-specific genomic information from datasets of both sexes when compared to the normal population. These contributions should allow a better understanding of the role of genetics, genomics, epigenetics, and specific candidate genes and their variants, along with environmental factors playing a role in ASD in relationship to multifactorial influences in family studies [38,112,114,115]. Confounding effects of clinical heterogeneity and diagnostic uncertainty are other complicating issues needing further characterization and evaluation to gain more experience in clinical assessment, genetics, and treatment approaches in autism spectrum disorder.

In addition, research with brain and tissue harvested and stored for structural DNA and RNA expression studies are needed on individuals with ASD having data from cognitive, behavioral, and ASD assessment tools and neuroimaging results while living. Coding and non-coding expression patterns and epigenetic (methylation) signals supplemented with WES and CNV data would be beneficial for a better understanding of the role of genetics in ASD, particularly with larger cohorts of individuals having similar genetic backgrounds, patterns, and ethnicity to identify large-effect pathogenic variants for facilitating genotype–phenotype correlations and allow comparisons. The biological processes, molecular functions with gene-interactions, and pathways that are more autism-specific may be identified through these analytical genetic studies. Currently, there are no molecular pathways known to be uniquely associated with ASD when disturbed. Some gene variants are more related to neurodevelopmental disorders and not specific for autism. Classification of gene variants that specifically cause ASD alone and not attributable to other neurodevelopmental or psychiatric disorders are under investigation as rare, large-effect mutations seen in ASD also influence cognition in a high proportion of individuals, complicating the degree of impact on the ASD phenotype vs. impact on cognitive function [42]. Certain neurodevelopmental gene variants may also impact gene function differently including neural circuits depending on an individual's genetic background differences.

Particular class of variants such as missense or nonsense changes may confer different effects at the protein level. Individual gene variants coding for specific amino acids may impact more important protein regions or domains with certain characteristics at specific amino acid positions, conferring mild consequences, while other amino acid positions may be more important for protein function. These areas of gene variant(s)-protein relationships will require more studies in ASD in the future using improved genetic technology, data collection, and analysis with genotype–phenotype correlations.

Brain tissue regions most often affected in ASD (e.g., hippocampus, cerebellum, etc.) may yield useful information if studied in those persons with documented autism, particularly with stored clinical and imaging data with CNVs and gene variants combined with expression patterns and methylation status in relationship to control subjects who are similarly studied. Mosaicism/tissue-specific gene expression should be considered and further studied in view of more males than females affected with

ASD, particularly X-linked genes. Additionally, hormonal-mediated gender influences or differential expression in the brain should be examined for dysregulation in ASD including methylation status of brain-expressed genes on the X chromosome and interaction with autosomal genes (e.g., X-linked FMR1 gene causing fragile X syndrome [116] and CYFIP1 gene at 15q11.2 involved with coding transporter for FMR1 protein [117]). These investigations will require more specialized methods with increased sensitivity such as droplet digital PCR [118].

6. Summary

On behalf of individuals living with ASD and their families and for the benefit of society as a whole, increased awareness and knowledge regarding autism spectrum disorder and commonly related neurobehavioral conditions with contribution of genetic differences are imperative for healthcare professionals who provide evaluation and treatment services for ASD. Early recognition, diagnosis, and treatment should increase the likelihood that affected individuals will achieve optimal long-term outcomes and improved quality of life. Genetic and epigenetic discoveries underlying causes, as well as factors impacting treatment, such as pharmacogenetic variability, have the potential to improve the overall health of individuals with ASD. Additional clinical research to improve the evidence base for various treatment interventions for ASD with related behavioral and psychiatric challenges is desperately needed.

Author Contributions: A.G. and M.G.B. designed and contributed to the study equally by reviewing the literature, writing and revising the manuscript and agreeing to publish the article. M.G.B. generated the figure. All authors have read and agreed to the published version of the manuscript.

Funding: This research received no external funding.

Acknowledgments: We thank Grace Graham for expert preparation of the manuscript.

Conflicts of Interest: The authors declare no conflict of interest.

References

1. Kanner, L. Autistic disturbances of affective contact. *Nervous Child.* **1943**, *32*, 217–253.
2. American Psychiatric Association. *Diagnostic and Statistical Manual of Mental Disorders (DSM-5)*, 5th ed.; American Psychiatric Association: Washington, DC, USA, 2013.
3. World Health Organization. *ICD-10: International Statistical Classification of Diseases and Related Health Problems: Tenth Revision*, 2nd ed.; World Health Organization: Geneva, Switzerland, 2004.
4. Hyman, S.L.; Levy, S.E.; Myers, S.M. AAP Council on Children with Disabilities, Section on Developmental and Behavioral Pediatrics. Identification, Evaluation, and Management of Children with Autism Spectrum Disorder. *Pediatrics* **2020**, *145*, e20193447. [CrossRef] [PubMed]
5. Rutter, M.; Le Couteur, A.; Lord, C. *ADI-R: Autism Diagnostic Interview-Revised (ADI-R)*; Western Psychological Services: Los Angeles, CA, USA, 2003.
6. Lord, C.; DiLavore, P.C.; Gotham, K.; Guthrie, W.; Luyster, R.J.; Risi, S.; Rutter, M. *Autism Diagnostic Observation Schedule: ADOS-2*; Western Psychological Services: Los Angeles, CA, USA, 2012.
7. Tordjman, S.; Cohen, D.; Anderson, G.M.; Botbol, M.; Banitano, R.; Coulon, N.; Roubertous, P.L. Reprint of "Reframing autism as a behavioral syndrome and not a specific mental disorder: Implications of genetic and phenotypic heterogeneity". *Neurosci. Biobehav. Rev.* **2018**, *89*, 132–150.
8. Miles, J.H.; Takahashi, T.N.; Bagby, S.; Sahota, P.K.; Vaslow, D.F.; Wang, C.H.; Hillman, R.E.; Farmer, J.E. Essential versus complex autism: Definition of fundamental prognostic subtypes. *Am. J. Med. Genet.* **2005**, *135*, 171–180. [CrossRef] [PubMed]
9. Cohen, D.; Pichard, N.; Tordjman, S.; Baumann, C.; Burglen, L.; Excoffier, E.; Lazar, G.; Mazet, P.; Pinquier, C.; Verloes, A.; et al. Specific genetic disorders and autism: Clinical contribution towards their identification. *J. Autism Dev. Disord.* **2005**, *35*, 103–116. [CrossRef] [PubMed]
10. Rapin, I. Autistic regression and disintegrative disorder: How important the role of epilepsy? *Semin. Pediatr. Neurol.* **1995**, *2*, 278–285. [CrossRef]

11. Miles, J.H.; Hillman, R.E. Value of a clinical morphology examination in autism. *Am. J. Med. Genet.* **2000**, *10*, 245–253. [CrossRef]
12. Fombonne, E.; Roge, B.; Claverie, J.; Courty, S.; Frémolle, J. Microcephaly and macrocephaly in autism. *J. Autism. Dev. Disord.* **1999**, *29*, 113–119. [CrossRef]
13. Miles, J.H. Autism spectrum disorders—A genetics review. *Genet Med.* **2011**, *13*, 278–294. [CrossRef]
14. Butler, M.G.; Dasouki, M.J.; Zhou, X.P.; Talebizadeh, Z.; Brown, M.; Takahashi, T.N.; Miles, J.H.; Wang, C.H.; Stratton, R.; Pilarski, R.; et al. Subset of individuals with autism spectrum disorders and extreme macrocephaly associated with germline PTEN tumour suppressor gene mutations. *J. Med. Genet.* **2005**, *42*, 318–321. [CrossRef]
15. Carper, R.A.; Courchesne, E. Inverse correlation between frontal lobe and cerebellum sizes in children with autism. *Brain* **2000**, *123*, 836–844. [CrossRef] [PubMed]
16. Carper, R.A.; Moses, P.; Tigue, Z.D.; Courchesne, E. Cerebral lobes in autism: Early hyperplasia and abnormal age effects. *Neuroimage* **2002**, *16*, 1038–1051. [CrossRef] [PubMed]
17. Mueller, S.; Keeser, D.; Reiser, M.F.; Teipel, S.; Meindl, T. Functional and structural MR imaging in neuropsychiatric disorders, part 2: Application in schizophrenia and autism. *AJNR Am. J. Neuroradiol.* **2012**, *33*, 2033–2037. [CrossRef] [PubMed]
18. Philip, R.C.; Daubermann, M.R.; Whalley, H.C.; Baynham, K.; Lawrie, S.M.; Stanfield, A.C. A systematic review and meta-analysis of the fMRI investigation of autism spectrum disorders. *Neurosci. Biobehav. Rev.* **2012**, *36*, 901–942. [CrossRef]
19. Kobayashi, A.; Yokota, S.; Takeuchi, H.; Asano, K.; Asano, M.; Sassa, Y.; Taki, Y.; Kawashima, R. Increased grey matter volume of the right superior temporal gyrus in healthy children with autistic cognitive style: A VBM study. *Brain Cogn.* **2020**, *139*, 105514. [CrossRef]
20. Gabrielli, A.P.; Manzardo, A.M.; Butler, M.G. GeneAnalytics pathways and profiling of shared autism and cancer genes. *Int. J. Mol. Sci.* **2019**, *20*, 1166. [CrossRef]
21. Butler, M.G.; Rafi, S.K.; Manzardo, A.M. High-resolution chromosome ideogram representation of currently recognized genes for Autism spectrum disorders. *Int. J. Mol Sci.* **2015**, *16*, 6464–6495. [CrossRef]
22. Tordjman, S.; Drapier, D.; Bonnot, O.; Graignic, R.; Fortes, S.; Cohen, D.; Millet, B.; Laurent, C.; Roubertoux, P.L. Animal models relevant to schizophrenia and autism: Validity and limitations. *Behav. Genet.* **2007**, *37*, 61–67. [CrossRef]
23. Walsh, P.; Elsabbagh, M.; Bolton, P.; Singh, I. In search of biomarkers for autism: Scientific, social and ethical challenges. *Nat. Rev. Neurosci.* **2011**, *2*, 603–612. [CrossRef]
24. Happé, F.; Ronald, A.; Plomin, R. Time to give up on a single explanation for Autism. *Nat. Neurosci.* **2006**, *9*, 1218–1220. [CrossRef]
25. Schaefer, G.B.; Mendelsohn, N.J.; Professional Practice Guidelines Committee. Clinical genetics evaluation in identifying the etiology of autism spectrum disorders. *Genet. Med.* **2008**, *10*, 301–305. [CrossRef] [PubMed]
26. Shen, Y.; Dies, K.A.; Holm, I.A.; Bridgemohan, C.; Sobeih, M.M.; Caronna, E.B.; Miller, K.J.; Frazier, J.A.; Silverstain, I.; Picker, J.; et al. Austism Consortium Clinical Genetics/DNA Diagnostics Collaboration. Clinical genetic testing for patients with autism spectrum disorders. *Pediatrics* **2010**, *125*, 727–735. [CrossRef] [PubMed]
27. Waye, M.M.Y.; Cheng, H.Y. Genetics and epigenetics of autism: A review. *Psychiatry Clin. Neurosci.* **2018**, *72*, 228–244. [CrossRef] [PubMed]
28. Howes, O.D.; Rogdaki, M.; Findon, J.L.; Wichers, R.H.; Charman, T.; King, B.H.; Loth, E.; McAlonan, G.M.; McCracker, J.T.; Parr, J.R.; et al. Autism spectrum disorder: Consensus guidelines on assessment, treatment and research from the British Association for Psychopharmacology. *J. Psychopharmacol.* **2018**, *32*, 3–29. [CrossRef] [PubMed]
29. Rosen, T.E.; Mazefsky, C.A.; Vasa, R.A.; Lerner, M.D. Co-occurring psychiatric conditions in autism spectrum disorder. *Int Rev. Psychiatry.* **2018**, *30*, 40–61. [CrossRef] [PubMed]
30. Butler, M.G.; Youngs, E.L.; Roberts, J.L.; Hellings, J.A. Assessment and treatment in autism spectrum disorders: A focus on genetics and psychiatry. *Autism Res. Treat.* **2012**, *2012*, 242537. [CrossRef]
31. Rice, C. Prevalence of Autism spectrum disorders—Autism and developmental disabilities monitoring network. *Morbid Mortal Wkly. Rep.* **2006**, *58*, 1–20.
32. Rose, S.; Niyazov, D.M.; Rossignol, D.A.; Golenthal, M.; Kahler, S.G.; Frye, R.E. Clinical and molecular characteristics of mitochondrial dysfunction in autism spectrum disorder. *Mol. Diagn. Ther.* **2018**, *22*, 571–593. [CrossRef]

33. Abrahams, B.S.; Geschwind, D.H. Advances in autism genetics: On the threshold of a new neurobiology. *Nat. Rev. Genet.* **2008**, *9*, 341–355. [CrossRef]

34. Schaefer, G.B.; Mendelsohn, N.J.; Professional Practice and Guidelines Committee. Clinical genetics evaluation in identifying the etiology of autism spectrum disorders: 2013 guideline revisions. *Genet. Med.* **2013**, *15*, 399–407. [CrossRef]

35. Sebat, J.; Lakshmi, B.; Malhotra, D.; Troge, J.; Lese-Martin, C.; Walsh, T.; Yamrom, B.; Yoon, S.; Krasnitz, A.; Kendall, J.; et al. Strong association of de novo copy number mutations with autism. *Science* **2007**, *316*, 445–449. [CrossRef] [PubMed]

36. Schaefer, G.B.; Starr, L.; Pickering, D.; Skar, G.; Dehaai, K.; Sanger, W.G. Array comparative genomic hybridization findings in a cohort referred for an autism evaluation. *J. Child. Neurol.* **2010**, *25*, 1498–1503. [CrossRef] [PubMed]

37. Wenger, T.L.; Kao, C.; McDonald-McGinn, D.M.; Zackair, E.H.; Bailey, A.; Schultz, R.T.; Morrow, B.E.; Emanuel, B.S.; Hakonarson, H. The role of mGluR copy number variation in genetic and environmental forms of syndromic autism spectrum disorder. *Sci. Rep.* **2016**, *6*, 19372. [CrossRef] [PubMed]

38. Hallmayer, J.; Cleveland, S.; Torres, A.; Phillips, J.; Cohen, B.; Torigoe, T.; Miller, J.; Fedele, A.; Collins, J.; Smith, K.; et al. Genetic heritability and shared environmental factors among twin pairs with autism. *Arch. Gen. Psychiatry* **2011**, *68*, 1095–1102. [CrossRef]

39. Tick, B.; Bolton, P.; Happe, F.; Rutther, M.; Rijsdijk, F. Heritability of autism spectrum disorders: A meta-analysis of twin studies. *J. Child Psychol. Psychiatry* **2016**, *57*, 585–595. [CrossRef]

40. Weinder, D.J.; Wigoder, E.M.; Riple, S.; Walters, R.K.; Kosmicki, J.A.; Grove, J.; Samocha, K.E.; Goldstein, J.I.; Okbay, A.; Bybjerg-Grauhom, J.; et al. Polygenic transmission disequlibirium confirms that common and rate vairation act additively to create risk for autism spectrum disorders. *Nat. Genet.* **2017**, *49*, 978–983. [CrossRef]

41. Pizzo, L.; Jensen, M.; Polyak, A.; Rosenfeld, J.A.; Mannik, K.; Krishnan, A.; McCready, E.; Pichon, O.; Le Caignec, C.; Van Dijck, A.; et al. Rare variants in the genetic background modulate cognitive and developmental phenotypes in individuals carryng disease-associated varients. *Genet Med.* **2019**, *21*, 816–825. [CrossRef]

42. Myers, S.M.; Challman, T.D.; Bernier, R.; Bourgeron, T.; Chung, W.K.; Constantinto, J.N.; Eichler, E.E.; Jacquemenot, S.; Miller, D.T.; Mitchell, K.J.; et al. Insufficient evidence for "Autism-Specific" genes. *Am. J. Hum. Genet.* **2020**, *106*, 587–595.

43. Vorstman, J.A.; Parr, J.R.; Moreno-De-Luca, D.; Anney, R.J.L.; Nurnberger, J.I.; Hallmayer, J.F. Autism genetics: Opportunities and challenges for clinical translation. *Nat. Rev. Genet.* **2017**, *18*, 362–376. [CrossRef]

44. Yenkoyan, K.; Griogryan, A.; Fereshetyan, K.; Ypremyan, D. Adances in understanding the pathophysiology of autism spectrum disorders. *Behav. Brain Res.* **2017**, *331*, 92–101. [CrossRef]

45. Srivastava, S.; Love-Nichols, J.A.; Dies, K.A.; Ledbetter, D.H.; Martin, C.L.; Chung, W.K.; Firth, H.V.; Frazier, T.; Hansen, R.L.; Prock, L.; et al. NDD exome scoping review work group. Meta-analysis and multidisciplinary consensus statement: Exome sequencing is a first-tier clinical diagnostic test for individuals with neurodevelopmental disorders. *Genet. Med.* **2019**, *27*, 2413–2421. [CrossRef] [PubMed]

46. Dhillon, S.; Hellings, J.A.; Butler, M.G. Genetics and mitochondrial abnormalities in autism spectrum disorders: A review. *Curr. Genom.* **2011**, *12*, 322–332. [CrossRef]

47. Ho, K.S.; Wassman, E.R.; Baxter, A.L.; Hensel, C.H.; Martin, M.M.; Prasad, A.; Twede, H.; Vanzo, R.J.; Butler, M.G. Chromosomal microarray analysis of consecutive individuals with autism spectrum disorders using an ultra-high resolution chromosomal microarray optimized for neurodevelopmental disorders. *Int. J. Mol. Sci.* **2016**, *17*, 2070. [CrossRef] [PubMed]

48. Woodbury-Smith, M.; Paterson, A.D.; O'Connor, I.; Zarrei, M.; Yuen, R.K.C.; Howe, J.L.; Thompson, A.; Parlier, M.; Fernandez, B.; Piven, J.; et al. A genome-wide linkage study of autism spectrum disorder and the broad autism phenotype in extended pedigrees. *J. Neurodev. Disord.* **2018**, *10*, 20. [CrossRef]

49. Fernandez, B.A.; Roberts, W.; Chung, B.; Weksberg, R.; Meyn, S.; Szatmari, P.; Joseph-George, A.M.; Mackay, S.; Whitten, K.; Nble, B.; et al. Phenotypic spectrum associated with de novo and inherited deletions and duplications at 16p11.2 in individuals ascertained for diagnosis of autism spectrum disorder. *J. Med. Genet.* **2010**, *47*, 195–203. [CrossRef] [PubMed]

50. Miller, D.T.; Shen, Y.; Weiss, L.A.; Korn, J.; Anselm, I.; Bridgemohan, C.; Cox, G.F.; Dickinson, H.; Gentile, J.; Harris, D.J.; et al. Microdeletion/duplication at 15q13.2q13.3 among individuals with features of autism and other neuropsychiatric disorders. *J. Med. Genet.* **2009**, *46*, 242–248. [CrossRef]

51. Rossi, M.; El-Khechen, D.; Black, M.H.; Hagmna, K.D.F.; Tang, S.; Powis, Z. Outcomes of diagnostic exome sequencing in patients with diagnosed or suspected autism spectrum disorders. *Pediatr. Neurol.* **2017**, *70*, 34–43. [CrossRef] [PubMed]

52. Tammimies, K.; Marshall, C.R.; Walker, S.; Kaur, G.; Thiruvahindrapuram, B.; Lionel, A.C.; Yuen, R.K.C.; Uddin, M.; Roberts, W.; Weksberg, R.; et al. Molecular diagnostic yield of chromosomal microarray analysis and whole-exome sequencing in children with autism spectrum disorder. *JAMA* **2017**, *314*, 895–903. [CrossRef] [PubMed]

53. Wang, K.; Zhang, H.; Ma, D.; Bucan, M.; Glessner, J.T.; Abrahams, B.S.; Salyakina, D.; Imielinski, M.; Bradfield, J.P.; Sleiman, P.M.A.; et al. Common genetic variants on 5p14.1 associate with autism spectrum disorders. *Nature* **2009**, *459*, 528–533. [CrossRef]

54. Delvin, B.; Scherer, S.W. Genetic architecture in autism spectrum disorder. *Curr. Opin. Genet. Dev.* **2012**, *22*, 229–237.

55. Geschwind, D.H.; State, M.W. Gene hunting in autism spectrum disorder: On the path to precision medicine. *Lancet Neurol.* **2015**, *14*, 1109–1120. [CrossRef]

56. Pinto, D.; Delaby, E.; Merico, D.; Barbosa, M.; Merikangas, A.; Klei, L.; Thiruvahindrapuram, B.; Xu, X.; Ziman, R.; Wang, Z.; et al. Convergence of genes and cellular pathways dysregulated in autism spectrum disorders. *Am. J. Hum. Genet.* **2014**, *94*, 677–694. [CrossRef] [PubMed]

57. Yuen, R.K.C.; Merico, D.; Bookman, M.; Howe, J.L.; Thiruvahindrapuram, B.; Patel, R.V.; Whitney, J.; Delaux, N.; Bingham, J.; Wang, Z.; et al. Whole genome sequencing resource identifies 18 new candidate genes for autism spectrum disorder. *Nat. Neurosci.* **2017**, *20*, 602–611. [CrossRef] [PubMed]

58. Glessner, J.T.; Wang, K.; Cai, G.; Korvatska, O.; Kim, C.E.; Wood, S.; Zhang, H.; Estes, A.; Brune, C.W.; Bradfield, J.P.; et al. Autism genome-wide copy number variation reveals ubiquitin and neuronal genes. *Nature* **2009**, *459*, 569–573. [CrossRef]

59. Holt, R.; Monaco, A.P. Links between genetics and pathophysiology in the autism spectrum disorders. *EMBO Molecul. Med.* **2011**, *3*, 438–450. [CrossRef] [PubMed]

60. Khanzada, N.S.; Butler, M.G.; Manzardo, A.M. GeneAnalytics pathway analysis and genetic overlap among autism spectrum disorder, bipolar disorder and schizophrenia. *Int. J. Mol Sci.* **2017**, *18*, 527. [CrossRef]

61. Chatterjee, M.; Schild, D.; Teunissen, C.E. Contactins in the central nervous system: Role in health and disease. *Neural. Regen. Res.* **2019**, *14*, 206–216.

62. Varga, N.A.; Pentelenyi, K.; Balicza, P.; Gezsi, A.; Remenyi, V.; Harsfalvi, V.; Bencsik, R.; Iles, A.; Prekop, C.; Molnar, M.J. Mitochondrial dysfunction and autism: Comprehensive genetic analyses of children with autism and mtDNA deletion. *Behav Brain Funct.* **2018**, *14*, 4. [CrossRef] [PubMed]

63. Wallace, D.C. Mitochondrial genes and disease. *Hosp. Pract.* **1986**, *21*, 77–92.

64. Wallace, D.C. Mitochondrial diseases in mand and mouse. *Science* **1999**, *283*, 1482–1488. [CrossRef]

65. Schon, E.A.; Manfredi, G. Neuronal degeneration and mitochondrial dysfunction. *J. Clin. Investig.* **2003**, *111*, 303–312. [CrossRef] [PubMed]

66. DiMauro, S.; Schon, E.A. Mitochondrial respiratory-chain diseases. *N. Engl. J. Med.* **2003**, *348*, 2656–2668. [CrossRef] [PubMed]

67. Pons, R.; Andreu, A.L.; Checcarelli, N.; Vila, M.R.; Engelstad, K.; Sue, C.M.; Shungu, D.; Haggerty, R.; de Vivo, D.C.; DiMauro, S. Mitochondrial DNA abnormalities and autistic spectrum disorders. *J. Pediatr.* **2004**, *144*, 81–85. [CrossRef] [PubMed]

68. Spelbrink, J.N. Functional organization of mammalian mitochondrial DNA in nucleotides: History, recent developments, and future challenges. *IUBMB* **2010**, *62*, 19–32.

69. Boyle, C.A.; Boulet, S.; Schieve, L.A.; Cohen, R.A.; Blumberg, S.J.; Yeargin-Allsopp, M.; Visser, S.; Kogan, M.D. Trends in the prevalence of developmental disabilities in the US children, 1997–2008. *Pediatrics* **2011**, *127*, 1034–1042. [CrossRef] [PubMed]

70. Heil, K.M.; Schaaf, C.P. The genetics of autism spectrum disorders—A guide for clinicians. *Curr. Psychiatry Rep.* **2013**, *15*, 334. [CrossRef]

71. Roberts, J.L.; Jovanes, K.; Dasouki, M.; Manzardo, A.M.; Butler, M.G. Chromosomal microarray analysis of consecutive individuals with autism spectrum disorders or learning disability presenting for genetic services. *Gene* **2014**, *535*, 70–78. [CrossRef]

72. Weitlauf, A.S.; McPheeters, M.L.; Peters, B.; Sathe, N.; Travis, R.; Aiello, R.; Williamson, E.; Veenstra-VanderWeele, J.; Krishnaswami, S.; Jerome, R.; et al. *Therapies for Children with Autism Spectrum Disorder: Behavioral Interventions Update*; Comparative Effectiveness Review No. 137. (Prepared by the Vanderbilt evidence-Based Practice Center Under Contract No. 290-2012-00009-I.) AHRQ Publication No. 14-EHC036-EF.; Agency for Healthcare Research and Quality: Rockville, MD, USA, 2014.

73. Tiura, M.; Kim, J.; Detmers, D.; Baldi, H. Predictors of longitudinal ABA treatment outcomes for children with autism: A growth curve analysis. *Res. Dev. Disabil.* **2017**, *70*, 185–197. [CrossRef]

74. Reichow, B.; Hume, K.; Barton, E.E.; Boyd, B.A. Early intensive behavioral intervention (EIBI) for young children with autism spectrum disorders (ASD). *Cochrane Database Syst. Rev.* **2018**, *5*, CD009260. [CrossRef]

75. Frankel, F.; Myatt, R.; Sugar, C. A randomized controlled study of parent-assisted children's friendship training with children having autism spectrum disorders. *J. Autism Dev. Disord.* **2010**, *40*, 827–842. [CrossRef]

76. National Institute for Clinical Excellence. Autism: Recognition, referral, diagnosis and management of adults on the autism spectrum. *Natl. Inst. Health Care Excell.* **2012**, *142*, 18.

77. Hillier, A.; Fish, T.; Cloppert, P. Outcomes of a social and vocational skills support group for adolescents and young adults on the autism spectrum. *Focus Autism Other Dev. Disabl.* **2007**, *22*, 107–115. [CrossRef]

78. Lang, R.; Regester, A.; Lauderdale, S. Treatment of anxiety in autism spectrum disorders using cognitive behaviour therapy: A systematic review. *Dev. Neurorehabil.* **2010**, *13*, 53–63. [CrossRef] [PubMed]

79. Accordino, R.E.; Kidd, C.; Politte, L.C.; Henry, C.A.; McDougle, C.J. Psychopharmacological interventions in autism spectrum disorder. *Expert Opin. Pharmacother.* **2016**, *17*, 937–952.

80. Madden, J.M.; Lakoma, M.D.; Lynch, F.L.; Rusinak, D.; Owen-Smith, A.A.; Coleman, K.J.; Quinn, V.P.; Yau, V.M.; Qian, Y.X.; Croen, L.A. Psychotropic medication use among insured children with autism spectrum disorder. *J. Autism Dev. Disord.* **2017**, *47*, 144–154. [CrossRef]

81. Stepanova, E.; Dowling, S.; Phelps, M.; Findling, R.L. Pharmacotherapy of emotional and behavioral symptoms associated with autism spectrum disorder in children and adolescents. *Dialogues Clin. Neurosci.* **2017**, *19*, 395–402.

82. Lamy, M.; Erickson, C.A. Pharmacological management of behavioral disturbances in children and adolescents with autism spectrum disorders. *Curr. Prob. Ped. Adolesc Health Care* **2012**, *48*, 250–264. [CrossRef] [PubMed]

83. Research Units on Pediatric Psychopharmacology (RUPP). Randomized, controlled, crossover trial of methylphenidate in pervasive developmental disorders with hyperactivity. *Arch. Gen. Psychiatry.* **2005**, *62*, 1266–1275. [CrossRef]

84. Reichow, B.; Volkmar, F.R.; Bloch, M.H. Systematic review and meta-analysis of pharmacological treatment of the symptoms of attention-deficit/hyperactivity disorder in children with pervasive developmental disorders. *J. Autism Dev. Disord.* **2013**, *43*, 2435–4241. [CrossRef]

85. Harfterkamp, M.; van de Loo-Neus, G.; Minderaa, R.B.; van der Gaag, R.-J.; Escobar, R.; Schacht, A.; Pamulapati, S.; Buietelaar, J.K.; Hoekstra, P.J. A randomized double-blind study of atomoxetine versus placebo for attention-deficit/hyperactivity disorder symptoms in children with autism spectrum disorders. *J. Am. Acad. Child Adol. Psychiatry* **2012**, *51*, 733–741. [CrossRef]

86. Guy, W. *ECDEU Assessment Manual for Psychopharmacology, Revised.*; Department of Health, Education, and Welfare Publication (ADM): National Institute of Mental Health: Rockville, MD, USA, 1976; pp. 76–338.

87. Scahill, L.; McCracken, J.T.; King, B.H.; Rockhill, C.; Shah, B.; Politte, L.; Sanders, R.; Minjarez, M.; Cowen, J.; Mullett, J.; et al. Research Unites on Pediatric Psychopharmacology Autism Network. Extended-release Guanfacine for hyperactivity in children with autism spectrum disorder. *Am. J. Psychiatry* **2015**, *172*, 1197–1206. [CrossRef] [PubMed]

88. Pandina, G.J.; Bossie, C.A.; Youssef, E.; Zhu, Y.; Dunbar, F. Risperidone improves behavioral symptoms in children with autism in a randomized, double-blind, placebo-controlled trial. *J. Autism Dev. Disord.* **2007**, *37*, 367–373. [CrossRef] [PubMed]

89. Aman, M.G.; Singh, N.N. *Aberrant Behavior Checklist Manual*; Slosson Publications: East Aurora, NY, USA, 1986.

90. Levine, S.Z.; Kodesh, A.; Goldberg, Y.; Reichenberg, A.; Furukawa, T.A.; Kolevzon, A.; Leucht, S. Initial severity and efficacy of risperidone in autism: Results from the RUPP trial. *Eur. Psychiatry.* **2016**, *32*, 16–20. [CrossRef]

91. Wink, L.K.; Early, M.; Schaefer, T.; Pottenger, A.; Horn, P.; MDougle, C.J.; Erickson, C.A. Body mass index change in autism spectrum disorders: Comparison of treatment with risperidone and aripiprazole. *J. Child Adolesc. Psychopharmacol.* **2014**, *24*, 78–82. [CrossRef]

92. Hollander, E.; Chaplin, W.; Soorya, L.; Wasserman, S.; Novotny, S.; Rusoff, J.; Feirsen, N.; Pepa, L.; Anagnostou, E. Divalproex sodium vs placebo for the treatment of irritability in children and adolescents with autism spectrum disorders. *Neuropsychopharmacol* **2010**, *35*, 990–998. [CrossRef]

93. Hellings, J.A.; Weckbaugh, M.; Nickel, E.J.; Cain, S.E.; Zarcone, J.R.; Reese, R.M.; Hall, S.; Ermer, D.J.; Tsai, L.Y.; Schroeder, S.R.; et al. A double-blind, placebo-controlled study of valproate for aggression in youth with pervasive developmental disorders. *J. Child Adolesc. Psychopharmacol.* **2005**, *15*, 682–692. [CrossRef] [PubMed]

94. Mazzone, L.; Ruta, L. Topiramate in children with autistic spectrum disorders. *Brain Dev.* **2006**, *28*, 668. [CrossRef] [PubMed]

95. Rezaei, V.; Mohammadi, M.R.; Ghanizadeh, A.; Sahraian, A.; Tabrizi, M.; Rezazadeh, S.-A.; Akhondzadeh, S. Double-blind, placebo-controlled trial of risperidone plus topiramate in children with autistic disorder. *Prog. Neuropsychopharmacol. Biol. Psychiatry* **2010**, *34*, 1269–1272. [CrossRef] [PubMed]

96. Swatzyna, R.J.; Boutros, N.N.; Genovese, A.C.; MacInerney, E.K.; Roark, A.J.; Kozlowski, G.P. Electroencephalogram (EEG) for children with autism spectrum disorder: Evidential considerations for routine screening. *Eur. Child Adolesc. Psychiatry* **2019**, *28*, 615–624. [CrossRef] [PubMed]

97. Hollander, E.; Soorya, L.; Chaplin, W.; Anagnostou, E.; Taylor, C.P.; Ferretti, C.J.; Wasserman, S.; Swanson, E.; Settipani, C. A double-blind placebo-controlled trial of fluoxetine for repetitive behaviors and global severity in adult autism spectrum disorders. *Am. J. Psychiatry* **2012**, *169*, 292–299. [CrossRef]

98. Williams, K.; Brignell, A.; Randall, M.; Silove, N.; Hazell, P. Selective serotonin reuptake inhibitors (SSRIs) for autism spectrum disorders (ASD). *Cochrane Database Syst. Rev.* **2013**, *8*, CD004677. [CrossRef] [PubMed]

99. Souders, M.C.; Zavodny, S.; Eriksen, W.; Sinko, R.; Connell, J.; Kerns, C.; Schaaf, R.; Pinto-Martin, J. Sleep in children with autism spectrum disorder. *Curr. Psychiatry Rep.* **2017**, *19*, 34. [CrossRef] [PubMed]

100. Blackmer, A.B.; Feinstein, J.A. Management of sleep disorders in children with neurodevelopmental disorders: A review. *Pharmacother* **2016**, *36*, 84–98. [CrossRef] [PubMed]

101. Ming, X.; Gordon, E.; Kang, N.; Wagner, G.C. Use of clonidine in children with autism spectrum disorders. *Brain Dev.* **2008**, *30*, 454–460. [CrossRef]

102. Butler, M.G. Pharmacogenetics and psychiatric care: A review and commentary. *J. Ment. Health Clin. Psychol.* **2018**, *2*, 17–24. [CrossRef]

103. Weinshilboum, R.M.; Wang, L. Pharmacogenetics and pharmacogenomics: Development, science and translation. *Annu Rev. Genom. Hum. Genet.* **2006**, *7*, 223–245. [CrossRef]

104. Weng, L.; Zhang, L.; Peng, Y.; Huang, R.S. Pharamcogenetics and pharmacogenomics: A bridge to individualized cancer therapy. *Pharmacogenomics* **2013**, *14*, 315–324. [CrossRef]

105. Kirchheiner, J.; Seeringer, A. Clinical implications of pharmacogenetics of cytochrome P450 drug metabolizing enzymes. *Biochim. Biophys. Acta* **2007**, *1770*, 489–494. [CrossRef]

106. Reynolds, K.S. Achieving the promise of personalized medicine. *Clin. Pharmacol. Ther.* **2012**, *92*, 401–405. [CrossRef]

107. Lee, J.W.; Aminken, F.; Bhavsar, A.P.; Shaw, K.; Carleton, B.C.; Hayden, M.R.; Ross, C.J.D. The emerging era of pharmacogenomics: Current successes, future potential, and challenges. *Clin. Genet.* **2014**, *86*, 21–28. [CrossRef]

108. Kalow, W. Human pharmacogenomics: The development of a science. *Hum. Genom.* **2004**, *1*, 375–380. [CrossRef] [PubMed]

109. Werck-Reichhart, D.; Feyereisen, R. Cytochromes P450: A success story. *Genome Biol.* **2000**, *1*, 3003. [CrossRef] [PubMed]

110. Samer, C.F.; Lorenzini, K.I.; Rollason, V.; Daali, Y.; Desmeues, J.A. Applications of CYP450 testing in the clinical setting. *Mol. Diagn. Ther.* **2013**, *17*, 165–184. [CrossRef]

111. Danielson, P.B. The cytochrome P450 superfamily: Biochemistry, evolution and drug metabolism in humans. *Curr. Drug Metab.* **2002**, *3*, 561–597. [CrossRef] [PubMed]

112. Chen, C.; Chen, Y.; Guan, M.X. A peep into mitochondrial disorder: Multifaceted from mitochondrial DNA mutations to nuclear gene modulation. *Protein Cell* **2015**, *6*, 862–870. [CrossRef] [PubMed]
113. Schaefer, G.B. Clinical genetic aspects of ASD spectrum disorders. *Int. J. Mol. Sci.* **2016**, *17*, 180. [CrossRef]
114. Oikonomakis, V.; Kosma, K.; Mitrakos, A.; Sofocleous, C.; Pervanidou, P.; Syrmou, A.; Pampanos, A.; Psoni, S.; Fryssira, H.; Kanavakis, E.; et al. Recurrent copy number variations as risk factors for autism spectrum disorders: Analysis of the clinical implications. *Clin. Genet.* **2016**, *89*, 708–718. [CrossRef]
115. Hall, L.; Kelley, E. The contribution of epigenetics to understanding genetic factors in autism. *Autism* **2014**, *18*, 872–881. [CrossRef]
116. Hagerman, R.J.; Berry-Kravis, E.; Hazlett, H.C.; Bailey, D.B., Jr.; Moine, H.; Kooy, R.F.; Tassone, F.; Gantois, I.; Sonenberg, N.; Mandel, J.L.; et al. Fragile X Syndrome. *Nat. Rev. Dis. Primers* **2017**, *29*, 17065. [CrossRef]
117. Rafi, S.K.; Butler, M.G. The 15q11.2 BP1-BP2 Microdeletion (*Burnside–Butler*) Syndrome: In Silico Analyses of the Four Coding Genes Reveal Functional Associations with Neurodevelopmental Phenotypes. *Int. J. Med. Sci.* **2020**, *21*, 3296. [CrossRef]
118. Hartin, S.M.; Hossain, W.A.; Butler, M.G.; Francis, D.; Godler, D.E.; Barkataki, S. Analysis of the Prader-Willi syndrome imprinting center using droplet digitcal PCR and Next-Generation whole-exome sequencing. *Mol. Genet. Genom. Med.* **2019**, *7*, e00575. [CrossRef] [PubMed]

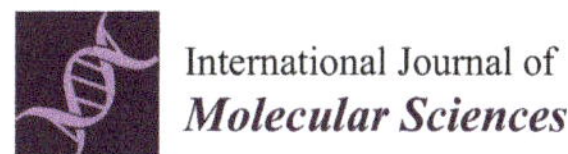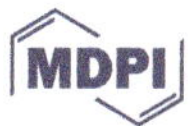

International Journal of
Molecular Sciences

Review

Proteomics and Metabolomics Approaches towards a Functional Insight onto AUTISM Spectrum Disorders: Phenotype Stratification and Biomarker Discovery

Maria Vittoria Ristori [1], Stefano Levi Mortera [2], Valeria Marzano [2], Silvia Guerrera [3], Pamela Vernocchi [2], Gianluca Ianiro [4], Simone Gardini [5], Giuliano Torre [6], Giovanni Valeri [3], Stefano Vicari [3,7], Antonio Gasbarrini [8,9] and Lorenza Putignani [1,*]

[1] Department of Laboratories, Unit of Parasitology and Area of Genetics and Rare Diseases, Unit of Human Microbiome, Bambino Gesù Children's Hospital, IRCCS, 00165 Rome, Italy; mvittoria.ristori@opbg.net

[2] Area of Genetics and Rare Diseases, Unit of Human Microbiome, Bambino Gesù Children's Hospital, IRCCS, 00165 Rome, Italy; stefano.levimortera@opbg.net (S.L.M.); valeria.marzano@opbg.net (V.M.); pamela.vernocchi@opbg.net (P.V.)

[3] Department of Neuroscience, Unit of Head Child & Adolescent Psychiatry, Bambino Gesù Children's Hospital, IRCCS, 00165 Rome, Italy; silvia.guerrera@opbg.net (S.G.); giovanni.valeri@opbg.net (G.V.); stefano.vicari@opbg.net (S.V.)

[4] Dipartimento di Gastroenterologia, Università Cattolica del Sacro Cuore, Fondazione Policlinico Universitario A. Gemelli IRCCS, Largo A. Gemelli 8, 00168 Rome, Italy; gianluca.ianiro@hotmail.it

[5] GENOMEUP S.R.L, Viale Pasteur 8, 00144 Rome, Italy; simone@genomeup.com

[6] Department of Specialist Pediatricians and Liver-Kidney Transplantation, Bambino Gesù Children's Hospital, IRCCS, 00165 Rome, Italy; giuliano.torre@opbg.net

[7] Department of Life Sciences and Public Health, Catholic University, 00153 Rome, Italy

[8] Istituto di Patologia Speciale Medica, Università Cattolica del Sacro Cuore, 00168 Rome, Italy; antonio.gasbarrini@unicatt.it

[9] UOC Medicina Interna e Gastroenterologia, Area Gastroenterologia ed Oncologia Medica, Dipartimento di Scienze Gastroenterologiche, Endocrino-Metaboliche e Nefro-Urologiche, Fondazione Policlinico Universitario A. Gemelli IRCCS, 00168 Rome, Italy

* Correspondence: lorenza.putigani@opbg.net; Tel.: +39-0668-59-4127

Received: 14 August 2020; Accepted: 27 August 2020; Published: 30 August 2020

Abstract: Autism spectrum disorders (ASDs) are neurodevelopmental disorders characterized by behavioral alterations and currently affect about 1% of children. Significant genetic factors and mechanisms underline the causation of ASD. Indeed, many affected individuals are diagnosed with chromosomal abnormalities, submicroscopic deletions or duplications, single-gene disorders or variants. However, a range of metabolic abnormalities has been highlighted in many patients, by identifying biofluid metabolome and proteome profiles potentially usable as ASD biomarkers. Indeed, next-generation sequencing and other omics platforms, including proteomics and metabolomics, have uncovered early age disease biomarkers which may lead to novel diagnostic tools and treatment targets that may vary from patient to patient depending on the specific genomic and other omics findings. The progressive identification of new proteins and metabolites acting as biomarker candidates, combined with patient genetic and clinical data and environmental factors, including microbiota, would bring us towards advanced clinical decision support systems (CDSSs) assisted by machine learning models for advanced ASD-personalized medicine. Herein, we will discuss novel computational solutions to evaluate new proteome and metabolome ASD biomarker candidates, in terms of their recurrence in the reviewed literature and laboratory medicine feasibility. Moreover, the way to exploit CDSS, performed by artificial intelligence, is presented as an effective tool to integrate omics data to electronic health/medical records (EHR/EMR), hopefully acting as added value in the near future for the clinical management of ASD.

Keywords: autism spectrum disorders (ASDs); proteomics; metabolomics; interactomics; disease biomarkers; clinical decision support systems (CDSSs)

---

1. Introduction

Autism spectrum disorders (ASDs) are a complex set of neurodevelopmental diseases, behaviourally diagnosed, that affect several spheres of mental development. They represent a panel of conditions that begin during the developmental period and result in impairments of personal, social, academic or occupational functioning (Figure 1) [1–3].

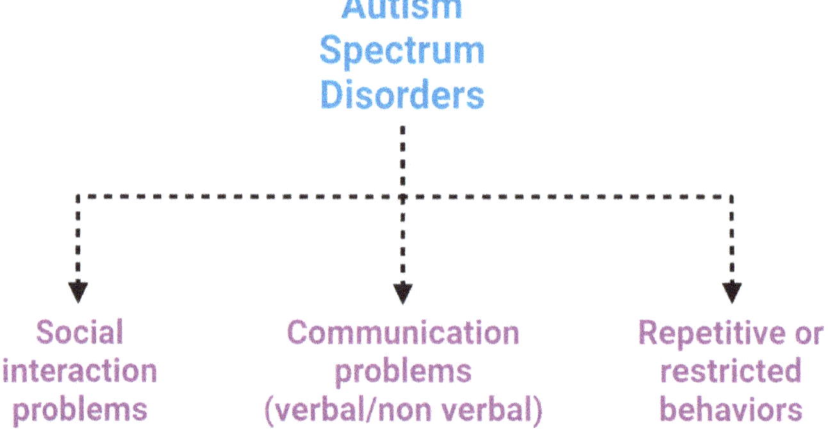

Figure 1. Neuropsychiatric features of autism spectrum disorder (ASD). ASD is characterized by impairments in social interaction, difficulty in adapting behaviour in various social contexts, or lack of interest in peers; communication problems, such as difficulty making eye contact, facial expressions, body postures, and difficulty understanding or using the gestures that regulate interaction with others; and restricted or repetitive behaviours, such as rituals that are conducted with a rigid manner or movements.

Comorbidity with intellectual disabilities, impaired motor coordination and gastrointestinal (GI) disorders are also often present [3,4]. An incidence of ASD of 1 in every 60 subjects is estimated in the United States, with a fourfold frequency for males with respect to females [5–7]. Clinical manifestations typically occur in the 2nd–3rd year of life, usually persist in adulthood, and influence various aspects of mental development [8]. The exact etiopathogenesis of ASDs is not yet well known but many studies have investigated both genetic and environmental factors [9,10]. In particular, gene inheritance has been found in around 60% [11,12] or 80% [13] of cases with significant heterogeneity concerning the genetic factors actually involved in ASD onset [14,15]. In a review of the literature, Higdon R. et al. found that many ASD patients have recurrent de novo disruptive mutations particularly affecting specific protein targets such as chromodomain helicase DNA binding protein 8 (CHD8), activity-dependent neuroprotector homeobox (ADNP), dual-specificity tyrosine phosphorylation-regulated kinase 1A (DYRK1A), and phosphatase and tensin homolog (PTEN). In particular, subjects with PTEN mutations showed abnormal brain white matter volumes in addition to autism symptoms; subjects with CHD8 mutations carried chronic GI complications, distinct facial dysmorphology and macrocephaly; those with DYRK1A mutations had a higher probability of microencephaly and early growth difficulties compared to healthy subjects; and patients carrying an ADNP-disruptive mutation were characterized by intellectual disability and dysmorphic features [16]. Interestingly, a recent study directed by Risch and his group found that ASD siblings showed a risk increment of 10.1% to develop ASD, compared to control siblings, hence confirming a genetic predisposition in the familial recurrence of ASD [10]. Additionally, oxidative stress, inflammation, mitochondrial dysfunction, and immune dysregulation, associated with changes in protein and metabolites pathways, have been reported in the literature in many ASD studies [17–19].

However, it is also well established that several factors involving the pre-, perinatal, or postnatal environment are associated with amplified risk of ASD [20] (Figure 2). Amongst these, the main factors of maternal infections, stress, and diabetes, also in addition to exposure to pesticides, air pollution, dietary habits, infections, inflammatory conditions, and consumption of antibiotics during pregnancy, which together make up the so-called exposome, combine to increase the ASD risk [21,22]. Indeed, environmental factors can influence genetic vulnerability [23] by modifying the development of neuronal circuits [24]. These alterations are heterogeneous and this can contribute to determining the complexity of the disorder in terms of neurobiology, symptomatology, and etiology [25]. In particular, GI comorbidity associated with an alteration in the microbiota composition is frequently reported in ASD groups. [21,26]. Indeed, many studies have investigated the association between autism severity and GI, showing positive correlations [26–30]. The increased presence of irritability [31], anxiety and affective disorders [3,32], dysregulation and externalizing problems [33], rigid/compulsive behaviors [34,35], increased sensory sensitivity [36], and sleep problems [33,37] have been reported in ASD subjects with concurrent GI symptoms compared to ASD subjects without. Significant GI symptoms are associated with chronic abdominal pain [3,4,26,33,38,39], chronic constipation [3,4,26,39,40], chronic diarrhea [3,39,41], and gastroesophageal reflux [26,38,42]. The existence of a complex bidirectional interaction between the central nervous system and the GI tract is currently more than a hypothesis and primarily involves the impact of ecology and function of the microbiota [43].

Targeted-metagenomics studies on the ecology of the microbiota, performed using next-generation sequencing (NGS), have revealed that specific signatures, such as *Prevotella*, *Enterococcus*, *Lactobacillus*, *Ruminococcus*, *Faecalibacterium prausnitzii*, *Sutterella*, and *Bifidobacterium*, are overrepresented in children with ASD compared to healthy controls [28,44–46]. Furthermore, metabolomics studies evidenced an involvement of the microbiota in the production of molecules, such as tryptophan, inflammatory cytokines, or cortisol, which exert a role in ASD disorders and GI-related symptoms, as recently reported by our group [47]. Therefore, an approach to the investigation of ASD based on omics or meta-omics disciplines is becoming crucial for both disease phenotype stratification and biomarker discovery. Given the large amount of data (i.e., big data) produced by a single omics or meta-omics discipline, an untargeted evaluation of data may provide substantial new models to properly stratify a multifactorial disease such as ASD, considering both host and microbiome profiling and producing integrated models to co-represent genomics/metagenomics, metabolomics/metametabolomics, and proteomics/metaproteomics profiling of the disease.

In particular, transcriptomics and proteomics may improve the existing gene models by profiling molecular phenotypes at transcriptionally active regions of the genome (the transcriptome) and protein abundance (the proteome) levels. Besides a proteomics profiling, post-translational modifications and protein–protein interactions can contribute to providing further specific information on pathways and molecular networks. Furthermore, metabolomics may provide information on the modulation of the host and microbiota metabolism. As previously reported, the diagnosis of ASD depends on clinical observation and procedures to evaluate behavioral, historical, and parent-report information [48]. These tools may involve a significant degree of host variability; hence, detecting metabolomics biomarkers may contribute to the advance of the diagnostics and clinical management of ASD, and may provide new biomarkers that could be used to improve the outcome of individualized interventions as personalized medicine tools.

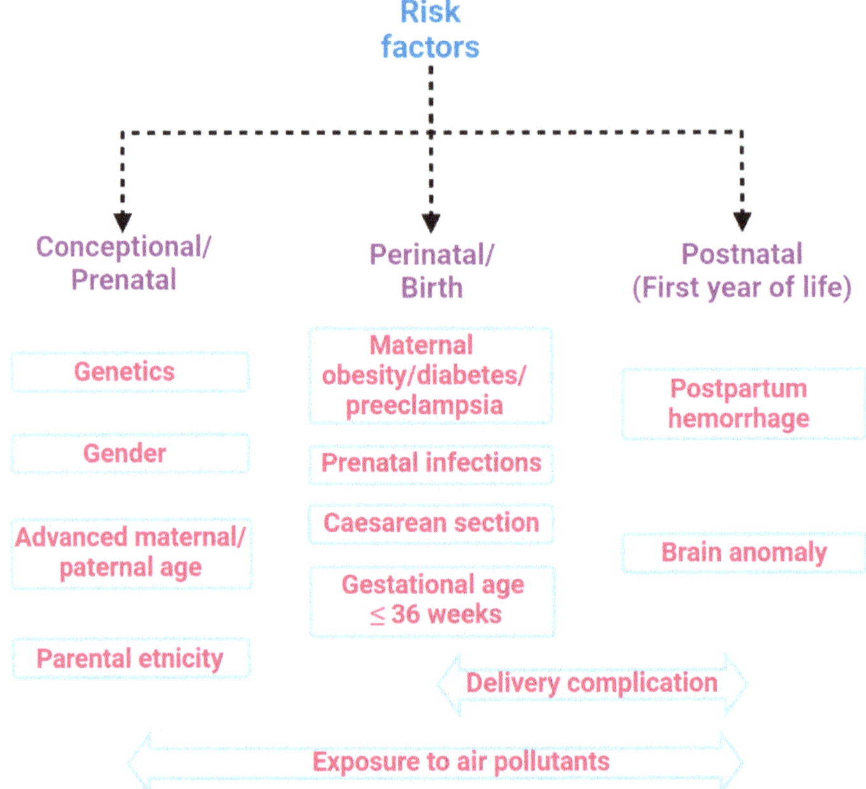

Figure 2. Risk factors associated with ASD: ASD is a multifactorial condition characterized by genetic and environmental factors, including prenatal and postnatal factors that increase the risk of disease. Among the main factors, genetic predisposition, parents' age, and exposures during pregnancy to air pollutants have been associated with poor cognitive outcomes in the perinatal age. Moreover, delivery complications or postpartum haemorrhage might also increase the risk of ASD. All these factors, globally constituting the exposome, may contribute to ASD, hence hampering the search for single biomarkers of the disease.

Given the growing interest in identifying new functional traits of the disease and novel biomarkers, big data obtained by metabolomics and proteomics approaches from blood, urine or saliva specimens should be collected and stored in open source digital biobanks available to omics scientists and clinicians for deep phenotyping. This system biology-based approach will allow multidimensional data to be integrated at cellular, tissue and organ organization levels, providing computational chemometric models concurring in the understanding of the pathophysiological mechanisms of diseases (i.e., onset and progression) [49]. In this paper, we introduce a new analysis of the data (i.e., ontology enrichment of protein and metabolites), based on the category "Biological Process" to highlight new possible biomarkers and metabolic pathways that could open new avenues to the study of ASD disease biomarkers based on proteomics and metabolomics. Moreover, novel biomarkers are discussed in terms of their added value in clinical decision support systems (CDSS), approached by artificial intelligence (AI), that represent a new way to integrate omics, multi-omics data and health/medical records (EHR/EMR). This may represent a novel tool to assist clinicians in the near future to approach ASD phenotype stratification and hopefully to disentangle the complexity of this disease due to multifactorial components.

2. Methods

2.1. Search Strategy

We conducted a review of the literature to evaluate the role of the proteomics and metabolomics disciplines, and data for disease phenotype stratification and biomarker discovery, in ASD patients. The research was conducted on PubMed, including papers from 2004 to 2019 and using the following terms: "autism" or "autism spectrum disorder" and "proteomics" or "interactome" or "metabolomics" or "protein" or "metabolites" and "omics". All articles providing enough information about the relationship between multi-omics data and ASD were included.

2.2. Selection Criteria

The inclusion criteria for study selection were the following: (1) observational prospective and retrospective studies, case–control studies, cohort studies, or systematic reviews; (2) studies involving proteomics- and metabolomics-based biomarker research in ASD; and (3) English written studies. All studies that did not meet the following criteria were excluded from the review process.

2.3. Analysis of Protein and Metabolites Highlighted in Tables 1 and 2

New "ontology enrichment" analyses, based on class, subclass, and biological processes were performed for both metabolites and proteins reported in Tables 1 and 2. The aim was to identify new potential biomarkers found in the literature that could be interpreted in a new way for appropriate evaluation in decision support systems (DSSs) through the framework discussed herein.

Table 1. Proteomics-based targets of ASD.

Reference	Matrix	N° of Subjects	Analytical Technique	Proteins Implicated and Pathways
[50] Junaid MA et al., 2004	Brain	8 ASD and 10 controls	2-DE, LC-MS/MS	Glo1 (osteoclastogenesis and ASD etiology)
[51] Broek JA et al., 2014	Brain	prefrontal cortex, 10 ASD and 10 controls; cerebellum, 16 ASD, 17 controls	SRM-MS	VIME, CKB, MAG, MBP, MOG, PLP1, DNM2, STX1A, STXBP1, GFAP, PACSIN1, SYN2, SYT1 (synaptic transmission and energy metabolism)
[52] Wingo et al., 2019	Brain	27 ASD, 76 controls	Large-scale proteome-wide association	VGF, SEPT5, DBI, MAPT, KIAA1045, DLD, ABHD10, VDAC1, NDUFV1, PDHB (cognitive stability)
[53] Corbett et al., 2007	Blood	69 ASD and 35 controls	LC-MS/MS	FHR1, C1Q, FN1, APOB-100 (indirect impact on brain development in ASD)
[54] Ngounou Wetie et al., 2014	Blood	7 ASD and 7 controls	one dimensional gel electrophoresis (1-DE), LC-MS/MS	APOA1, APOA4, PON1 (Lipid metabolism - paraoxonase activity)
[55] Steeb et al., 2014	Blood	30 ASD and 29 controls	Immunoassay, LC-MS/MS	ADIPO, ARMC3, APOA1, APOE, APOC2, BMP6, CHGA, CLC4K, CTGF, EPO, FETUB, GLCE, ICAM1, IL3, IGA, IL16, IL12A, MRRP1, RGPD4, SHBG, PAP, PTPA, RN149, TENA, TLE1, TNF, TF, TRIPB, ZC3HE (Lipid metabolism, cell growth, inflammation)
[56] Yang et al., 2018	Blood	68 ASD and 80 controls	MALDI-TOF MS	APOC1, AFP, CPB2, FAPB1, FGA, PF4, SERPINA5, TAAR6 (lipid metabolism)
[57] Cortelazzo et al., 2016	Blood	30 ASD and 30 controls	2-DE, LC-MS/MS	A1AT, A2M, HPT, FIBB, FIBG, APOA1, APOA4, APOJ, ALBU, IGHA1, IGHAG (acute inflammatory and lipid metabolism)
[58] Feng et al., 2017	Blood	15 ASD and 15 controls	2-DE, Western blot/protein carbonylation and MALDI-TOF	C8A, IGKC (Immune system)
[59] Shen et al., 2018	Blood	30 ASD and 30 controls	Proteo-Miner protein enrichment, iTRAQ, LC-M S/MS	ACTG1, ACTN1, AGT, APOE, CALM1, CALR, C3, C5, EHD3, ENO1, FERMT3, FBLN1, FN1, IGFALS, ITGA2B, MAPRE2, PARVB, SERPINA1, SERPIN4A, THBS1, TLN1, VCL, VCP, VTN (complement system, platelet function, focal adhesions, cytoskeleton, motility and migration and synaptogenesis)

Table 1. *Cont.*

Reference	Matrix	N° of Subjects	Analytical Technique	Proteins Implicated and Pathways
[60] Castagnola et al., 2008	Saliva	27 ASD and 23 controls	LC-MS/MS	HTN1, PRP, STATH (Antimicrobial peptides and central nervous system)
[61] Ngounou Wetie et al., 2015	Saliva	6 ASD and 6 controls	2-DE, LC-MS/MS	AMY1A, AZGP1, CREBBP, CST5, FRAT1, GRTP1, KIF14, ITGA6, HERC1, MRP14, MUC16, PLG, PSP, PIP, TF, ZG16 (immune and inflammation response, lipid metabolism, oxidative stress)
[62] Ngounou Wetie et al., 2015	Saliva	6 ASD and 6 controls	LC-MS/MS	DMBT1, ELANE, HTN1, IGKC, IGHG1, IGLC2, LTF, PIGR, PIP, PRH1, STATH (Inflammation and Immune response)
[63] Suganya et al., 2015	Urine	30 ASD and 30 controls	2-DE, MALDI-TOF MS	IGHG1, KNG1, MASP2 (Inflammation, coagulation and complement system)
[64] Pichitpunpong et al., 2019	lymphoblastoid cell lines	Not available	2-DE, LC-MS/MS, Western blotting	DLD, IDH2, TPT1, ANXA5, CCT5, COX5A, LGALS1, GSTP1, HNRNPA1, PGAM1, TUBB, H3F3C, DBI, AHSG, ERH, CLTA, CALM1, ENO1 (Neurological functions and inflammation)

Table 2. Metabolomics-based targets of ASD.

Reference	Matrix	N of Subjects	Analytical Technique	Metabolite Implicated and Metabolic Process
[65] Graham et al., 2016	Brain	11 ASD and 11 controls	LC-LTQ Orbitrap MS	3-methoxytyramine, 5,6-dihydrouridine, N-carboxyethyl-γ-aminobutyric acid (dopamine, nucleotide metabolism and cell growth and proliferation)
[66] Kurochkin et al., 2019	Brain	32 ASD and 40 controls	UPLC–MS/MS	5-oxoproline, glutathione disulfide, Glutathione, l-γ-glutamyl-cysteine, l-cysteinyl-glycine (glutathione; purine; pyruvate; propanoate; TCA cycle; galactose; starch and sucrose; nicotinate and nicotinamide; cysteine and methionine; arginine and proline metabolism)
[67] Kuwabara et al., 2013	Blood	25 ASD and 28 controls	CE-TOF MS	arginine, taurine, 5-Oxoproline, lactic acid (oxidative stress and mitochondrial dysfunction)
[68] West et al., 2014	Blood	52 ASD and 30 controls	LC-MS and GC-MS	aspartate, DHEA-S, glutaric acid, serine, succinic acid citrate, creatinine, isoleucine, hydroxyphenyllactate, glutamate (energy production, mitochondrial disease or dysfunction and oxidative stress)
[69] Wang et al., 2016	Blood	173 ASD and 163 controls	UPLC/Q–TOF– MS/MS	decanoylcarnitine, pregnanetriol, adrenic acid, docosahexaenoic acid, sphingosine-1-phosphate, uric acid (β-oxidation, fatty acid and mitochondrial dysfunction)
[70] Rangel-Huerta et al., 2019	Blood	20 ASD and 30 controls	UPLC–MS/MS	1-methylnicotinamide, 3-Indoxyl sulfate, 4-methyl-2-oxopetane, 5-bromotryptophan, 6-hydroxyindole sulfate, cortisone, methionine, tryptophan, γ-glutamylmethionine, ursodeoxycholate, sphingomyelins, kynurenine, choline phosphate, decanoylcarnitine, 2-keto-3-deoxyglutamate, arachidate, behenate, fructose, sebacate, dodecanedioate, glutamate, aspartate, orotate, galactitol, N-acetyl-aspartyl glutamate (amino acid, lipid, nicotinamide)
[71] Kelly RS et al., 2019	Blood	403 children of which 52 ASD	UPLC-MS / MS	trimethylamine N-oxide, cinnamoylglycine, linoleoyl ethanolamide, palmitoyl ethanolamide, erythritol, docosahexaenoylcarnitine, prolylhydroxyproline, alpha-ketobutyrate, serotonin, oleoyl ethanolamide, N-formylphenylalanine, 5-Hydroxyindoleacetate, pyrraline, sphingomyelin, N-formylanthranilic acid (Endocannabinoid metabolism, Xenobiotics, Tryptophan metabolism, Urea cycle, Amino acid mebolism, Fatty acid metabolism, Phospholipid metabolism, Sphingolipid metabolism)
[72] Yap et al., 2010	Urine	39 ASD and 34 controls	^{1}H-NMR	N-methylnicotinamide, N-methylnicotinic acid, dimethylamine, succinic acid, taurine, N-methyl-2-pyridone-5-carboxamide, hippurate, phenylacetylglutamine, platelet serotonin (gut microbiota and gastrointestinal dysfunction)

Table 2. *Cont.*

Reference	Matrix	N of Subjects	Analytical Technique	Metabolite Implicated and Metabolic Process
[73] Ming et al., 2012	Urine	48 ASD and 53 controls	UPLC–MS/MS and GC-MS	trans-Urocanate, glutaroylcarnitine, 3-methylglutaroylcarnitine, β-alanine, alanine, carnosine, glycine, histidine, serine, threonine, taurine, uric acid (oxidative stress; amino acid; mammalian microbial co-metabolism)
[74] Mavel et al., 2013	Urine	30 ASD and 28 controls	2D-NMR	serotonin, glycine, β-alanine, taurine, succinic acid, creatine, 3-methylhistidine (dopaminergic, serotonergic, synapse, tryptophan, oxidation, amino acids metabolism)
[75] Emond et al., 2013	Urine	26 ASD and 24 controls	GC-MS	succinic acid, glycolic acid, hippurate, phosphate, palmitate, stearate, 3-methyladipate (gut microbiota)
[76] Noto et al., 2014	Urine	21 ASD and 21 controls	GC-MS	3,4-dihydroxybutyric acid, glycolic acid, homovanillic acid, tryptophan 1,2,3-butanetriol, fructose, propylene glycol (interactions among diet, gut microbiota and host genetics)
[77] Diémé et al., 2015	Urine	30 ASD and 32 controls	^{1}H-NMR, 2D-HSQC NMR, LC-HRMS	N-acetylarginine, indoxyl, indoxylsulfate, dihydroxy-1H-indole glucuronide, methylguanidine, desaminotyrosine, dihydrouracil (gut microbiota)
[78] Bitar et al., 2018	Urine	40 ASD and 40 controls	^{1}H-NMR, 2D-HSQC NMR and LC-HRMS	5-amino-imidazole-4-carboxamide, chalice acid, glutamic acid, N-phosphoserine, nicotinamide ribonucleotide, glycerol-3-phosphate, trigonelline, riboflavin, 2-hydroxybutyric acid, 5-oxoproline, acetylcarnitine, cysteic acid, citric acid, threonine, creatine, serine, N-acetylphenylalanine;tyrosine, hydroxybenzoic acid, hydroxyproline, lactic acid, guanine, N-amidino aspartic acid, methyl acetoacetic acid, urocanic acid (amino acids; carbohydrates and oxidative stress)
[79] Barone et al., 2018	Dried Blood	83 ASD and 79 controls	ESI-Tandem MS/MS system	citrulline, acetylcarnitine, methylmalonyl/3-OH isovalerylcarnitine, decanoylcarnitine, dodecanoylcarnitine, tetradecadienoylcarnitine, hexadecanoylcarnitine, octadecenoylcarnitine (amino acids, fatty acid, gastrointestinal disturbances and mitochondrial dysfunction)

To be precise, we analyzed 140 proteins, as shown in Table 1:

1. we downloaded all the information from the UniProt database [80], via a Perl script;
2. we analyzed all of the Gene Ontology terms for "Biological Process" (GOTERM-BP) [81];
3. we calculated the terms found through ad hoc scripts in bash;
4. we designed a bubble chart by taking GOTERM-BP with the source "Traceable author statement" (e.g., TAS: Reactome) starting from the highest value (count) and then descending ending the list of proteins. Thus, we clustered all of the proteins for GOTERM-BP with at least one term.

Some proteins were not included in the analysis because we did not find the associated GOTERM-BP TAS.

We have analyzed 119 metabolites, as shown in Table 2:

1. we started from the complete Human Metabolome Database (HMDB) [82];
2. we selected our metabolites, analyzed the classes, subclasses and all terms under the Ontology category and Biochemical Pathway terms, such as biological process and physiological effect, via an ad hoc script in Python;
3. we calculated the terms found through ad hoc scripts in Python;
4. we designed a bubble chart by taking all of the associated biological processes.

Some metabolites were not included in the analysis because we did not find the associated ontology terms in HMDB.

3. Stratification of Complex Disease Phenotypes, Early Interventions and Omics-Generated Biomarkers

There is high variability in ASD symptoms and severity, principally focused on a general deficit in interpersonal interactions, due to reduced or absent verbal communication, or difficulty in communicating with other people [83]. This heterogeneity could result from a combination of many molecular mechanisms and environmental issues and an integrative approach could be a new strategy for ASD deep profiling, possibly allowing behavioural intervention as quickly as possible. Indeed, some studies showed a significant improvement when therapies started before 24 months of age, at which time the neural system is still extremely mouldable [84]. Early interventions would probably reduce the cognitive abnormalities of subjects and help in preventing the onset of an autistic condition [85]. Thus, early diagnosis and prediction are essential for ASD and could be achieved due to the study of molecules involved in the etiopathogenesis of the ASD phenotype. Subgroups can be individuated in ASD patient cohorts, including functioning levels based on different parameters such as IQ values, language, and/or reading impairment, and this could help in the identification of gene/protein candidates or molecular mechanisms that can be associated with one or more of these subpopulations. This type of approach could be useful for the diagnosis and prognosis of the disease and/or for the choice of the therapy to be applied [86–90].

Omics and meta-omics disciplines currently allow deep investigation of ASD starting from a wide panel of samples, ranging from biological fluids to tissues. Omics sciences originate from a holistic vision of the system under study, thus overcoming the classical genetic/biochemical studies based on single or few target molecules. The strength of omics approaches resides in their ability to provide complete profiles of biological "features" (genes/transcripts/proteins/metabolites) to obtain a broad description of a biological system by the so-called systems biology. A non-targeted and high-throughput search of the genetic scaffold (DNA) and functional reservoir (RNA, proteins, metabolites) is key to decoding the pathophysiology of systems as complex as biological systems without any "a priori" statement on the descriptive variable of the systems, hence providing the most appropriate stratification of the disease or identification of novel biomarkers.

These new approaches are possible due to high-throughput technological platforms that have been developed with unprecedented specificity and sensitivity, fused to modern data processing based on the most recent bioinformatics and computational tools, and capable of processing the big data produced. Indeed, the current challenges of the omics technologies rely on the harmonization and integration of the big data generated by the different technologies [91].

A multi-omics approach that combines and integrates the results of more than a single discipline is becoming crucial to understand the pathophysiology of ASD and to identify new diagnostic and prognostic biomarkers from blood, saliva, urine, faeces, or other body fluids [19]. Different matrices can be treated for the direct extraction of DNA, proteins, peptides, or metabolites, or preliminarily processed for fractionation and isolation of cells or bacteria (Figure 3). Genomics or metagenomics follow a single path, starting with the DNA extraction from any matrix and finishing with the genome sequencing and the following bioinformatics' pipeline. Proteins can also be extracted from a wide range of samples and analysed by liquid chromatography and mass spectrometry (LC-MS). Gel electrophoresis alone does not provide the same performance in biomarker discovery and is often used as a further preliminary fractionation step before LC-MS. In this sense, interactomics is a powerful tool for focusing on a potential target and its relationships with other proteins in promoting or inhibiting important functions related to ASD. Faeces and saliva are the most frequently used matrices for bacterial protein extraction, which is a crucial step in microbiota metaproteomics. The subsequent analytical procedure does not differ from that of a study on a single proteome but everything concerning data analysis or taxonomic assessments must rely on huge computational efforts for the individuation of a microbial biomarker or a functional signature of the microbiota or of the host co-metabolism. Metabolites can be easily extracted from faeces along with all biological fluids and analysed with different techniques on the basis of the chemical–physical features of molecules. The volatile fraction of metabolites can be detected by gas chromatography-mass spectrometry (GC-MS) experiments for both untargeted profiling and targeted quantitative analysis. Other small molecules can be analysed by NMR, LC-MS, or even direct infusion in MS.

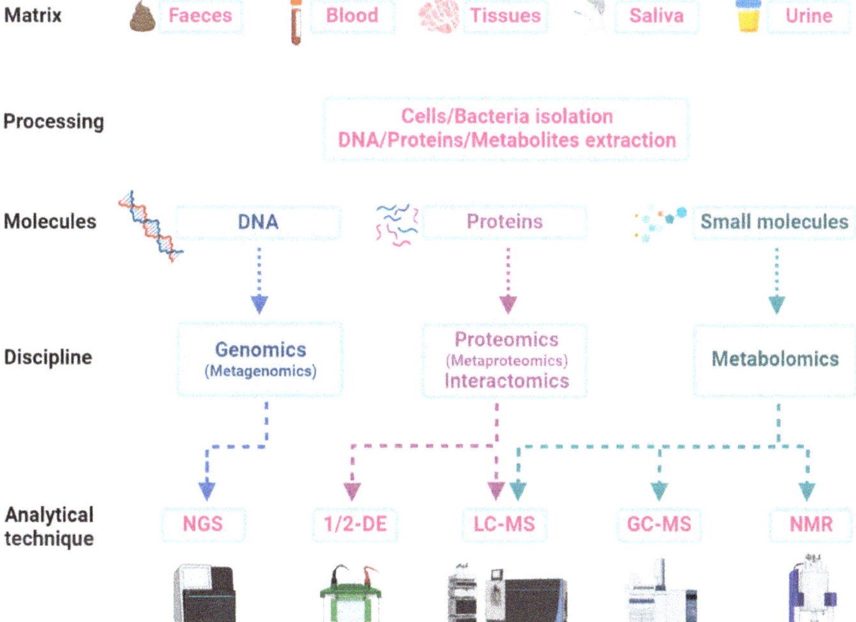

Figure 3. Scheme of the paths from matrices to analytical techniques in a multi-omics approach: An integrative approach could be a new strategy for ASD deep profiling, which combines data from genome sequencing (next-generation sequencing—NGS) with those from proteomics and metabolomics

by one or two-dimensional gel electrophoresis (1/2-DE), liquid-chromatography and gas-chromatography mass spectrometry (LC-MS or GC-MS), or even from metabolomics data obtained by nuclear magnetic resonance (NMR) experiments.

A crucial point regards "sample size" computation (i.e., statistical power) for big data that cannot be predicted based on "basic" statistics but rather uses multivariate and univariate analyses for multi-step reduction of multidimensional data. Indeed, big data are usually produced by considering an order of tens or hundreds of samples, but this point (i.e., the number of samples) can be established for each produced chemometric model using different multivariate statistical methods (e.g., Hotelling T2, number of misclassifications (NMC), area under the receiver operating characteristics curves (AUROC), and discriminant Q2; in the case of the latter, in contrast to NMC and AUROC, PLS-DA models with low complexity compared to PLS models are preferred). Therefore, each integrated model based on omics-derived data needs to be validated for each sample set under analysis [92–95].

Integrated multi-omics approaches usually involve metabolomics in conjunction with genomics or metagenomics. However, the coupling of metabolomics and proteomics, in which both yield information about the functional aspects of ASD, appears to be even more promising. Thus, this review mainly focuses on these disciplines.

Computational Models Used to Generate Proteomics and Metabolomics Single and Fused Data

Regarding computational pipelines ("dry laboratories") able to process big data generated from omics platforms ("wet laboratories"), the analysis of single and fused multidimensional data requires several steps of multi-step reiterated reduction supported by multivariate and univariate models. The variables under study may be the number of subjects (i.e., healthy or patients) and their omics "features" (i.e., proteins, metabolites), represented by worksheets that, overall, represent the system under study; such a system can be represented by a different number of features expressible by different percentages (e.g., 80–50–20%). Hence, the representativeness of the system (e.g., subjects and omics variables) can be evaluated by considering the most appropriate percentages to depict the entire system. Therefore, the starting raw data matrix (big data) becomes reduced to a new data matrix (smart data), the latter ready to be harmonized and integrated into a fused omics data model with data coming from different omics platforms. Then, the reduced and integrated data can be analyzed by chemometric models based on different multivariate statistical methods, as previously described [96]. In this way, the integrated generated model can be validated for each type of sample set (e.g., row data from GC-MS, LC-MS, ^{1}H-NMR, etc.) and for each patient and/or reference subject dataset (e.g., phenomics data) [92–95].

4. Translational and Clinical Proteomics

The rapid expansion of proteomics in recent decades has provided powerful tools to undertake investigations of biological systems, aimed at identifying biomarkers for clinical diagnosis, monitoring the stage of diseases, studying the pathogenetic molecular mechanism, and choosing appropriate treatments.

Translational proteomics is a crucial component of a picture in which other omics and meta-omics disciplines (genomics, metabolomics/lipidomics, transcriptomics, and microbiomics), contribute to complex workflows producing both qualitative and quantitative relevant outcomes.

Under the approach of omics research, molecular profiles, combined with clinical profiles of patients, can be managed to drive clinical decisions, and, hence, advanced treatments. However, a key challenge is to overcome technical bottlenecks and to bridge the gap between early-stage discovery (translational research) and the subsequent stage, which is represented by routine quantitative searching and the determination of biomarker candidates in clinical research settings. Moreover, to accelerate the discovery of clinically actionable biomarkers, the focus must be switched from identification (ID) to quantitation. That is, precision proteomics must converge with precision medicine, in addition to other omics sciences.

For this purpose, the major issue of quantitation and calibration in mass spectrometry (MS) must be correctly addressed. During the past decade, numerous experimental strategies have been developed and refined, together with tools and analytical kits, to provide researchers with a number of solutions for different proteomic approaches, on the basis of sample complexity and matrix variability. These approaches are difficult because a series of factors must be considered for both relative and absolute proteomics quantification [97]. Given the ascertained performance of MS in the absolute quantification of proteins, as a strong alternative to immunoassays, the principal needs currently appear to be focused on the calibration methods, not only to improve the measurement precision but also to make data interchangeable by laboratories globally. Synthetic stable isotope labelled (SIL) proteins and peptides, used as internal standards (IS), present both advantages and drawbacks, due to availability, cost, reproducibility of biological features, and accuracy [98]. An open question is how recombinant SIL proteins, synthetic labelled tryptic peptides (tSIL), or even the so-called "flanked" or "winged" peptides, could be used with reasonable confidence to provide the best accuracy as an internal calibration (IC) in bottom-up experiments [99]. Furthermore, new strategies for external calibration (EC), by means of external reference (molecules), are needed for selected or multiple reaction monitoring experiments (SRM/MRM), to correct bias coming from instrumental variance and sample preparation workflows [100]. Concerning protein ID, due to the continuous growth of public repositories of MS datasets, the use of spectral libraries is increasingly mined compared to classical peptide sequences matching with protein databases (DB). Data-independent acquisition (DIA) approaches appear particularly promising for future applications in biomarker discovery in proteomics. SWATH (Sequential Window Acquisition of all Theoretical Mass Spectra) analysis is currently employed for large scale ID and quantitation in proteomics, with the aim of exploiting the increasing number of spectral libraries available, considerably reducing computational time and space [101]. Applications in metaproteomics remain limited but the desire to identify alternative paths for protein detection and inference, overcoming the bias of conventional sequence databases, makes this an intriguing analytical strategy for faster identification/quantitation [102,103].

The extension to metabolomics continues to suffer from a lack of public libraries, but also appears to be a powerful approach. A new tool has recently been developed to match MS and MS/MS spectra searching for identical or analogous features in public repositories of metabolomics data [104].

Fewer proteomics studies on ASD have been published than those based on other disciplines, such as genomics or transcriptomics. Many of them rely on post-mortem brain tissues [50–52], serum [53–56], plasma [57–59], urine [63], saliva [60–62] direct samples or lymphoblastoid cell lines [64] (Table 1).

The first study on brain tissues was conducted by Junaid et al. [50]. Post-mortem brain samples from 8 ASD patients and 10 controls were analysed using two-dimensional gel electrophoresis (2-DE) followed by liquid chromatography-tandem mass spectrometry (LC-MS/MS) analysis; the glyoxalase 1 (Glo1) protein showed a shift in net charge allowing a polymorphic form of the protein in the brain of ASD patients to be characterized. Furthermore, they found that isoform have reduced enzyme activity and its variant was found to be increased in ASD patients with respect to control cases. The authors suggested that the homozygosity of a Glo1 variant could be one of the susceptibility factors in the etiology of autism. In another study of post-mortem brain tissue, the authors studied the prefrontal cortex of 10 ASD individuals and the cerebellum of 16 ASD patients versus control subjects. The results showed that the proteins, found in the brain tissue of ASD patients, are involved in processes of synaptic vesicle regulation, myelination, and energy metabolism [51]. Recently, Wingo et al. recruited 104 participants who were followed for up to 14 years, and 27% of the cohort were finally diagnosed as ASD. They studied proteins to identify new processes underlying variation in cognitive modification, by label-free LC-MS/MS experiments and found 579 proteins associated with cognitive trajectory after meta-analysis. Moreover, they found 38 proteins related to cognitive trajectory independently of β-amyloid plaques and neurofibrillary tangles [52]. Studies conducted on non-neurological tissues highlighted changes in quantities of proteins associated with inflammation or regulation of the immune system, including some interleukins [50,51,105–108]. Interestingly, most proteomic studies investigating ASD identified proteins involved in lipid metabolism and differentially expressed in ASD [51,55,57,105,106,109,110]. As an example, Corbett et al. identified differentially expressed peptides using LC-MS/MS, which allowed for the recognition of complement factor H-related protein (FHR1), apolipoprotein (APO) B-100, fibronectin 1 (FN1), and complement C1q as dysregulated proteins in children with ASD compared to control subjects [53]. In another study, apolipoproteins involved in cholesterol metabolism were found to be increased in an ASD cohort with respect to the control subjects [54]. In addition, two studies reported an alteration in proteins implicated in lipid metabolism, in the inflammation process and cell growth [55,56] (Table 1).

The study of Cortelazzo evidenced a total of 12 dysregulated proteins, associated primarily with acute inflammatory response [57]; despite irregularities of lipid metabolism shown in ASD tissues, the authors could not characterize primary or secondary occurrence in ASD pathophysiology. In the study by Pichitpunpong et al., ASD patients were subdivided into subgroups using the Autism Diagnostic Interview-Revised (ADI-R) method, and subsequently, dysregulated genes were identified by studying transcriptome profiles of individuals with ASD and control subjects. They profiled protein from lymphoblastoid cell lines using 2-DE followed by LC-MS/MS. Subsequently, proteins were compared to the dysregulated transcripts. Selected proteins were also analysed by Western blotting [64]. The authors reported 82 proteins linked to subjects with ASD and with severe language impairment and, among these, 14 were correlated with inflammation and neurological functions. Moreover, the diazepam-binding inhibitor (DBI) protein was notably reduced in the subgroup with severe language impairment. Furthermore, its expression levels were matched with the ADI-R items [64]. Recently, Shen et al. used the iTRAQ-based proteomics approach to compare plasma protein profiles of ASD compared with healthy subjects. They identified 24 differentially expressed proteins expressed in different pathways associated with ASDs [59] (Table 1). This evidence supports the thesis that synapsis growth, the complement system, cytoskeleton-related activities and cell adhesion are all involved in ASD. Moreover, using ELISA (enzyme-linked immune-adsorbent assay) and ROC (receiver operating characteristic) analysis, the authors found five proteins as possible biomarkers to discriminate ASD from controls [59]. Interestingly, they identified focal adhesion, cell adhesion molecules, and leukocyte trans-endothelial migration pathways that were correlated with ADS in a Chinese cohort [111].

Saliva, urine, and blood samples have also been taken into consideration. In particular, saliva-based studies showed an alteration in the processes involved in antimicrobial peptides, immune response, and inflammation at the mucosal level [60–62].

Overall, a large number of studies highlighted abnormalities in synapse biology in ASD patients, showing a prevalence of proteins related to neural tissue, and evidencing a limitation in the application of non-neural tissues in proteomics studies of ASD.

Indeed, due to the blood–brain barrier (BBB), it can be difficult to find proteins associated with ASD in peripheral blood, as possible disease-specific protein markers, despite the ease of use, cost-effectiveness, and low invasiveness of blood collection. Moreover, a study highlighted high intestinal and BBB permeability in ASD patients; indeed, ASD shows a reduced expression of occluding, tricellulin, claudin-1, and increased pore-forming claudins, which are part of gut barrier-forming "tight junction" (TJ) components [108]. Furthermore, it was found that a protein (zonulin) involved in intestinal permeability increased in ASD patients compared with controls, particularly with respect to the Childhood Autism Rating Scale score. [109]. Thus, possible blood biomarkers could be proteins associated with intestinal and BBB permeability.

We conducted an in-depth analysis of the protein data found in the reviewed studies, as reported in Table 1. For the 140 proteins (Table S1), we first undertook an analysis based on the matrix (e.g., blood, brain, saliva, urine, and lymphoblastoid cell lines) and on the number of times (frequency) that the protein was reported in all of the analyzed articles. The analysis showed a major presence of the apolipoproteins (APOE and APOA1 proteins) and fibronectin (FN1). Then, we analyzed all of the biological pathways associated with the proteins and clustered all of the proteins according to the biological process (BP). Interestingly, the results showed that the two major biological processes associated with ASD were platelet degranulation and lipid metabolism (Figure 4).

Indeed, platelets play a safe role in the pathophysiology of thrombogenesis and atherogenesis, and this connection may also be due to an increase in Body Mass Index in ASD children [112]. In addition, serotonin is also present in the platelet, and stimulates aggregation by exercising the vasoconstrictor and thrombogenic effect in response to lesions of the basal endothelium. In fact, it is now known that many ASD patients have hyperserotonemia or elevated serotonin levels in whole blood (5-hydroxytryptamine, 5-HT). Despite decades of study, the mechanisms behind this well-replicated biomarker and the contributions of the serotonergic system to ASD remain unclear and further studies are necessary [113]. Almost all whole blood 5-HT is found in the platelet and the serotonin 5-HT2A receptor improves platelet functions induced by adenosine diphosphate (ADP) signaling, with exposure to phosphotidylserine (PS) and receptor activation fibrinogen.

Overall, the 5-HT2A receptor improves platelet aggregation. Thus, this suggests some level of mutual regulation. Remarkably, this link with the serotonin 5-HT2 receptor has been extensively studied in ASD [114]. Although the importance of fats in the correct development and maintenance of cells of the nervous system is now recognized, lipids may actually play a role in regulating inflammation.

Overall, proteomics studies of ASD remain limited and vary between different technological approaches, focusing on various matrices. However, blood may be promising for diagnostic purposes, and because the data produced from the analysis are more accessible. Finally, faeces represents an intriguing matrix, mostly concerning the strong relationship between ASD and GI symptoms; however, in this case, the gut bacterial proteome/metaproteome [102] could be involved in the investigation even though, to the best of our knowledge, no metaproteomics studies have been published to date.

i.Matrix

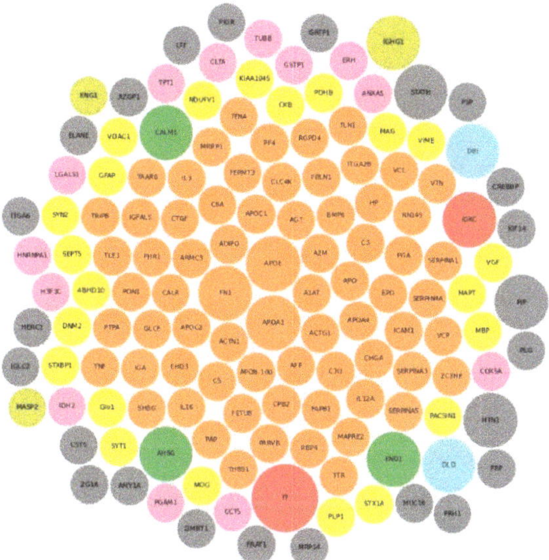

Figure 4. *Cont.*

ii.Biological Process

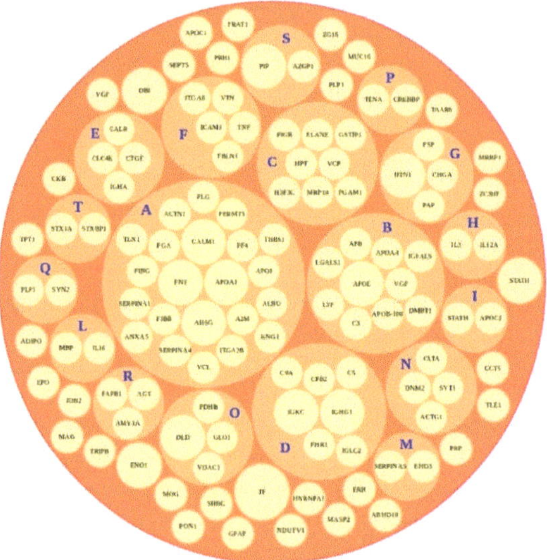

Figure 4. Protein analysis as a tool for the decision support system (DSS). In box (**i**), we grouped the proteins highlighted in Table 1 and Table S1 according to the matrix in which the proteins were studied, such as blood (**orange**), blood and urine (**lawn green**), brain (**red**), dried blood (**brown**), urine (**pink**), and brain biopsies, urine and blood (**lilac**). The size of the bubbles indicates the number of times the protein was found in that matrix in the different studies taken into consideration. In box (**ii**), we analyzed the data for the biological process and clustered the protein. Legend code: (A) platelet degranulation (GO:0002576); (B) cellular protein metabolic process (GO:0044267); (C) neutrophil degranulation (GO:0043312); (D) regulation of complement activation (GO:0030449); (E) receptor-mediated endocytosis (GO:0006898); (F) extracellular matrix organization (GO:0030198); (G) antimicrobial humoral response (GO:0019730); (H) cytokine-mediated signaling pathway (GO:0019221); (I) retinoid metabolic process (GO:0001523); (L) immune response (GO:0006955); (M) blood coagulation (GO:0007596); (N) membrane organization (GO:0061024); (O) pyruvate metabolic process (GO:0006090); (P) signal transduction (GO:0007165); (Q) chemical synaptic transmission (GO:0007268); (R) regulation of lipid metabolic process (GO:0019216); (S) transmembrane transport (GO:0055085); (T) glutamate secretion (GO:0014047).

5. Metabolomics

Metabolomics is an approach to understand the metabolic pathways and metabolic network regulation of a biological system. There are therefore many fields of application of this discipline, including medicine and biology [115].

Metabolomics has been studied to identify possible biomarkers in the serum or urine samples of patients with obesity [116], diabetes [117], and coronary heart diseases [118]. Recently, it has been evidenced that perturbations of metabolic pathways could affect the pathogenesis of central nervous system disorders [119].

Thus, metabolomics provides a powerful tool to map these perturbations and their relationship to disease and response to therapy. In fact, some studies have been carried out to investigate metabolomics biomarkers in the brain [65,66], plasma [67,68,70], dried blood [79] and urine [72–78] samples of ASD patients (Table 2). Yap and coworkers used a proton nuclear magnetic resonance (^{1}H-NMR) spectroscopy method that showed increased levels of taurine and low content of glutamate in urine samples of ASD patients [72]. Ming et al. used a combination of liquid chromatography (LC-) and gas chromatography (GC-)-based MS, and revealed abnormal amino acid metabolism and increased oxidative stress in urinary specimens of ASD patients [73].

Mavel et al. identified more than 150 metabolites in urine, comparing 30 ASD children with 28 neurotypical subjects. Increased levels of succinate, taurine, β-alanine, and glycine were found in ASD subjects [74]. In another study, a statistically significant increase of homovanillic acid, tryptophan, glycolic acid, and 3,4-dihydroxybutyric acid was detected [76]. The authors supposed that the increase in glycolate was linked with primary oxaluria type I, and that the phenomenon was also related to yeast overgrowth.

Tryptophan and homovanillic acid have been indicated as metabolites of neurotransmission probably involved in neurodevelopmental disorders. Although 3,4-dihydroxybutyric acid may be a typical component of human urine, its increase has been highlighted in cases of succinic semialdehyde dehydrogenase deficiency, which represents a disorder in patients that could also show ASD features [120]. Recently, Dieme et al. detected increased levels of indoxyl, indoxyl sulfate and *N*-acetylarginine, and decreased levels of methylguanidine and other compounds, such as desaminotyrosine and dihydrouracil [77]. Bitar et al., in a group of 40 ASD children and 40 age-matched controls, highlighted perturbations in various compounds [78], including 2-hydroxybutyrate, glutamate, creatine, and tyrosine. In addition, the authors also identified metabolites, including cysteic acid, guanine and trigonelline. These results showed abnormalities in carbohydrate and amino acid metabolisms, in addition to differences in oxidative stress pathways [78].

Furthermore, by using a GC-MS approach in urine sample analysis, it has been possible to build a multivariate statistical model that captures global biochemical signatures of autistic individuals, thus enabling patients to be distinguished from healthy children [75]. To investigate metabolites potentially related to the ASD disorder, it is possible to also study metabolites in plasma samples. The analysis of these metabolites tended to approximately support the results noted in urine, although specific gaps exist due to differences in renal clearance for some compounds.

Plasma fatty acids were recognized as diagnostic markers for ASD, specifically as an increase in the most saturated fatty acids and a decrease in polyunsaturated fatty acids, such as valeric, hexanoic and stearidonic acids [121]. Kuwabara et al. identified diverged levels of plasma metabolites connected with mitochondrial dysfunction and oxidative stress in ASD patients [67]. In a study by Wang et al., a cohort of ASD patients and participants without autism were analyzed using ultra-performance LC quadrupole time-of-flight tandem MS (UPLC/Q-TOF MS/MS) to identify metabolic variations in serum. In particular, the authors identified 17 metabolites, two of which were associated with ASD and could be significant predictors of autism: sphingosine 1-phosphate (S1P) and docosahexaenoic acid (DHA) [69].

West et al. used LC-MS/GC-MS to recognize significant concentrations in aspartate, dehydroepiandrosterone sulfate (DHEA-S), glutaric acid, serine, and succinic acid. Decreased levels of citrate, creatinine, glutamate, hydroxyphenyllactate and isoleucine were detected, thus indicating the roles of altered abnormal mitochondrial energy production (succinic acid, DHEA-S, citrate, aspartate, glutamate) and branched-chain amino acid metabolism (isoleucine, hydroxyphenyllactate) [68].

Rangel-Huerta et al. used untargeted metabolomics (HPLC–MS/MS) of plasma samples from 30 ASD children and 30 age-matched controls. In this study, ASD patients were subdivided into two groups: with (AR) and without (ANR) neurologic regression. The metabolic intermediates were detected in the aspartate, beta-alanine, glucose–alanine cycle, malate–aspartate shuttle, urea cycle, and tryptophan breakdown pathways showing significant statistical differences between controls and ASD patients. In addition, within the two subgroups, significant statistical differences were also highlighted in the levels of the fatty acids decanoylcarnitine, laurate, arachidate, myristate, octanoylcarnitine, quinate, and 7-methylurate [70]. Rachel S. Kelly et al. highlighted differences in tyrosine metabolism, tryptophan biosynthesis and endocannabinoid metabolism in a cohort of children, 13% of whom had ASDs. In addition, they hypothesized that metabolomic biomarkers could help to identify children with poor communication skills [71].

A recent study investigated the metabolic profile by extracting molecules from dried blood spots (DBSs) and performing a targeted analysis on a panel of 45 metabolites [79]. The level of nine of these molecules (20%) was significantly higher in ASD patients with respect to controls, including citrulline and acyl-carnitines C2. The results suggested that the mitochondrial fatty acid β-oxidation pathway was less active, revealing hidden molecular mechanisms related to ASD. Thus, this non-invasive methodology was shown to be suitable for a screening of newborn subjects to emphasize modifications in metabolic profiles during development [79].

Moreover, it is possible to analyze the metabolomes derived from brain tissue, for example, using LC-MS analyses for untargeted metabolomics analysis. As reported by Graham (106), in brain tissue from 11 deceased subjects with ASD, compared to 11 controls, a group of statistically significant compounds, such as 3-methoxytyramine, 5,6-dihydrouridine and *N*-carboxyethyl-γ-aminobutyric acid, was detected [65].

Post-mortem prefrontal cortex samples were analyzed by Kurochkin et al. in a cohort of 32 ASD subjects and 40 controls. The study identified increased levels of glutathione disulfide and 5-oxoproline and, on the contrary, decreased levels of glutathione, L- γ-glutamyl-cysteine and l-cysteinyl-glycine. All of these metabolites were involved in their respective metabolic pathways and in others such as pyruvate metabolism, starch and sucrose metabolism, arginine and proline metabolism and TCA cycle [66].

Regarding proteins, we performed a bubble analysis of the metabolites (Figure 5). For the 119 metabolites (Table 2 and Table S1), the first analyses based on the matrix showed a major presence of glutamate, decanoyl carnitine, and tryptophan, clustered in the major BP lipid metabolism pathway, confirming the data from the proteins. In addition, another implicated BP was the tryptophan metabolism, which was implicated in the gut–brain axis because of an increased 5′-HT, leading to tryptophan depletion and contributing to hyperserotonemia, which is associated with GI symptoms and neurodevelopmental disorders [47].

i.Matrix

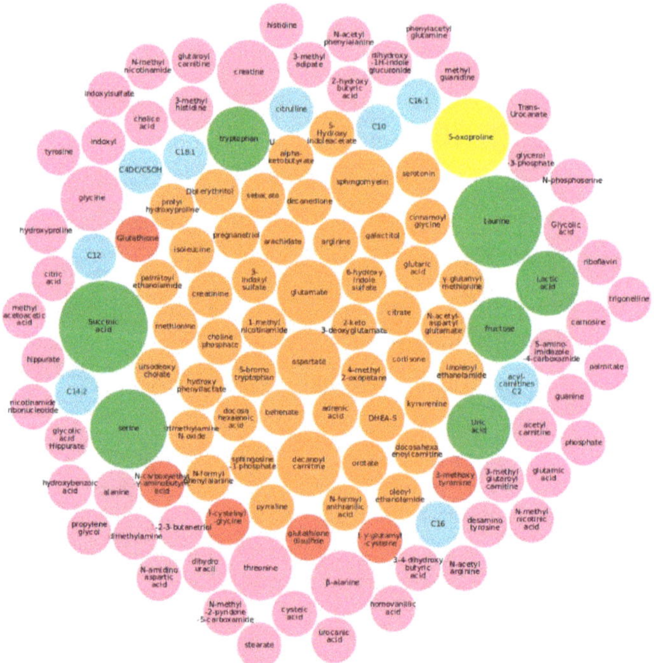

Figure 5. *Cont.*

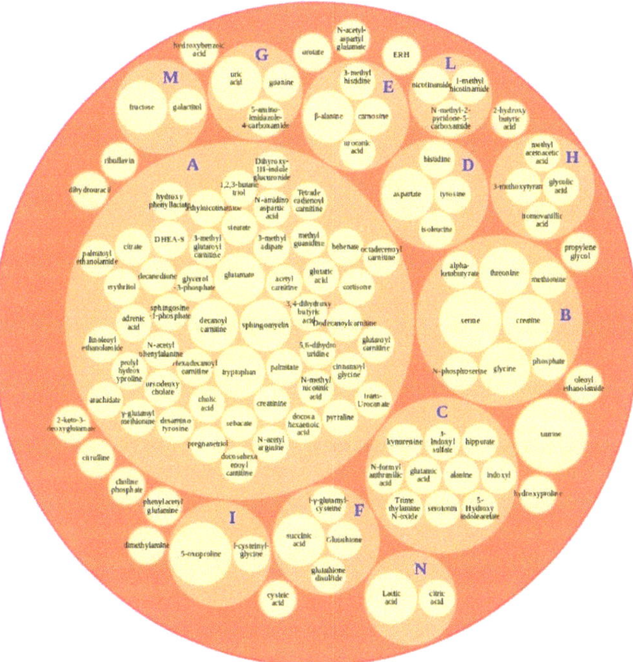

Figure 5. Metabolites analysis as a tool for the decision support system (DSS). In box (**i**), we grouped the metabolites highlighted in Table 2 and Table S1 according to the matrix in which the metabolites were studied, such as blood (orange), blood and urine (lawn green), brain (red), dried blood (brown), urine (pink), and brain, urine and blood (lilac). The size of the bubbles indicates the number of times the metabolites were found in that matrix in the different studies taken into consideration. We analyzed the data for the biological process (box (**ii**) and clustered the metabolites. Legend code: A: Lipid Metabolism Pathway; B: Glycine and Serine Metabolism; C: Tryptophan Metabolism; D: Transcription/Translation; E: Histidine Metabolism; F: Glutamate Metabolism; G: Thioguanine Action Pathway; H: Tyrosine Metabolism; I: Glutathione Metabolism; L: Nicotinate and Nicotinamide Metabolism; M: Galactose metabolism; N: Glutaminolysis and Cancer.

The study of the metabolites in the ASD subjects provides an understanding of the complexity of the system in terms of the main metabolic interactions between metabolites, with particular reference to their relationship with ASD.

6. Interactome in ASD

In the context of a multi-omics functional approach, the identification of proteins related to ASD, together with their functional annotation, correlations, and association to biological pathways, can be related to the metabolomics outcome, to depict a comprehensive picture of the functions involved in the ASD pathogenesis or in the identification of ASD-related biomarkers.

In this sense, interactomics, namely the ensemble of all of the molecular interactions that could take place in a group of proteins involved in a biological function, is furthermore key for data interpretation. Currently, more than 650,000 protein–protein interactions (PPIs) have been reported and found to constitute the human interactome. [122,123]. Furthermore, it was found that PPIs have been involved in most diseases, such as neurodegenerative disorders, leukemia, cervical cancer, and bacterial infection [122]. In fact, many human diseases involve the loss of an essential interaction or formation

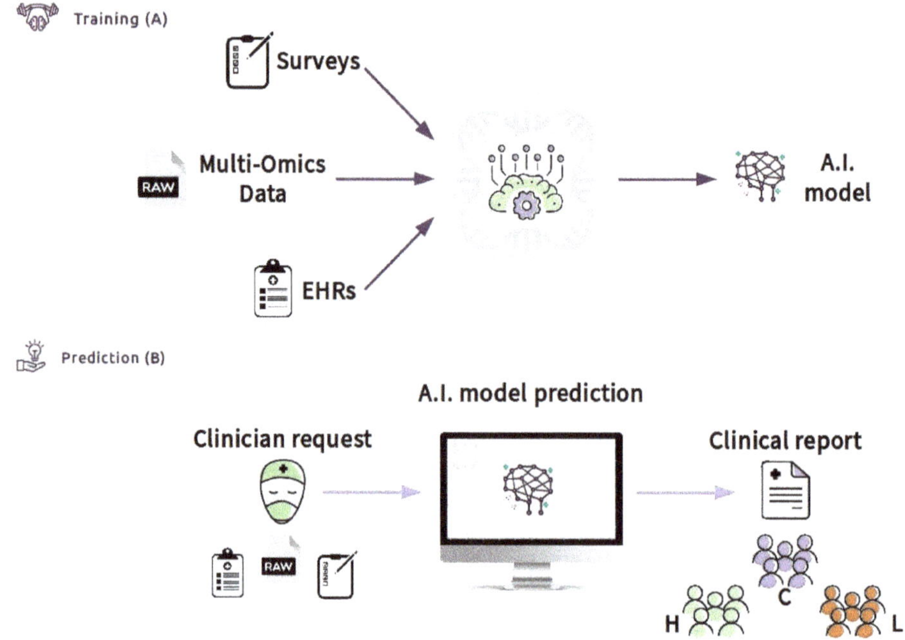

Figure 6. Clinical decision support system (CDSS) as a new approach to ASD children to screen and improve the age of diagnosis: Box (**A**) (training) shows the flowchart including all data used (survey, such as Child Health Improvement through Computer Automation system (CHICA), omics data and electronic medical records (EHR)) by machine learning model to classify patients. Once the model has been constructed with good accuracy, the clinician (box (**B**)) (prediction) will upload the patient data. An A.I. model will predict the class with an actionable result summarized in the clinical report. The result will generate subgroups based on the patient's features, for example, high functioning (H), low functioning (L), and control group (C). This system might be used by clinicians to improve early diagnosis because it provides significant information about the features of the ASD patient.

8. Discussion and Future Prospects

It is clear that the etiology of ASD is given by a combination of genetic and environmental factors, and the only therapy for ASD that has been demonstrated to be effective is behavior analysis. Furthermore, genetic and environmental factors are implicated in changes in the brain and metabolism, such as mitochondrial dysfunction, neurotransmitters alteration, abnormal neuron development, neuroinflammation and immune dysregulation and oxidative stress. In addition, the diagnosis of ASD currently depends on clinical observation and procedures to evaluate behavioral, historical, and parent-report information [48].

There are also important ASD-related considerations to be taken into account, namely, ASD's etiological heterogeneity, varied comorbidities, and the complexity of the brain as the centrally affected organ. In addition, there have been relatively few omics-based studies of ASD thus far. These aspects may involve significant variability, therefore, detecting proteomics and metabolomics biomarkers that look at the functional aspect may contribute to the advance of the clinical diagnosis of ASD and find new tools that could be used to estimate the outcome of individualized interventions. Results produced from proteomics-approaches show that differential expression of mitochondrial bioenergetics (involving NDUV1 protein), inflammation and immune function (MBP protein), proteins of lipid metabolism (APOB-100) and synaptic biology (SYT1 protein) are crucial in the pathogenesis and progression of the ASD. In fact, synaptic degeneration and mitochondria dysfunction are examples of the cellular events that could be correlated with ASD and cognitive impairment.

The altered metabolites are mainly associated with fatty acid metabolism (decanoyl-L-carnitine), oxidative stress (e.g., glutathione), mitochondrial dysfunction (e.g., arginine), amino acid metabolism, cholesterol metabolism, energy metabolism (e.g., Succinic acid), intestinal microbiota (e.g., tryptophan) and neurotransmitters (e.g., γ-aminobutyric acid).

Therefore, the results highlighted by metabolomics confirm that mitochondrial dysfunction may be a risk factor for autism; it could also be a target to find a possible biomarker to identify ASD patients and to show different expressions in subgroups of patients. All of these results may influence social and cognitive deficits in autism. In addition to elucidating the ASD pathobiology, multi-omics approaches could lead to the identification of novel biomarkers for improved diagnosis and therapeutic monitoring and diagnosis; hence the ultimate aim is to find biomarkers that are simple, inexpensive, and noninvasive, in accessible tissues and body fluids such as the blood or, preferably, urine (Figure 7).

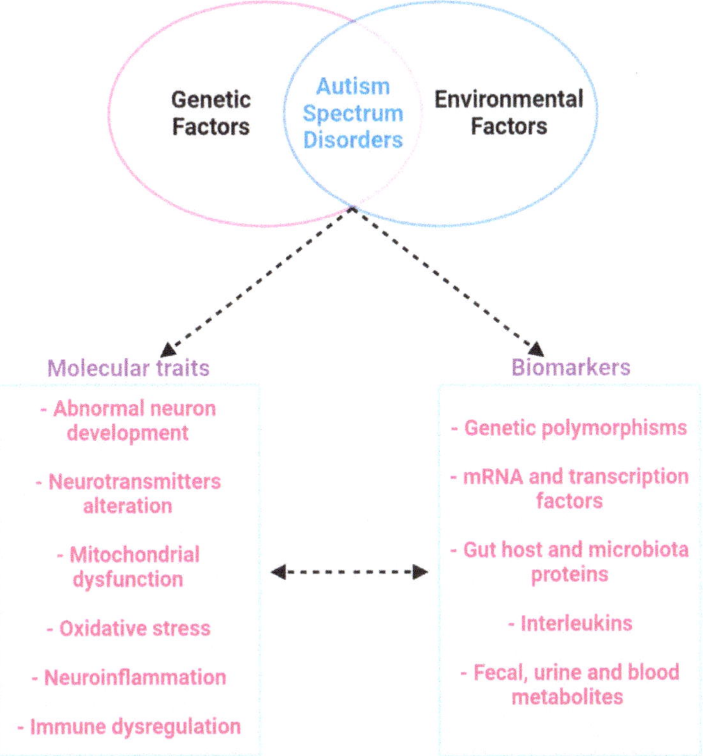

Figure 7. Multi-omics approach to ASD. ASD is a multifactor disease that includes genetic and environmental factors. The phenotype of ASD determines abnormal neurodevelopment with alteration in neurotransmitters. Furthermore, ASD is characterized by mitochondrial dysfunction, oxidative stress, inflammation and abnormal immune regulation. All of these dysfunctions produce possible biomarkers that could be identified by a new multi-omics approach to studying ASD.

Currently, the main limits are due to the lack of uniformity in the collection of clinical phenotypes with homogeneous methods; moreover, few studies have addressed the degree of correlation between different biomarkers or evaluated multiple biomarkers or endophenotypes in parallel. Furthermore, studies are limited in their evaluation of biomarkers by comparisons of patients with ASD and healthy controls, without considering the family and specific characteristics of the pathology. Often, the sample cohort is also highly limited. From the point of view of omics data, the biggest limit is that all of the data from the omics are not considered and the data are not integrated with collected clinical data.

Thus, this big data approach will be essential for the early detection of ASD and the possibility of developing more precise medicine to design and optimizing the pathway for diagnosis, therapeutic intervention, and prognosis using omics data that are able to highlight individual variability between ASD patients.

In this context, proteomics and metabolomics offer the best possibility of viewing changes in the functional pathways associated with the disease, such as increases or decreases in the expression of proteins or metabolites markers. These markers can be differently expressed in different patient cohorts thus helping improve diagnostics accuracy, ASD population stratification, and the development of effective personalized treatments.

Supplementary Materials: The following are available online at http://www.mdpi.com/1422-0067/21/17/6274/s1, Table S1: Table of all proteins with UniProt code with associated matrix.

Author Contributions: Conceptualization, M.V.R. and L.P.; methodology, M.V.R. and L.P.; investigation, M.V.R. and L.P.; writing—original draft preparation, M.V.R. and L.P.; writing—review and editing, M.V.R., S.L.M., V.M., S.G. (Silvia Guerrera), P.V., G.I., S.G. (Simone Gardini), G.T., G.V., S.V., A.G. and L.P.; supervision, A.G. and L.P. All authors have read and agreed to the published version of the manuscript.

Funding: This research was funded by Fondazione Bambino Gesù, Grant number 201903_FBG, and Ministry of Italian Health, Ricerca Corrente grant number 201905_genetica, to L.P.

Conflicts of Interest: The authors declare no conflict of interest.

Abbreviations

1-DE	one-dimensional gel electrophoresis
2-DE	two-dimensional gel electrophoresis
5'-HT	5-hydroxytryptamine
ADI-R	Autism Diagnostic Interview-Revised
ANR	without neurologic regression
APO	apolipoprotein
AR	neurologic regression
ASD	Autism Spectrum Disorders
AUC	area under the ROC curve
BBB	Blood–brain barrier
CDSS	Clinical decision support system
CHD8	chromodomain helicase DNA binding protein 8
CHICA	Child Health Improvement Trough Computer Automation
CNTNAP2	Contactin associated protein-like 2
DB	protein databases
DBI	diazepam-binding inhibitor
DBS	dried blood spots
DHA	docosahexaenoic acid
DHEA-S	Dehydroepiandrosterone sulfate
DIA	Data-independent analysis
DISC1	Disrupted in Schizophrenia 1
DSS	Decision support systems
EC	external calibration
EHR	electronic health record
ELISA	enzyme-linked immunoadsorbent assay
FHR1	complement factor H-related protein
FN1	fibronectin 1
GC	gas chromatography
GI	Gastrointestinal symptoms
Glo1	glyoxalase 1

GSH	glutathione
^{1}H-NMR	proton nuclear magnetic resonance spectroscopy
HPLC-MS/MS	high-performance liquid chromatography with tandem mass spectrometry
IC	internal calibration
ID	identification
IPA	Ingenuity Pathway Analysis
IS	internal standards
LC	liquid chromatography
LC-MS/MS	liquid chromatography-tandem mass spectrometry
MS	mass spectrometry
NGS	Next-generation sequencing
NMR	nuclear magnetic resonance spectroscopy
PPIs	Protein–protein interactions
ROC	receiver operating characteristic
S1P	sphingosine 1-phosphate
SH3	SRC Homology 3 Domain
SHANK 3	SH3 and multiple ankyrin repeat domain 3
SIL	Synthetic stable isotope labelled
SRM-MS	selected reaction monitoring mass spectrometry
SRM/MRM	selected reaction monitoring/multiple reaction monitoring
SRS	Social Responsiveness Scale
SWATH	Sequential Window Acquisition of all Theoretical Mass Spectra
TJ	tight junction
TSC	tuberous sclerosis complex
TSC1	tuberous sclerosis 1
TSC2	tuberous sclerosis 2
tSIL	synthetic labeled tryptic peptides
UPLC/Q-TOF MS/MS	ultra-performance liquid chromatography quadrupole time-of-flight tandem mass tandem mass spectrometry

References

1. Nomi, J.S.; Uddin, L.Q. Developmental changes in large-scale network connectivity in autism. *Neuroimage Clin.* **2015**, *7*, 732–741. [CrossRef]
2. Uddin, L.Q.; Supekar, K.; Menon, V. Reconceptualizing functional brain connectivity in autism from a developmental perspective. *Front. Hum. Neurosci.* **2013**, *7*, 458. [CrossRef]
3. Fulceri, F.; Morelli, M.; Santocchi, E.; Cena, H.; Del Bianco, T.; Narzisi, A.; Calderoni, S.; Muratori, F. Gastrointestinal symptoms and behavioral problems in preschoolers with Autism Spectrum Disorder. *Dig. Liver Dis.* **2016**, *48*, 248–254. [CrossRef]
4. Prosperi, M.; Santocchi, E.; Balboni, G.; Narzisi, A.; Bozza, M.; Fulceri, F.; Apicella, F.; Igliozzi, R.; Cosenza, A.; Tancredi, R.; et al. Behavioral phenotype of ASD preschoolers with gastrointestinal symptoms or food selectivity. *J. Autism. Dev. Disord.* **2017**, *47*, 3574–3588. [CrossRef]
5. Erratum: Vol. 67, No. SS-6. *MMWR Morb. Mortal. Wkly. Rep.* **2018**, *67*, 564. [CrossRef] [PubMed]
6. Baio, J.; Wiggins, L.; Christensen, D.L.; Maenner, M.J.; Daniels, J.; Warren, Z.; Kurzius-Spencer, M.; Zahorodny, W.; Robinson Rosenberg, C.; White, T.; et al. Prevalence of autism spectrum disorder among children aged 8 years—autism and developmental disabilities monitoring network, 11 sites, United States, 2014. *MMWR Surveill. Summ.* **2018**, *67*, 1–23. [CrossRef] [PubMed]
7. Fombonne, E.; Quirke, S.; Hagen, A. Prevalence and interpretation of recent trends in rates of pervasive developmental disorders. *Mcgill J. Med.* **2009**, *12*, 73. [PubMed]
8. Kupfer, D.J.; Regier, D.A.; Narrow, W.E.; American Psychiatric Association. *Diagnostic and Statistical Manual of Mental Disorders*, 5th ed.; American Psychiatric Association: Philadelphia, PA, USA, 2013; ISBN 978-0-89042-555-8.
9. Doernberg, E.; Hollander, E. Neurodevelopmental disorders (ASD and ADHD): DSM-5, ICD-10, and ICD-11. *CNS Spectr.* **2016**, *21*, 295–299. [CrossRef] [PubMed]

10. Risch, N.; Hoffmann, T.J.; Anderson, M.; Croen, L.A.; Grether, J.K.; Windham, G.C. Familial recurrence of autism spectrum disorder: Evaluating genetic and environmental contributions. *Am. J. Psychiatry* **2014**, *171*, 1206–1213. [CrossRef] [PubMed]

11. Gaugler, T.; Klei, L.; Sanders, S.J.; Bodea, C.A.; Goldberg, A.P.; Lee, A.B.; Mahajan, M.; Manaa, D.; Pawitan, Y.; Reichert, J.; et al. Most genetic risk for autism resides with common variation. *Nat. Genet.* **2014**, *46*, 881–885. [CrossRef]

12. Huguet, G.; Ey, E.; Bourgeron, T. The genetic landscapes of autism spectrum disorders. *Annu. Rev. Genom. Hum. Genet.* **2013**, *14*, 191–213. [CrossRef] [PubMed]

13. Sandin, S.; Lichtenstein, P.; Kuja-Halkola, R.; Hultman, C.; Larsson, H.; Reichenberg, A. The heritability of autism spectrum disorder. *JAMA* **2017**, *318*, 1182–1184. [CrossRef]

14. Durand, C.M.; Betancur, C.; Boeckers, T.M.; Bockmann, J.; Chaste, P.; Fauchereau, F.; Nygren, G.; Rastam, M.; Gillberg, I.C.; Anckarsäter, H.; et al. Mutations in the gene encoding the synaptic scaffolding protein SHANK3 are associated with autism spectrum disorders. *Nat. Genet.* **2007**, *39*, 25–27. [CrossRef] [PubMed]

15. Griswold, A.J.; Ma, D.; Cukier, H.N.; Nations, L.D.; Schmidt, M.A.; Chung, R.-H.; Jaworski, J.M.; Salyakina, D.; Konidari, I.; Whitehead, P.L.; et al. Evaluation of copy number variations reveals novel candidate genes in autism spectrum disorder-associated pathways. *Hum. Mol. Genet.* **2012**, *21*, 3513–3523. [CrossRef] [PubMed]

16. Higdon, R.; Earl, R.K.; Stanberry, L.; Hudac, C.M.; Montague, E.; Stewart, E.; Janko, I.; Choiniere, J.; Broomall, W.; Kolker, N.; et al. The promise of multi-omics and clinical data integration to identify and target personalized healthcare approaches in autism spectrum disorders. *OMICS* **2015**, *19*, 197–208. [CrossRef] [PubMed]

17. Shen, L.; Liu, X.; Zhang, H.; Lin, J.; Feng, C.; Iqbal, J. Biomarkers in autism spectrum disorders: Current progress. *Clin. Chim. Acta* **2020**, *502*, 41–54. [CrossRef]

18. Shen, L.; Zhao, Y.; Zhang, H.; Feng, C.; Gao, Y.; Zhao, D.; Xia, S.; Hong, Q.; Iqbal, J.; Liu, X.K.; et al. Advances in biomarker studies in autism spectrum disorders. *Adv. Exp. Med. Biol.* **2019**, *1118*, 207–233. [CrossRef]

19. Ruggeri, B.; Sarkans, U.; Schumann, G.; Persico, A.M. Biomarkers in autism spectrum disorder: The old and the new. *Psychopharmacology* **2014**, *231*, 1201–1216. [CrossRef]

20. de Theije, C.G.M.; Wu, J.; da Silva, S.L.; Kamphuis, P.J.; Garssen, J.; Korte, S.M.; Kraneveld, A.D. Pathways underlying the gut-to-brain connection in autism spectrum disorders as future targets for disease management. *Eur. J. Pharmacol.* **2011**, *668*, S70–S80. [CrossRef]

21. Lai, M.-C.; Lombardo, M.V.; Baron-Cohen, S. Autism. *Lancet* **2014**, *383*, 896–910. [CrossRef]

22. Raz, R.; Roberts, A.L.; Lyall, K.; Hart, J.E.; Just, A.C.; Laden, F.; Weisskopf, M.G. Autism spectrum disorder and particulate matter air pollution before, during, and after pregnancy: A nested case-control analysis within the Nurses' Health Study II Cohort. *Environ. Health Perspect.* **2015**, *123*, 264–270. [CrossRef] [PubMed]

23. Modabbernia, A.; Velthorst, E.; Reichenberg, A. Environmental risk factors for autism: An evidence-based review of systematic reviews and meta-analyses. *Mol. Autism* **2017**, *8*, 13. [CrossRef] [PubMed]

24. Geschwind, D.H.; Levitt, P. Autism spectrum disorders: Developmental disconnection syndromes. *Curr. Opin. Neurobiol.* **2007**, *17*, 103–111. [CrossRef] [PubMed]

25. Hegarty, J.P.; Lazzeroni, L.C.; Raman, M.M.; Pegoraro, L.F.L.; Monterrey, J.C.; Cleveland, S.C.; Hallmayer, J.F.; Wolke, O.N.; Phillips, J.M.; Reiss, A.L.; et al. Genetic and environmental influences on lobar brain structures in twins with autism. *Cereb. Cortex* **2019**. [CrossRef] [PubMed]

26. Gorrindo, P.; Williams, K.C.; Lee, E.B.; Walker, L.S.; McGrew, S.G.; Levitt, P. Gastrointestinal dysfunction in autism: Parental report, clinical evaluation, and associated factors. *Autism Res.* **2012**, *5*, 101–108. [CrossRef] [PubMed]

27. Adams, J.B.; Johansen, L.J.; Powell, L.D.; Quig, D.; Rubin, R.A. Gastrointestinal flora and gastrointestinal status in children with autism—comparisons to typical children and correlation with autism severity. *BMC Gastroenterol.* **2011**, *11*. [CrossRef]

28. Wang, L.W.; Tancredi, D.J.; Thomas, D.W. The prevalence of gastrointestinal problems in children across the United States with autism spectrum disorders from families with multiple affected members. *J. Dev. Behav. ediatr.* **2011**, *32*, 351–360. [CrossRef]

29. Chaidez, V.; Hansen, R.L.; Hertz-Picciotto, I. Gastrointestinal problems in children with autism, developmental delays or typical development. *J. Autism Dev. Disord* **2014**, *44*, 1117–1127. [CrossRef]

30. Tomova, A.; Husarova, V.; Lakatosova, S.; Bakos, J.; Vlkova, B.; Babinska, K.; Ostatnikova, D. Gastrointestinal microbiota in children with autism in Slovakia. *Physiol. Behav.* **2015**, *138*, 179–187. [CrossRef]

31. Bresnahan, M.; Hornig, M.; Schultz, A.F.; Gunnes, N.; Hirtz, D.; Lie, K.K.; Magnus, P.; Reichborn-Kjennerud, T.; Roth, C.; Schjølberg, S.; et al. Association of maternal report of infant and toddler gastrointestinal symptoms with autism: Evidence from a prospective birth cohort. *JAMA Psychiatry* **2015**, *72*, 466–474. [CrossRef]
32. Valicenti-McDermott, M.; McVicar, K.; Rapin, I.; Wershil, B.K.; Cohen, H.; Shinnar, S. Frequency of gastrointestinal symptoms in children with autistic spectrum disorders and association with family history of autoimmune disease. *J. Dev. Behav. Pediatr.* **2006**, *27*, S128–S136. [CrossRef]
33. Horvath, K.; Perman, J.A. Autistic disorder and gastrointestinal disease. *Curr. Opin. Pediatr.* **2002**, *14*, 583–587. [CrossRef] [PubMed]
34. Peters, B.; Williams, K.C.; Gorrindo, P.; Rosenberg, D.; Lee, E.B.; Levitt, P.; Veenstra-VanderWeele, J. Rigid-compulsive behaviors are associated with mixed bowel symptoms in autism spectrum disorder. *J. Autism Dev. Disord* **2014**, *44*, 1425–1432. [CrossRef] [PubMed]
35. Marler, S.; Ferguson, B.J.; Lee, E.B.; Peters, B.; Williams, K.C.; McDonnell, E.; Macklin, E.A.; Levitt, P.; Margolis, K.G.; Beversdorf, D.Q.; et al. Association of rigid-compulsive behavior with functional constipation in autism spectrum disorder. *J. Autism Dev. Disord* **2017**, *47*, 1673–1681. [CrossRef]
36. Mazurek, M.O.; Vasa, R.A.; Kalb, L.G.; Kanne, S.M.; Rosenberg, D.; Keefer, A.; Murray, D.S.; Freedman, B.; Lowery, L.A. Anxiety, sensory over-responsivity, and gastrointestinal problems in children with autism spectrum disorders. *J. Abnorm. Child. Psychol.* **2013**, *41*, 165–176. [CrossRef] [PubMed]
37. Maenner, M.J.; Arneson, C.L.; Levy, S.E.; Kirby, R.S.; Nicholas, J.S.; Durkin, M.S. Brief report: Association between behavioral features and gastrointestinal problems among children with autism spectrum disorder. *J. Autism Dev. Disord* **2012**, *42*, 1520–1525. [CrossRef] [PubMed]
38. Molloy, C.A.; Manning-Courtney, P. Prevalence of chronic gastrointestinal symptoms in children with autism and autistic spectrum disorders. *Autism* **2003**, *7*, 165–171. [CrossRef]
39. Parracho, H.M.R.T.; Bingham, M.O.; Gibson, G.R.; McCartney, A.L. Differences between the gut microflora of children with autistic spectrum disorders and that of healthy children. *J. Med. Microbiol.* **2005**, *54*, 987–991. [CrossRef]
40. Taylor, B.; Miller, E.; Lingam, R.; Andrews, N.; Simmons, A.; Stowe, J. Measles, mumps, and rubella vaccination and bowel problems or developmental regression in children with autism: Population study. *BMJ* **2002**, *324*, 393–396. [CrossRef]
41. Fombonne, E.; Chakrabarti, S. No evidence for a new variant of measles-mumps-rubella-induced autism. *Pediatrics* **2001**, *108*, E58. [CrossRef]
42. Xue, M.; Brimacombe, M.; Chaaban, J.; Zimmerman-Bier, B.; Wagner, G.C. Autism spectrum disorders: Concurrent clinical disorders. *J. Child. Neurol.* **2008**, *23*, 6–13. [CrossRef]
43. Stilling, R.M.; Bordenstein, S.R.; Dinan, T.G.; Cryan, J.F. Friends with social benefits: Host-microbe interactions as a driver of brain evolution and development? *Front. Cell Infect. Microbiol.* **2014**, *4*, 147. [CrossRef] [PubMed]
44. de Angelis, M.; Piccolo, M.; Vannini, L.; Siragusa, S.; de Giacomo, A.; Serrazzanetti, D.I.; Cristofori, F.; Guerzoni, M.E.; Gobbetti, M.; Francavilla, R. Fecal microbiota and metabolome of children with autism and pervasive developmental disorder not otherwise specified. *PLoS ONE* **2013**, *8*, e76993. [CrossRef]
45. Kang, D.-W.; Park, J.G.; Ilhan, Z.E.; Wallstrom, G.; Labaer, J.; Adams, J.B.; Krajmalnik-Brown, R. Reduced incidence of Prevotella and other fermenters in intestinal microflora of autistic children. *PLoS ONE* **2013**, *8*, e68322. [CrossRef]
46. Williams, B.L.; Hornig, M.; Buie, T.; Bauman, M.L.; Cho Paik, M.; Wick, I.; Bennett, A.; Jabado, O.; Hirschberg, D.L.; Lipkin, W.I. Impaired carbohydrate digestion and transport and mucosal dysbiosis in the intestines of children with autism and gastrointestinal disturbances. *PLoS ONE* **2011**, *6*, e24585. [CrossRef] [PubMed]
47. Ristori, M.V.; Quagliariello, A.; Reddel, S.; Ianiro, G.; Vicari, S.; Gasbarrini, A.; Putignani, L. Autism, gastrointestinal symptoms and modulation of gut microbiota by nutritional interventions. *Nutrients* **2019**, *11*. [CrossRef]
48. Falkmer, T.; Anderson, K.; Falkmer, M.; Horlin, C. Diagnostic procedures in autism spectrum disorders: A systematic literature review. *Eur. Child. Adolesc. Psychiatry* **2013**, *22*, 329–340. [CrossRef]
49. Putignani, L.; Gasbarrini, A.; Dallapiccola, B. Potential of multiomics technology in precision medicine. *Curr. Opin. Gastroenterol.* **2019**, *35*, 491–498. [CrossRef]

50. Junaid, M.A.; Kowal, D.; Barua, M.; Pullarkat, P.S.; Sklower Brooks, S.; Pullarkat, R.K. Proteomic studies identified a single nucleotide polymorphism in glyoxalase I as autism susceptibility factor. *Am. J. Med. Genet. A* **2004**, *131*, 11–17. [CrossRef]
51. Broek, J.A.; Guest, P.C.; Rahmoune, H.; Bahn, S. Proteomic analysis of post mortem brain tissue from autism patients: Evidence for opposite changes in prefrontal cortex and cerebellum in synaptic connectivity-related proteins. *Mol. Autism* **2014**, *5*, 41. [CrossRef]
52. Wingo, A.P.; Dammer, E.B.; Breen, M.S.; Logsdon, B.A.; Duong, D.M.; Troncosco, J.C.; Thambisetty, M.; Beach, T.G.; Serrano, G.E.; Reiman, E.M.; et al. Large-scale proteomic analysis of human brain identifies proteins associated with cognitive trajectory in advanced age. *Nat. Commun.* **2019**, *10*, 1619. [CrossRef] [PubMed]
53. Corbett, B.A.; Kantor, A.B.; Schulman, H.; Walker, W.L.; Lit, L.; Ashwood, P.; Rocke, D.M.; Sharp, F.R. A proteomic study of serum from children with autism showing differential expression of apolipoproteins and complement proteins. *Mol. Psychiatry* **2007**, *12*, 292–306. [CrossRef] [PubMed]
54. Ngounou, W.A.G.; Wormwood, K.; Thome, J.; Dudley, E.; Taurines, R.; Gerlach, M.; Woods, A.G.; Darie, C.C. A pilot proteomic study of protein markers in autism spectrum disorder. *Electrophoresis* **2014**, *35*, 2046–2054. [CrossRef] [PubMed]
55. Steeb, H.; Ramsey, J.M.; Guest, P.C.; Stocki, P.; Cooper, J.D.; Rahmoune, H.; Ingudomnukul, E.; Auyeung, B.; Ruta, L.; Baron-Cohen, S.; et al. Serum proteomic analysis identifies sex-specific differences in lipid metabolism and inflammation profiles in adults diagnosed with Asperger syndrome. *Mol. Autism* **2014**, *5*, 4. [CrossRef] [PubMed]
56. Yang, J.; Chen, Y.; Xiong, X.; Zhou, X.; Han, L.; Ni, L.; Wang, W.; Wang, X.; Zhao, L.; Shao, D.; et al. Peptidome analysis reveals novel serum biomarkers for children with autism spectrum disorder in china. *Proteomics Clin. Appl.* **2018**, *12*, e1700164. [CrossRef]
57. Cortelazzo, A.; de Felice, C.; Guerranti, R.; Signorini, C.; Leoncini, S.; Zollo, G.; Leoncini, R.; Timperio, A.M.; Zolla, L.; Ciccoli, L.; et al. Expression and oxidative modifications of plasma proteins in autism spectrum disorders: Interplay between inflammatory response and lipid peroxidation. *Proteomics Clin. Appl.* **2016**, *10*, 1103–1112. [CrossRef]
58. Feng, C.; Chen, Y.; Pan, J.; Yang, A.; Niu, L.; Min, J.; Meng, X.; Liao, L.; Zhang, K.; Shen, L. Redox proteomic identification of carbonylated proteins in autism plasma: Insight into oxidative stress and its related biomarkers in autism. *Clin. Proteomics* **2017**, *14*, 2. [CrossRef]
59. Shen, L.; Zhang, K.; Feng, C.; Chen, Y.; Li, S.; Iqbal, J.; Liao, L.; Zhao, Y.; Zhai, J. iTRAQ-based proteomic analysis reveals protein profile in plasma from children with autism. *Proteomics Clin. Appl.* **2018**, *12*. [CrossRef]
60. Castagnola, M.; Messana, I.; Inzitari, R.; Fanali, C.; Cabras, T.; Morelli, A.; Pecoraro, A.M.; Neri, G.; Torrioli, M.G.; Gurrieri, F. Hypo-phosphorylation of salivary peptidome as a clue to the molecular pathogenesis of autism spectrum disorders. *J. Proteome Res.* **2008**, *7*, 5327–5332. [CrossRef]
61. Ngounou, W.A.G.; Wormwood, K.L.; Charette, L.; Ryan, J.P.; Woods, A.G.; Darie, C.C. Comparative two-dimensional polyacrylamide gel electrophoresis of the salivary proteome of children with autism spectrum disorder. *J. Cell. Mol. Med.* **2015**, *19*, 2664–2678. [CrossRef]
62. Ngounou, W.A.G.; Wormwood, K.L.; Russell, S.; Ryan, J.P.; Darie, C.C.; Woods, A.G. A Pilot proteomic analysis of salivary biomarkers in autism spectrum disorder. *Autism Res.* **2015**, *8*, 338–350. [CrossRef] [PubMed]
63. Suganya, V.; Geetha, A.; Sujatha, S. Urine proteome analysis to evaluate protein biomarkers in children with autism. *Clin. Chim. Acta* **2015**, *450*, 210–219. [CrossRef] [PubMed]
64. Pichitpunpong, C.; Thongkorn, S.; Kanlayaprasit, S.; Yuwattana, W.; Plaingam, W.; Sangsuthum, S.; Aizat, W.M.; Baharum, S.N.; Tencomnao, T.; Hu, V.W.; et al. Phenotypic subgrouping and multi-omics analyses reveal reduced diazepam-binding inhibitor (DBI) protein levels in autism spectrum disorder with severe language impairment. *PLoS ONE* **2019**, *14*, e0214198. [CrossRef] [PubMed]
65. Graham, S.F.; Chevallier, O.P.; Kumar, P.; Türkoğlu, O.; Bahado-Singh, R.O. High resolution metabolomic analysis of ASD human brain uncovers novel biomarkers of disease. *Metabolomics* **2016**, *12*, 62. [CrossRef]
66. Kurochkin, I.; Khrameeva, E.; Tkachev, A.; Stepanova, V.; Vanyushkina, A.; Stekolshchikova, E.; Li, Q.; Zubkov, D.; Shichkova, P.; Halene, T.; et al. Metabolome signature of autism in the human prefrontal cortex. *Commun. Biol.* **2019**, *2*, 234. [CrossRef] [PubMed]

67. Kuwabara, H.; Yamasue, H.; Koike, S.; Inoue, H.; Kawakubo, Y.; Kuroda, M.; Takano, Y.; Iwashiro, N.; Natsubori, T.; Aoki, Y.; et al. Altered metabolites in the plasma of autism spectrum disorder: A capillary electrophoresis time-of-flight mass spectroscopy study. *PLoS ONE* **2013**, *8*, e73814. [CrossRef] [PubMed]

68. West, P.R.; Amaral, D.G.; Bais, P.; Smith, A.M.; Egnash, L.A.; Ross, M.E.; Palmer, J.A.; Fontaine, B.R.; Conard, K.R.; Corbett, B.A.; et al. Metabolomics as a tool for discovery of biomarkers of autism spectrum disorder in the blood plasma of children. *PLoS ONE* **2014**, *9*, e112445. [CrossRef]

69. Wang, H.; Liang, S.; Wang, M.; Gao, J.; Sun, C.; Wang, J.; Xia, W.; Wu, S.; Sumner, S.J.; Zhang, F.; et al. Potential serum biomarkers from a metabolomics study of autism. *J. Psychiatry Neurosci.* **2016**, *41*, 27–37. [CrossRef]

70. Rangel-Huerta, O.D.; Gomez-Fernández, A.; de la Torre-Aguilar, M.J.; Gil, A.; Perez-Navero, J.L.; Flores-Rojas, K.; Martín-Borreguero, P.; Gil-Campos, M. Metabolic profiling in children with autism spectrum disorder with and without mental regression: Preliminary results from a cross-sectional case-control study. *Metabolomics* **2019**, *15*, 99. [CrossRef]

71. Kelly, R.S.; Boulin, A.; Laranjo, N.; Lee-Sarwar, K.; Chu, S.H.; Yadama, A.P.; Carey, V.; Litonjua, A.A.; Lasky-Su, J.; Weiss, S.T. Metabolomics and communication skills development in children; evidence from the ages and stages questionnaire. *Metabolites* **2019**, *9*. [CrossRef]

72. Yap, I.K.S.; Angley, M.; Veselkov, K.A.; Holmes, E.; Lindon, J.C.; Nicholson, J.K. Urinary metabolic phenotyping differentiates children with autism from their unaffected siblings and age-matched controls. *J. Proteome Res.* **2010**, *9*, 2996–3004. [CrossRef] [PubMed]

73. Ming, X.; Stein, T.P.; Barnes, V.; Rhodes, N.; Guo, L. Metabolic perturbance in autism spectrum disorders: A metabolomics study. *J. Proteome Res.* **2012**, *11*, 5856–5862. [CrossRef] [PubMed]

74. Mavel, S.; Nadal-Desbarats, L.; Blasco, H.; Bonnet-Brilhault, F.; Barthélémy, C.; Montigny, F.; Sarda, P.; Laumonnier, F.; Vourc'h, P.; Andres, C.R.; et al. 1H-13C NMR-based urine metabolic profiling in autism spectrum disorders. *Talanta* **2013**, *114*, 95–102. [CrossRef] [PubMed]

75. Emond, P.; Mavel, S.; Aïdoud, N.; Nadal-Desbarats, L.; Montigny, F.; Bonnet-Brilhault, F.; Barthélémy, C.; Merten, M.; Sarda, P.; Laumonnier, F.; et al. GC-MS-based urine metabolic profiling of autism spectrum disorders. *Anal. Bioanal. Chem.* **2013**, *405*, 5291–5300. [CrossRef] [PubMed]

76. Noto, A.; Fanos, V.; Barberini, L.; Grapov, D.; Fattuoni, C.; Zaffanello, M.; Casanova, A.; Fenu, G.; de Giacomo, A.; De Angelis, M.; et al. The urinary metabolomics profile of an Italian autistic children population and their unaffected siblings. *J. Matern. Fetal. Neonatal. Med.* **2014**, *27*, 46–52. [CrossRef] [PubMed]

77. Diémé, B.; Mavel, S.; Blasco, H.; Tripi, G.; Bonnet-Brilhault, F.; Malvy, J.; Bocca, C.; Andres, C.R.; Nadal-Desbarats, L.; Emond, P. Metabolomics study of urine in autism spectrum disorders using a multiplatform analytical methodology. *J. Proteome Res.* **2015**, *14*, 5273–5282. [CrossRef]

78. Bitar, T.; Mavel, S.; Emond, P.; Nadal-Desbarats, L.; Lefèvre, A.; Mattar, H.; Soufia, M.; Blasco, H.; Vourc'h, P.; Hleihel, W.; et al. Identification of metabolic pathway disturbances using multimodal metabolomics in autistic disorders in a Middle Eastern population. *J. Pharm. Biomed. Anal.* **2018**, *152*, 57–65. [CrossRef]

79. Barone, R.; Alaimo, S.; Messina, M.; Pulvirenti, A.; Bastin, J.; Ferro, A.; Frye, R.E.; Rizzo, R.; MIMIC-Autism Group. A subset of patients with autism spectrum disorders show a distinctive metabolic profile by dried blood spot analyses. *Front. Psychiatry* **2018**, *9*, 636. [CrossRef]

80. UniProt Consortium. UniProt: A worldwide hub of protein knowledge. *Nucleic Acids Res.* **2019**, *47*, D506–D515. [CrossRef]

81. The Gene Ontology Consortium. The Gene Ontology Resource: 20 years and still GOing strong. *Nucleic Acids Res.* **2019**, *47*, D330–D338. [CrossRef]

82. Wishart, D.S.; Feunang, Y.D.; Marcu, A.; Guo, A.C.; Liang, K.; Vázquez-Fresno, R.; Sajed, T.; Johnson, D.; Li, C.; Karu, N.; et al. HMDB 4.0: The human metabolome database for 2018. *Nucleic Acids Res.* **2018**, *46*, D608–D617. [CrossRef] [PubMed]

83. DiCicco-Bloom, E.; Lord, C.; Zwaigenbaum, L.; Courchesne, E.; Dager, S.R.; Schmitz, C.; Schultz, R.T.; Crawley, J.; Young, L.J. The developmental neurobiology of autism spectrum disorder. *J. Neurosci.* **2006**, *26*, 6897–6906. [CrossRef] [PubMed]

84. Zachor, D.A. Autism spectrum disorders–a syndrome on the rise: Risk factors and advances in early detection and intervention. *Harefuah* **2012**, *151*, 162–164. [PubMed]

85. Dawson, G. Early behavioral intervention, brain plasticity, and the prevention of autism spectrum disorder. *Dev. Psychopathol.* **2008**, *20*, 775–803. [CrossRef] [PubMed]

86. Saeliw, T.; Tangsuwansri, C.; Thongkorn, S.; Chonchaiya, W.; Suphapeetiporn, K.; Mutirangura, A.; Tencomnao, T.; Hu, V.W.; Sarachana, T. Integrated genome-wide Alu methylation and transcriptome profiling analyses reveal novel epigenetic regulatory networks associated with autism spectrum disorder. *Mol. Autism* **2018**, *9*, 27. [CrossRef]

87. Talebizadeh, Z.; Arking, D.E.; Hu, V.W. A novel stratification method in linkage studies to address inter and intra-family heterogeneity in autism. *PLoS ONE* **2013**, *8*, e67569. [CrossRef]

88. Hu, V.W.; Frank, B.C.; Heine, S.; Lee, N.H.; Quackenbush, J. Gene expression profiling of lymphoblastoid cell lines from monozygotic twins discordant in severity of autism reveals differential regulation of neurologically relevant genes. *BMC Genom.* **2006**, *7*, 118. [CrossRef]

89. Hu, V.W.; Sarachana, T.; Kim, K.S.; Nguyen, A.; Kulkarni, S.; Steinberg, M.E.; Luu, T.; Lai, Y.; Lee, N.H. Gene expression profiling differentiates autism case-controls and phenotypic variants of autism spectrum disorders: Evidence for circadian rhythm dysfunction in severe autism. *Autism Res.* **2009**, *2*, 78–97. [CrossRef]

90. Hu, V.W.; Lai, Y. Developing a predictive gene classifier for autism spectrum disorders based upon differential gene expression profiles of phenotypic subgroups. *North. Am. J. Med. Sci.* **2013**, *6*. [CrossRef]

91. Karahalil, B. Overview of systems biology and omics technologies. *Curr. Med. Chem.* **2016**, *23*, 4221–4230. [CrossRef]

92. del Chierico, F.; Nobili, V.; Vernocchi, P.; Russo, A.; de Stefanis, C.; Gnani, D.; Furlanello, C.; Zandonà, A.; Paci, P.; Capuani, G.; et al. Gut microbiota profiling of pediatric nonalcoholic fatty liver disease and obese patients unveiled by an integrated meta-omics-based approach. *Hepatology* **2017**, *65*, 451–464. [CrossRef] [PubMed]

93. Vernocchi, P.; del Chierico, F.; Russo, A.; Majo, F.; Rossitto, M.; Valerio, M.; Casadei, L.; La Storia, A.; de Filippis, F.; Rizzo, C.; et al. Gut microbiota signatures in cystic fibrosis: Loss of host CFTR function drives the microbiota enterophenotype. *PLoS ONE* **2018**, *13*, e0208171. [CrossRef] [PubMed]

94. del Chierico, F.; Vernocchi, P.; Petrucca, A.; Paci, P.; Fuentes, S.; Praticò, G.; Capuani, G.; Masotti, A.; Reddel, S.; Russo, A.; et al. Phylogenetic and metabolic tracking of gut microbiota during perinatal development. *PLoS ONE* **2015**, *10*, e0137347. [CrossRef] [PubMed]

95. Miccheli, A.; Capuani, G.; Marini, F.; Tomassini, A.; Praticò, G.; Ceccarelli, S.; Gnani, D.; Baviera, G.; Alisi, A.; Putignani, L.; et al. Urinary (1)H-NMR-based metabolic profiling of children with NAFLD undergoing VSL#3 treatment. *Int. J. Obes.* **2015**, *39*, 1118–1125. [CrossRef]

96. Szymańska, E.; Saccenti, E.; Smilde, A.K.; Westerhuis, J.A. Double-check: Validation of diagnostic statistics for PLS-DA models in metabolomics studies. *Metabolomics* **2012**, *8*, 3–16. [CrossRef]

97. Domon, B.; Aebersold, R. Options and considerations when selecting a quantitative proteomics strategy. *Nat. Biotechnol.* **2010**, *28*, 710–721. [CrossRef] [PubMed]

98. Oeckl, P.; Steinacker, P.; Otto, M. Comparison of internal standard approaches for srm analysis of alpha-synuclein in cerebrospinal fluid. *J. Proteome Res.* **2018**, *17*, 516–523. [CrossRef]

99. Shuford, C.M.; Walters, J.J.; Holland, P.M.; Sreenivasan, U.; Askari, N.; Ray, K.; Grant, R.P. Absolute protein quantification by mass spectrometry: Not as simple as advertised. *Anal. Chem.* **2017**, *89*, 7406–7415. [CrossRef]

100. Pino, L.K.; Searle, B.C.; Huang, E.L.; Noble, W.S.; Hoofnagle, A.N.; MacCoss, M.J. Calibration using a single-point external reference material harmonizes quantitative mass spectrometry proteomics data between platforms and laboratories. *Anal. Chem.* **2018**, *90*, 13112–13117. [CrossRef]

101. Schubert, O.T.; Gillet, L.C.; Collins, B.C.; Navarro, P.; Rosenberger, G.; Wolski, W.E.; Lam, H.; Amodei, D.; Mallick, P.; MacLean, B.; et al. Building high-quality assay libraries for targeted analysis of SWATH MS data. *Nat. Protoc.* **2015**, *10*, 426–441. [CrossRef]

102. Levi Mortera, S.; Soggiu, A.; Vernocchi, P.; del Chierico, F.; Piras, C.; Carsetti, R.; Marzano, V.; Britti, D.; Urbani, A.; Roncada, P.; et al. Metaproteomic investigation to assess gut microbiota shaping in newborn mice: A combined taxonomic, functional and quantitative approach. *J. Proteom.* **2019**, *203*, 103378. [CrossRef] [PubMed]

103. Slavomíra, N.; Zdeno, Š.; Andrej, K.; vana, F.; Gábor, B.; Maksym, D. Corrigendum to "Cucumber mosaic virus resistance: Comparative proteomics of contrasting Cucumis sativus cultivars after long-term infection". *J. Proteom.* **2020**, *214*, 103674. [CrossRef]

104. Wang, M.; Jarmusch, A.K.; Vargas, F.; Aksenov, A.A.; Gauglitz, J.M.; Weldon, K.; Petras, D.; da Silva, R.; Quinn, R.; Melnik, A.V.; et al. Mass spectrometry searches using MASST. *Nat. Biotechnol.* **2020**, *38*, 23–26. [CrossRef]

105. Kalsner, L.; Twachtman-Bassett, J.; Tokarski, K.; Stanley, C.; Dumont-Mathieu, T.; Cotney, J.; Chamberlain, S. Genetic testing including targeted gene panel in a diverse clinical population of children with autism spectrum disorder: Findings and implications. *Mol. Genet. Genomic Med.* **2018**, *6*, 171–185. [CrossRef] [PubMed]

106. Won, H.; Mah, W.; Kim, E. Autism spectrum disorder causes, mechanisms, and treatments: Focus on neuronal synapses. *Front. Mol. Neurosci.* **2013**, *6*, 19. [CrossRef] [PubMed]

107. Wang, P.; Mokhtari, R.; Pedrosa, E.; Kirschenbaum, M.; Bayrak, C.; Zheng, D.; Lachman, H.M. CRISPR/Cas9-mediated heterozygous knockout of the autism gene CHD8 and characterization of its transcriptional networks in cerebral organoids derived from iPS cells. *Mol. Autism* **2017**, *8*, 11. [CrossRef]

108. Fiorentino, M.; Sapone, A.; Senger, S.; Camhi, S.S.; Kadzielski, S.M.; Buie, T.M.; Kelly, D.L.; Cascella, N.; Fasano, A. Blood-brain barrier and intestinal epithelial barrier alterations in autism spectrum disorders. *Mol. Autism* **2016**, *7*, 49. [CrossRef] [PubMed]

109. Esnafoglu, E.; Cırrık, S.; Ayyıldız, S.N.; Erdil, A.; Ertürk, E.Y.; Daglı, A.; Noyan, T. Increased serum zonulin levels as an intestinal permeability marker in autistic subjects. *J. Pediatr.* **2017**, *188*, 240–244. [CrossRef]

110. Hayashi-Takagi, A.; Vawter, M.P.; Iwamoto, K. Peripheral biomarkers revisited: Integrative profiling of peripheral samples for psychiatric research. *Biol. Psychiatry* **2014**, *75*, 920–928. [CrossRef]

111. Skafidas, E.; Testa, R.; Zantomio, D.; Chana, G.; Everall, I.P.; Pantelis, C. Predicting the diagnosis of autism spectrum disorder using gene pathway analysis. *Mol. Psychiatry* **2014**, *19*, 504–510. [CrossRef]

112. Yorbik, O.; Mutlu, C.; Tanju, I.A.; Celik, D.; Ozcan, O. Mean platelet volume in children with attention deficit hyperactivity disorder. *Med. Hypotheses* **2014**, *82*, 341–345. [CrossRef] [PubMed]

113. Muller, C.L.; Anacker, A.M.J.; Veenstra-Vanderweele, J. The serotonin system in autism spectrum disorder: From biomarker to animal models. *Neuroscience* **2016**, *321*, 24–41. [CrossRef] [PubMed]

114. Aaron, E.; Montgomery, A.; Ren, X.; Guter, S.; Anderson, G.; Carneiro, A.M.D.; Jacob, S.; Mosconi, M.; Pandey, G.N.; Cook, E.; et al. Whole blood serotonin levels and platelet 5-HT2A binding in autism spectrum disorder. *J. Autism Dev. Disord* **2019**, *49*, 2417–2425. [CrossRef]

115. The Handbook of Metabonomics and Metabolomics—1st Edition. Available online: https://www.elsevier.com/books/the-handbook-of-metabonomics-and-metabolomics/lindon/978-0-444-52841-4 (accessed on 3 December 2019).

116. Serkova, N.J.; Jackman, M.; Brown, J.L.; Liu, T.; Hirose, R.; Roberts, J.P.; Maher, J.J.; Niemann, C.U. Metabolic profiling of livers and blood from obese Zucker rats. *J. Hepatol.* **2006**, *44*, 956–962. [CrossRef] [PubMed]

117. Gloyn, A.L.; Faber, J.H.; Malmodin, D.; Thanabalasingham, G.; Lam, F.; Ueland, P.M.; McCarthy, M.I.; Owen, K.R.; Baunsgaard, D. Metabolic profiling in Maturity-onset diabetes of the young (MODY) and young onset type 2 diabetes fails to detect robust urinary biomarkers. *PLoS ONE* **2012**, *7*, e40962. [CrossRef] [PubMed]

118. Brindle, J.T.; Antti, H.; Holmes, E.; Tranter, G.; Nicholson, J.K.; Bethell, H.W.L.; Clarke, S.; Schofield, P.M.; McKilligin, E.; Mosedale, D.E.; et al. Rapid and noninvasive diagnosis of the presence and severity of coronary heart disease using 1H-NMR-based metabonomics. *Nat. Med.* **2002**, *8*, 1439–1444. [CrossRef]

119. Kaddurah-Daouk, R.; Krishnan, K.R.R. Metabolomics: A global biochemical approach to the study of central nervous system diseases. *Neuropsychopharmacology* **2009**, *34*, 173–186. [CrossRef]

120. Pearl, P.L.; Gibson, K.M.; Acosta, M.T.; Vezina, L.G.; Theodore, W.H.; Rogawski, M.A.; Novotny, E.J.; Gropman, A.; Conry, J.A.; Berry, G.T.; et al. Clinical spectrum of succinic semialdehyde dehydrogenase deficiency. *Neurology* **2003**, *60*, 1413–1417. [CrossRef]

121. El-Ansary, A.K.; Bacha, A.G.B.; Al-Ayadhi, L.Y. Plasma fatty acids as diagnostic markers in autistic patients from Saudi Arabia. *Lipids Health Dis.* **2011**, *10*, 62. [CrossRef]

122. Ryan, D.P.; Matthews, J.M. Protein-protein interactions in human disease. *Curr. Opin. Struct. Biol.* **2005**, *15*, 441–446. [CrossRef]

123. Stumpf, M.P.H.; Thorne, T.; de Silva, E.; Stewart, R.; An, H.J.; Lappe, M.; Wiuf, C. Estimating the size of the human interactome. *Proc. Natl. Acad. Sci. USA* **2008**, *105*, 6959–6964. [CrossRef] [PubMed]

124. Careaga, M.; Van de Water, J.; Ashwood, P. Immune dysfunction in autism: A pathway to treatment. *Neurotherapeutics* **2010**, *7*, 283–292. [CrossRef] [PubMed]

125. Malki, K.; Pain, O.; Tosto, M.G.; Du Rietz, E.; Carboni, L.; Schalkwyk, L.C. Identification of genes and gene pathways associated with major depressive disorder by integrative brain analysis of rat and human prefrontal cortex transcriptomes. *Transl. Psychiatry* **2015**, *5*. [CrossRef]

126. Nascimento, J.M.; Martins-de-Souza, D. The proteome of schizophrenia. *NPJ Schizophr.* **2015**, *1*, 14003. [CrossRef] [PubMed]

127. Kilpinen, H.; Ylisaukko-Oja, T.; Hennah, W.; Palo, O.M.; Varilo, T.; Vanhala, R.; Nieminen-von Wendt, T.; von Wendt, L.; Paunio, T.; Peltonen, L. Association of DISC1 with autism and Asperger syndrome. *Mol. Psychiatry* **2008**, *13*, 187–196. [CrossRef]

128. Camargo, L.M.; Collura, V.; Rain, J.-C.; Mizuguchi, K.; Hermjakob, H.; Kerrien, S.; Bonnert, T.P.; Whiting, P.J.; Brandon, N.J. Disrupted in Schizophrenia 1 Interactome: Evidence for the close connectivity of risk genes and a potential synaptic basis for schizophrenia. *Mol. Psychiatry* **2007**, *12*, 74–86. [CrossRef]

129. Sakai, Y.; Shaw, C.A.; Dawson, B.C.; Dugas, D.V.; Al-Mohtaseb, Z.; Hill, D.E.; Zoghbi, H.Y. Protein interactome reveals converging molecular pathways among autism disorders. *Sci. Transl. Med.* **2011**, *3*, 86ra49. [CrossRef]

130. Vignoli, A.; La Briola, F.; Peron, A.; Turner, K.; Vannicola, C.; Saccani, M.; Magnaghi, E.; Scornavacca, G.F.; Canevini, M.P. Autism spectrum disorder in tuberous sclerosis complex: Searching for risk markers. *Orphanet J. Rare Dis.* **2015**, *10*, 154. [CrossRef]

131. Alfieri, A.; Sorokina, O.; Adrait, A.; Angelini, C.; Russo, I.; Morellato, A.; Matteoli, M.; Menna, E.; Boeri Erba, E.; McLean, C.; et al. Synaptic interactome mining reveals p140Cap as a new hub for PSD proteins involved in psychiatric and neurological disorders. *Front. Mol. Neurosci.* **2017**, *10*, 212. [CrossRef]

132. Qiu, S.; Lu, Z.; Levitt, P. MET receptor tyrosine kinase controls dendritic complexity, spine morphogenesis, and glutamatergic synapse maturation in the hippocampus. *J. Neurosci.* **2014**, *34*, 16166–16179. [CrossRef]

133. Han, K.; Holder, J.L.; Schaaf, C.P.; Lu, H.; Chen, H.; Kang, H.; Tang, J.; Wu, Z.; Hao, S.; Cheung, S.W.; et al. SHANK3 overexpression causes manic-like behaviour with unique pharmacogenetic properties. *Nature* **2013**, *503*, 72–77. [CrossRef] [PubMed]

134. Boeckers, T.M.; Bockmann, J.; Kreutz, M.R.; Gundelfinger, E.D. ProSAP/Shank proteins a family of higher order organizing molecules of the postsynaptic density with an emerging role in human neurological disease. *J. Neurochem.* **2002**, *81*, 903–910. [CrossRef] [PubMed]

135. Naisbitt, S.; Kim, E.; Tu, J.C.; Xiao, B.; Sala, C.; Valtschanoff, J.; Weinberg, R.J.; Worley, P.F.; Sheng, M. Shank, a novel family of postsynaptic density proteins that binds to the NMDA receptor/PSD-95/GKAP complex and cortactin. *Neuron* **1999**, *23*, 569–582. [CrossRef]

136. Lee, Y.; Kim, S.G.; Lee, B.; Zhang, Y.; Kim, Y.; Kim, S.; Kim, E.; Kang, H.; Han, K. Striatal transcriptome and interactome analysis of shank3-overexpressing mice reveals the connectivity between shank3 and mTORC1 signaling. *Front. Mol. Neurosci.* **2017**, *10*, 201. [CrossRef] [PubMed]

137. Wyatt, J.; Spiegelhalter, D. Field trials of medical decision-aids: Potential problems and solutions. *Proc. Annu. Symp. Comput. Appl. Med. Care.* **1991**, 3–7.

138. Amarasingham, R.; Plantinga, L.; Diener-West, M.; Gaskin, D.J.; Powe, N.R. Clinical information technologies and inpatient outcomes: A multiple hospital study. *Arch. Intern. Med.* **2009**, *169*, 108–114. [CrossRef]

139. Institute of Medicine (US). *Committee on Quality of Health Care in America Crossing the Quality Chasm: A New Health System for the 21st Century*; National Academies Press (US): Washington, DC, USA, 2001; ISBN 978-0-309-07280-9.

140. Jaspers, M.W.M.; Smeulers, M.; Vermeulen, H.; Peute, L.W. Effects of clinical decision-support systems on practitioner performance and patient outcomes: A synthesis of high-quality systematic review findings. *J. Am. Med. Inform. Assoc.* **2011**, *18*, 327–334. [CrossRef]

141. Ingraham, A.M.; Cohen, M.E.; Bilimoria, K.Y.; Dimick, J.B.; Richards, K.E.; Raval, M.V.; Fleisher, L.A.; Hall, B.L.; Ko, C.Y. Association of surgical care improvement project infection-related process measure compliance with risk-adjusted outcomes: Implications for quality measurement. *J. Am. Coll. Surg.* **2010**, *211*, 705–714. [CrossRef]

142. Kuperman, G.J.; Bobb, A.; Payne, T.H.; Avery, A.J.; Gandhi, T.K.; Burns, G.; Classen, D.C.; Bates, D.W. Medication-related clinical decision support in computerized provider order entry systems: A review. *J. Am. Med. Inform. Assoc.* **2007**, *14*, 29–40. [CrossRef]

143. Kaushal, R.; Kern, L.M.; Barrón, Y.; Quaresimo, J.; Abramson, E.L. Electronic prescribing improves medication safety in community-based office practices. *J. Gen. Intern. Med.* **2010**, *25*, 530–536. [CrossRef]

144. Bates, D.W.; Cohen, M.; Leape, L.L.; Overhage, J.M.; Shabot, M.M.; Sheridan, T. Reducing the frequency of errors in medicine using information technology. *J. Am. Med. Inform. Assoc.* **2001**, *8*, 299–308. [CrossRef] [PubMed]

145. Bryan, C.; Boren, S.A. The use and effectiveness of electronic clinical decision support tools in the ambulatory/primary care setting: A systematic review of the literature. *Inform. Prim. Care* **2008**, *16*, 79–91. [CrossRef] [PubMed]

146. Eslami, S.; Abu-Hanna, A.; de Keizer, N.F. Evaluation of outpatient computerized physician medication order entry systems: A systematic review. *J. Am. Med. Inform. Assoc.* **2007**, *14*, 400–406. [CrossRef] [PubMed]

147. Pearson, S.-A.; Moxey, A.; Robertson, J.; Hains, I.; Williamson, M.; Reeve, J.; Newby, D. Do computerised clinical decision support systems for prescribing change practice? A systematic review of the literature (1990-2007). *BMC Health Serv. Res.* **2009**, *9*, 154. [CrossRef] [PubMed]

148. Shojania, K.G.; Jennings, A.; Mayhew, A.; Ramsay, C.R.; Eccles, M.P.; Grimshaw, J. The effects of on-screen, point of care computer reminders on processes and outcomes of care. *Cochrane Database Syst. Rev.* **2009**, CD001096. [CrossRef]

149. Anand, V.; Carroll, A.E.; Biondich, P.G.; Dugan, T.M.; Downs, S.M. Pediatric decision support using adapted Arden Syntax. *Artif. Intell. Med.* **2018**, *92*, 15–23. [CrossRef] [PubMed]

150. Anand, V.; Carroll, A.E.; Downs, S.M. Automated primary care screening in pediatric waiting rooms. *Pediatrics* **2012**, *129*, e1275–e1281. [CrossRef]

151. Downs, S.M.; Bauer, N.S.; Saha, C.; Ofner, S.; Carroll, A.E. Effect of a computer-based decision support intervention on autism spectrum disorder screening in pediatric primary care clinics: A cluster randomized clinical trial. *JAMA Netw. Open* **2019**, *2*, e1917676. [CrossRef]

152. Cancer Genome Atlas Research Network. Comprehensive genomic characterization defines human glioblastoma genes and core pathways. *Nature* **2008**, *455*, 1061–1068. [CrossRef]

153. Higdon, R.; Stewart, E.; Stanberry, L.; Haynes, W.; Choiniere, J.; Montague, E.; Anderson, N.; Yandl, G.; Janko, I.; Broomall, W.; et al. MOPED enables discoveries through consistently processed proteomics data. *J. Proteome Res.* **2014**, *13*, 107–113. [CrossRef]

154. Kolker, E.; Higdon, R.; Haynes, W.; Welch, D.; Broomall, W.; Lancet, D.; Stanberry, L.; Kolker, N. MOPED: Model organism protein expression database. *Nucleic Acids Res.* **2012**, *40*, D1093–D1099. [CrossRef] [PubMed]

155. Montague, E.; Janko, I.; Stanberry, L.; Lee, E.; Choiniere, J.; Anderson, N.; Stewart, E.; Broomall, W.; Higdon, R.; Kolker, N.; et al. Beyond protein expression, MOPED goes multi-omics. *Nucleic Acids Res.* **2015**, *43*, D1145–D1151. [CrossRef] [PubMed]

156. Montague, E.; Stanberry, L.; Higdon, R.; Janko, I.; Lee, E.; Anderson, N.; Choiniere, J.; Stewart, E.; Yandl, G.; Broomall, W.; et al. MOPED 2.5—An integrated multi-omics resource: Multi-omics profiling expression database now includes transcriptomics data. *OMICS* **2014**, *18*, 335–343. [CrossRef] [PubMed]

157. Hall, D.; Huerta, M.F.; McAuliffe, M.J.; Farber, G.K. Sharing heterogeneous data: The national database for autism research. *Neuroinformatics* **2012**, *10*, 331–339. [CrossRef] [PubMed]

158. Wright, A.; Sittig, D.F.; Ash, J.S.; Feblowitz, J.; Meltzer, S.; McMullen, C.; Guappone, K.; Carpenter, J.; Richardson, J.; Simonaitis, L.; et al. Development and evaluation of a comprehensive clinical decision support taxonomy: Comparison of front-end tools in commercial and internally developed electronic health record systems. *J. Am. Med. Inform. Assoc.* **2011**, *18*, 232–242. [CrossRef] [PubMed]

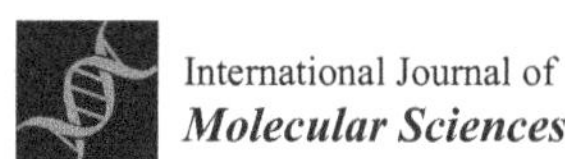 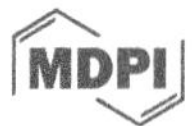

International Journal of
Molecular Sciences

Article

Phenotypic Subtyping and Re-Analysis of Existing Methylation Data from Autistic Probands in Simplex Families Reveal ASD Subtype-Associated Differentially Methylated Genes and Biological Functions

Elizabeth C. Lee [†] and Valerie W. Hu *

Department of Biochemistry and Molecular Medicine, The George Washington University, School of Medicine and Health Sciences, Washington, DC 20037, USA; elee171@jhu.edu
* Correspondence: valhu@gwu.edu; Tel.: +1-202-994-8431
† Current address: W. Harry Feinstone Department of Molecular Microbiology and Immunology,
  Johns Hopkins Bloomberg School of Public Health, Baltimore, MD 21205, USA.

Received: 25 August 2020; Accepted: 17 September 2020; Published: 19 September 2020

Abstract: Autism spectrum disorder (ASD) describes a group of neurodevelopmental disorders with core deficits in social communication and manifestation of restricted, repetitive, and stereotyped behaviors. Despite the core symptomatology, ASD is extremely heterogeneous with respect to the severity of symptoms and behaviors. This heterogeneity presents an inherent challenge to all large-scale genome-wide omics analyses. In the present study, we address this heterogeneity by stratifying ASD probands from simplex families according to the severity of behavioral scores on the Autism Diagnostic Interview-Revised diagnostic instrument, followed by re-analysis of existing DNA methylation data from individuals in three ASD subphenotypes in comparison to that of their respective unaffected siblings. We demonstrate that subphenotyping of cases enables the identification of over 1.6 times the number of statistically significant differentially methylated regions (DMR) and DMR-associated genes (DAGs) between cases and controls, compared to that identified when all cases are combined. Our analyses also reveal ASD-related neurological functions and comorbidities that are enriched among DAGs in each phenotypic subgroup but not in the combined case group. Moreover, relational gene networks constructed with the DAGs reveal signaling pathways associated with specific functions and comorbidities. In addition, a network comprised of DAGs shared among all ASD subgroups and the combined case group is enriched in genes involved in inflammatory responses, suggesting that neuroinflammation may be a common theme underlying core features of ASD. These findings demonstrate the value of phenotype definition in methylomic analyses of ASD and may aid in the development of subtype-directed diagnostics and therapeutics.

Keywords: phenotypic subgroups stratified by ASD severity; simplex families; DNA methylation; subgroup-associated genes and biological functions

---

1. Introduction

Autism spectrum disorder (ASD) is a complex neurodevelopmental disorder characterized by impaired social communication and repetitive behaviors [1]. Tremendous phenotypic and symptomatic heterogeneity exists within the ASD population, thereby presenting a challenge to diagnosis and treatment. The wide range of clinical presentation in ASD is attributed to different underlying etiologies, which include both genetic and environmental influences. One area that bridges the genetics–environment gap is epigenetic variation, which has been proposed to play a role in

ASD [2–6]. It has been shown that DNA methylation is dysregulated in ASD in multiple studies involving both peripheral and brain tissues, principally from individuals with ASD from the multiplex population [7–15]. However, published DNA methylation studies of ASD have produced inconsistent findings, including variable reporting of differentially methylated sites. This inconsistency may be explained not only by the different tissues used but also in part by the wide phenotypic heterogeneity intrinsic to ASD.

Previous findings from our laboratory showed that reduction of ASD clinical heterogeneity by classifying patients into subphenotypes based on cluster analyses of severity scores from the Autism Diagnostic Interview-Revised (ADI-R) diagnostic instrument [16] results in increased ability to detect statistically significant subphenotype-specific transcriptomic as well as genetic differences, which were otherwise undetectable in an aggregate analysis of all individuals with ASD [17–20]. Based on these previous studies that demonstrate the value of subphenotyping in genome-wide omics analyses and the growing body of evidence implicating a link between ASD and epigenetic modification, we hypothesized that the stratification of individuals with ASD by phenotypic severity will result in the identification of subphenotype-dependent DNA methylation differences between cases and controls that achieve statistical significance.

The present study involves re-analyzing existing Illumina HumanMethylation27K BeadChip data from lymphoblastoid cell lines (LCLs) derived from blood lymphocytes of 292 male ASD probands from the Simons Simplex Collection (SSC) after stratification into three distinct subgroups based on ADI-R symptom severity profiles (mild, intermediate, and severely language-impaired). The main goals of this research are to: (1) identify statistically significant differences in DNA methylation between cases and typically developing sibling controls for each of the three ASD subphenotypes, (2) examine the impact of decreasing phenotypic heterogeneity on the ability to detect statistically significant differentially methylated regions and associated genes (DAGs) by comparing results with and without subphenotyping, and (3) identify biological functions, signaling pathways, and disorders associated with DAGs from each subgroup analysis.

2. Results and Discussion

2.1. DAGs Associated with ASD Subphenotypes and the Combined Case Group

Hierarchical clustering (HCL) and principal components analysis (PCA) using scores on the ADI-R diagnostic scoresheets from each of the probands were performed as previously described [16]. These cluster analyses confirmed that the 292 cases in this methylation study could be separated into three phenotypic subgroups based on their severity scores from the ADI-R. A heatmap depicting clinical severity across 123 scores on 63 ADI-R items for individuals in each subgroup is shown in Figure 1, together with PCA plots from the data reduction analysis confirming the separation of cases into three distinguishable subgroups according to integrated severity profiles. Notably, the first three principal components (represented by the x, y, and z-axes of the 3-d PCA plot) account for 85.72% of the variability among all probands based on the 123 ADI-R scores.

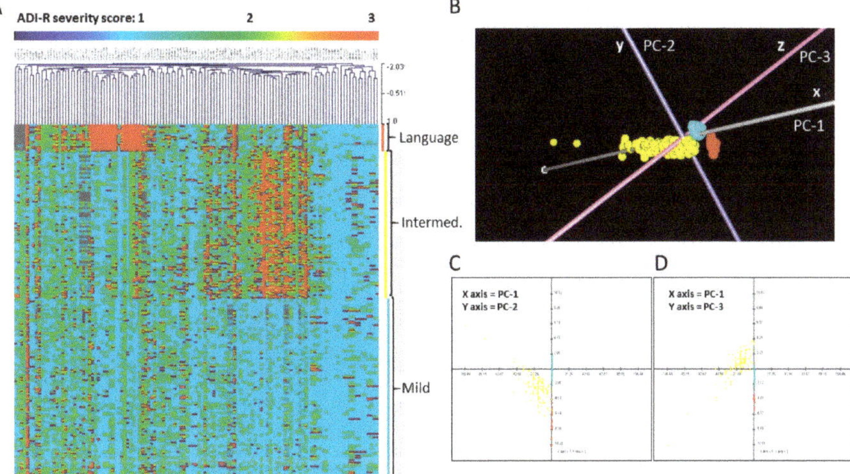

Figure 1. Separation of probands into three phenotypic subgroups based on cluster analyses of 123 scores on 63 Autism Diagnostic Interview-Revised (ADI-R) items for each individual. (**A**) Hierarchical clustering (HCL) analysis, (**B–D**) Principal components analysis (PCA) in 3-d (**B**) and 2-d projections showing PC-1 and PC-2 (C) and PC-1 and PC-3 (D). For the heatmap in (**A**), each row represents an individual, while each column represents a score from the ADI-R diagnostic. The range of severity scores (1–3) for each ADI-R item is represented in the color bar above the heatmap, with light blue indicating a score of 1, green-yellow indicating a score of 2, and red indicating a score of 3, which represents the most severe autism spectrum disorder (ASD) manifestation. The three ASD subgroups are identified by the vertical colored bars along the right side of the heatmap, with red indicating the severely language-impaired subgroup, yellow indicating the intermediate subgroup, and turquoise indicating the mild subgroup. This latter set of colors also applies to the subgroups shown in the PCA plots in which each point represents an individual. Note: In the heatmap (**A**), the large block of red columns associated with the severely language-impaired subgroup primarily corresponds to items involving spoken language on the ADI-R diagnostic.

Using GenomeStudio Methylation Module software, CpG sites across the genome were identified that exhibited statistically significant differential methylation with False Discovery Rate (FDR)-adjusted p-values < 0.05. For the severely language-impaired subgroup (n = 22 cases and 22 controls), 266 unique DAGs were mapped to the CpGs (Table S1). The intermediate subgroup (n = 121 cases and 121 controls) exhibited 360 unique DAGs (Table S2), and the mild subgroup (n = 149 cases and 149 controls) exhibited 4073 unique DAGs (Table S3). Among the three ASD subgroups, a total of 4155 unique DAGs with FDR-adjusted p-values < 0.05 were identified, with some DAGs shared among the subgroups. The volcano plots for each subgroup illustrate distinct differences in the number, distribution, and methylation profiles of significant DAGs in each subgroup (Figure 2). For example, the majority of the DAGs in the severely language-impaired subgroup show reduced methylation (negative delta β values), while the majority of the DAGs in the intermediate subgroup show increased methylation (positive delta β values) (Figure 2A). Although the majority of DAGs in the mild subgroup show decreased methylation as observed in the severely language-impaired subgroup, the mild subgroup has a much greater number of significant DAGs (Figure 2B). In addition, while all the DAGs in the mild subgroup exhibit delta β values < |±0.05|, a fraction of the DAGs associated with the severely language-impaired subgroup exceeds these absolute delta β values, indicating larger methylation differences between cases and controls, which are also reflected by larger fold-change values (see Figure S1). These data suggest that the three ASD subgroups can be distinguished from each other by their differential DNA methylation profiles.

To examine the impact of decreasing phenotypic heterogeneity on the ability to detect statistically significant DAGs, differential methylation analysis of the 27K BeadChip data using Illumina's GenomeStudio Methylation Module was also performed without stratification into phenotypic subtypes, i.e., combined case group (n = 292 cases and 292 controls). Without subgrouping, a total of 2570 unique DAGs with FDR-adjusted p-values < 0.05 were identified in the combined case group (Table S4). The volcano plot of DAGs for the combined case group is shown in

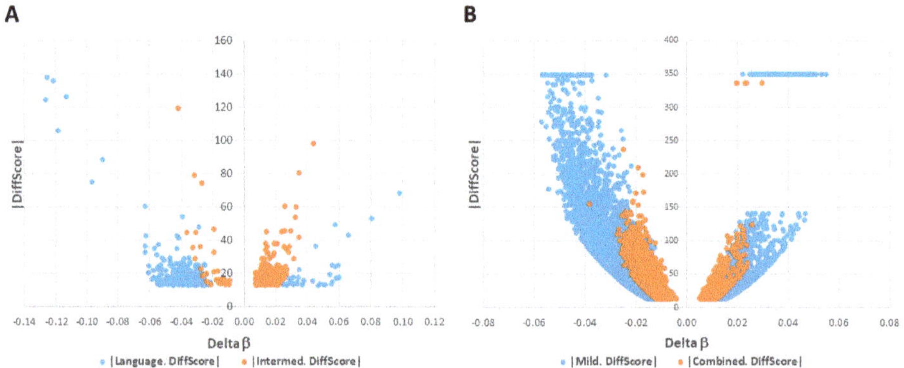

Figure 2. Volcano plots of significant differentially methylated regions and associated genes (DAGs) among subgroups and combined cases. |DiffScore| versus Delta β plots for significant DAGs in: (**A**) severely language-impaired (blue) and intermediate (red) subgroups; (**B**) mild subgroup (blue) and combined cases (red). Note: A |DiffScore| of 13 is roughly equivalent to a p-value of 0.05.

Figure 2B in comparison to that of the mild subgroup. It is notable that there are fewer significant DAGs in the combined case group compared to that of the mild subgroup (2570 vs. 4073), despite the larger number of individuals in the combined case group (292 vs. 149 case-control pairs). Figure 3 summarizes the location of the differentially methylated CpG sites relative to the transcription start site (TSS) for each case group and also the proportion of hypermethylated or hypomethylated sites in each group. In brief, more than 90% of CpG sites in all case groups were found within 1000 bp of the TSS, with the remainder less than 1500 bp away, suggesting that the majority of these sites are likely to be involved in the regulation of transcription. There are also noticeable quantitative differences in the methylation profiles among the case groups. For example, the severely language-impaired subgroup exhibits the greatest proportion of hypomethylated genes (86.8%) and the greatest proportion of CpGs (72.4%) that are closest (≤500 bp) to the TSS. By contrast, the intermediate subgroup exhibits the greatest proportion of hypermethylated genes (91.6%), while the location of the CpGs relative to the TSS is very similar to that of the mild and combined subgroups. Table S5 lists the map positions of the differentially methylated CpGs (and associated genes) in each subtype and the combined case group.

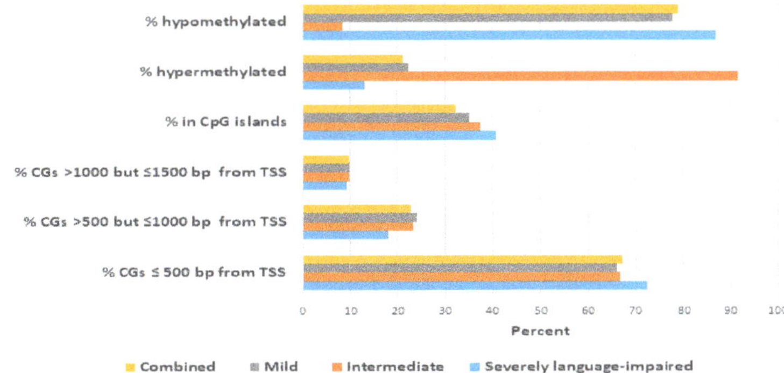

Figure 3. Summary of the proportions of differentially methylated CpG sites at different distances relative to the transcription start site (TSS) of the closest gene and the proportion of hypermethylated and hypomethylated sites in each ASD case group.

The Venn diagram in Figure 4A shows that there are 67 significant DAGs shared among the three subgroups and the combined case group, while Figure 4B shows volcano plots representing the relative distribution of these 67 DAGs in each group's differential methylation profile. The differences in the distribution of these overlapping DAGs in each of the four groups reflect the differences that were revealed in Figure 2, with the majority of DAGs in the intermediate subgroup showing increased methylation, while these same DAGs in the severely language-impaired, mild, and combined groups show decreased methylation, as shown quantitatively in Figure 3.

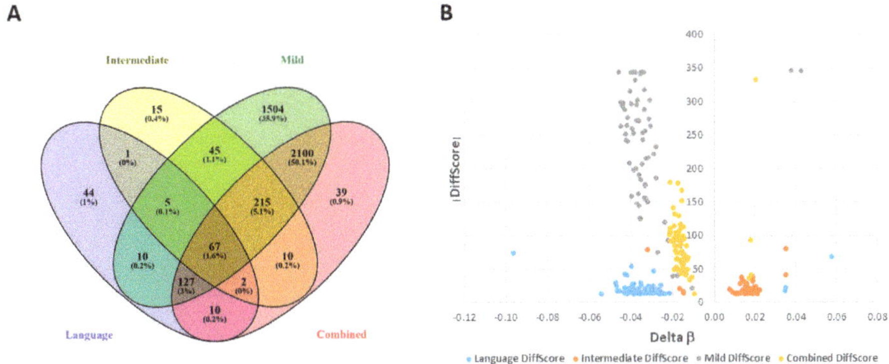

Figure 4. Stratification of ASD patients (*n* = 292) into distinct subphenotypes results in increased discovery of significant DAGs. (**A**) The Venn diagram shows unique significant DAGs that were identified using GenomeStudio Methylation Module v1.8 software with subphenotyping into three groups (mild, intermediate, and severely language-impaired) or without subphenotyping (combined case group) (FDR-adjusted *p*-values < 0.05). (**B**) Volcano plots for the 67 overlapping DAGs from each group, identified by color in the accompanying legend.

Not surprisingly, the |DiffScore| values (inversely related to *p*-values) for these DAGs are much greater in the mild subgroup than those for the severely language-impaired subgroup, which is likely the result of the larger number of samples in the mild subgroup (149 vs. 22 case-control pairs). On the other hand, despite having the largest number of cases and controls, the combined case group has smaller |DiffScore| and delta β values in comparison to the mild subgroup. This finding may reflect the increased heterogeneity underlying the combined case group in which the conglomeration of disparate cases dampens the average methylation differences (i.e., delta β) between the cases and controls. Hence, the present study demonstrates that phenotypic subtyping by clinical severity of ADI-R scores is a productive path for discovering a greater number of statistically significant DAGs between ASD cases and controls as well as differences in DNA methylation profiles among the subgroups.

2.2. Network Prediction Analyses of Subgroup-Associated DAGs

Ingenuity Pathway Analysis (IPA) was used to conduct functional analysis of the DAGs from each of the ASD subgroups as well as from the combined case group. Neurological functions enriched among DAGs in each subgroup and the combined case group are shown in Table 1. The specific DAGs associated with each function are included in Table S6. As shown, the severely language-impaired subgroup exhibits more functions known to be associated with ASD, such as: neuritogenesis, size and branching of neurites, and maturation of synapse and dendritic spines [21–25]. Figure S2 shows that axon guidance signaling and CXCR4 signaling are canonical pathways involved in the top network of genes involved in neuritogenesis. The intermediate subgroup is notably enriched in DAGs associated with the activation of neuroglia and astrocytes, suggesting inflammatory processes known to be involved in ASD [26,27]. Figure S3 shows that the neuroinflammation signaling pathway as well as the glucocorticoid signaling pathway are implicated by the genes involved in the abnormal morphology of neurons in the intermediate subgroup.

Table 1. Significantly over-represented neurological functions among DAGs from three phenotypic subgroups of ASD and a combined case group.

Nervous System Development and Function Severely Language Impaired ($n = 22$)	p-Value *	Number of Genes
Abnormal morphology of neurons	2.21×10^{-4}	19
Sensorimotor integration	3.39×10^{-3}	2
Neuritogenesis	3.52×10^{-3}	19
Maturation of synapse	4.25×10^{-3}	3
Size of neurites	6.09×10^{-3}	2
Branching of neurites	6.31×10^{-3}	11
Maturation of dendritic spines	7.15×10^{-3}	2
Development of neurons	9.24×10^{-3}	22
Intermediate ($n = 121$)		
Activation of neuroglia	7.35×10^{-5}	11
Activation of astrocytes	4.77×10^{-4}	6
Abnormal morphology of neurons	1.22×10^{-3}	21
Abnormal morphology of axons	1.27×10^{-3}	7
Abnormal morphology of neurites	1.48×10^{-3}	9
Loss of neurites	2.91×10^{-3}	4
Mild ($n = 149$)		
Abnormal morphology of nervous system	4.34×10^{-15}	297
Sensory system development	7.77×10^{-15}	194
Combined ($n = 292$)		
Abnormal morphology of nervous system	4.37×10^{-11}	194
Sensory system development	6.17×10^{-9}	121
Abnormal morphology of neurons	2.26×10^{-8}	121
Activation of neuroglia	4.27×10^{-8}	45

* Fisher exact p-value representing the probability that the indicated function is not over-represented among the DAGs for each group, using all genes in IPA's Knowledgebase as the reference gene set.

The mild subgroup is enriched in DAGs involved in sensory system development. Figure S4 shows that the top network of genes enriched for sensory system development is associated with axon guidance, transforming growth factor-β (TGFβ), and bone morphogenetic protein (BMP) signaling pathways. Interestingly, many individuals with ASD exhibit abnormal sensory responses, such as hypersensitivity to certain sounds, visual stimuli, taste, and textures [28–30]. Thus, it is not surprising that many genes related to the sensory system are affected. The nervous system functions associated with DAGs in the combined case group reflect those identified for the intermediate and mild subgroups but not for the severely language-impaired subgroup, which comprises just 7.5% of the total number of cases.

With respect to neurological disorders (see Table 2, Table S7), DAGs in the severely language-impaired subgroup are enriched for genes contributing to comorbidities in ASD, such as cognitive impairment [31–34] and motor dysfunction [35,36]. While axon guidance and synaptogenesis signaling is implicated by the top network of genes associated with cognitive impairment (Figure S5), calcium signaling and dendritic cell maturation are indicated by the top network of genes involved in motor dysfunction (Figure S6). On the other hand, DAGs in the intermediate and mild subgroups as well as the combined case group are over-represented with respect to schizophrenia genes. Figure S7 shows that the neuroinflammation signaling pathway as well as the cAMP and G-protein coupled receptor signaling pathways are involved in schizophrenia in the intermediate subgroup, while synaptogenesis, GABA receptor, and CREB signaling in neurons are involved in the top network of genes in the mild subgroup (Figure S8). Genes associated with motor dysfunction and movement disorders are also over-represented among DAGs in the mild subgroup. Interestingly, only the severely language-impaired subgroup exhibits DAGs explicitly enriched for ASD or intellectual disability (ID), a comorbidity that presents more frequently in individuals with deficits in spoken language.

Table 2. Significantly over-represented neurological and developmental disorders among DAGs from the three phenotypic subgroups of ASD and the combined case group.

Neurological Diseases	p-Value *	Number of Genes
Severely language impaired		
Cognitive impairment	1.32×10^{-5}	26
Syndromic X-linked mental retardation	2.99×10^{-4}	6
Mental retardation	4.13×10^{-3}	14
Motor dysfunction or movement disorder	7.75×10^{-3}	29
Autosomal dominant mental retardation type 11	9.94×10^{-3}	1
Intermediate		
Schizophrenia	7.73×10^{-4}	20
Demyelination of nerves	4.59×10^{-3}	4
Mild		
Schizophrenia	1.18×10^{-16}	184
Motor dysfunction or movement disorder	5.98×10^{-14}	393
Movement Disorders	3.93×10^{-13}	384
Combined		
Schizophrenia	1.81×10^{-7}	106
Developmental Disorders (Severely Language Impaired Only)	p-Value *	Number of Genes
Autism or intellectual disability	3.31×10^{-3}	15
Autism spectrum disorder or intellectual disability	3.67×10^{-3}	17
Dystrophy of muscle	5.51×10^{-3}	10

* Fisher exact p-value representing the probability that the indicated disorder is not over-represented among the DAGs for each group, using all genes in IPA's Knowledgebase as the reference gene set.

Figure 5 shows that one of the two networks of genes that are associated with ASD/ID includes *FMR1*, the gene responsible for fragile X syndrome, a genetic condition that is frequently associated with both intellectual disability and ASD. In a hierarchical layout of the network (Figure S9), *FMR1* is placed at the top of the network, highlighting its influence on the downstream genes, which include *UBE3A*, an E2 ubiquitin conjugating enzyme involved in cognitive disability, and *SLC1A7*, a glutamate transporter that is involved in pervasive developmental disorder (also used to describe ASD), social anxiety, and fragile X.

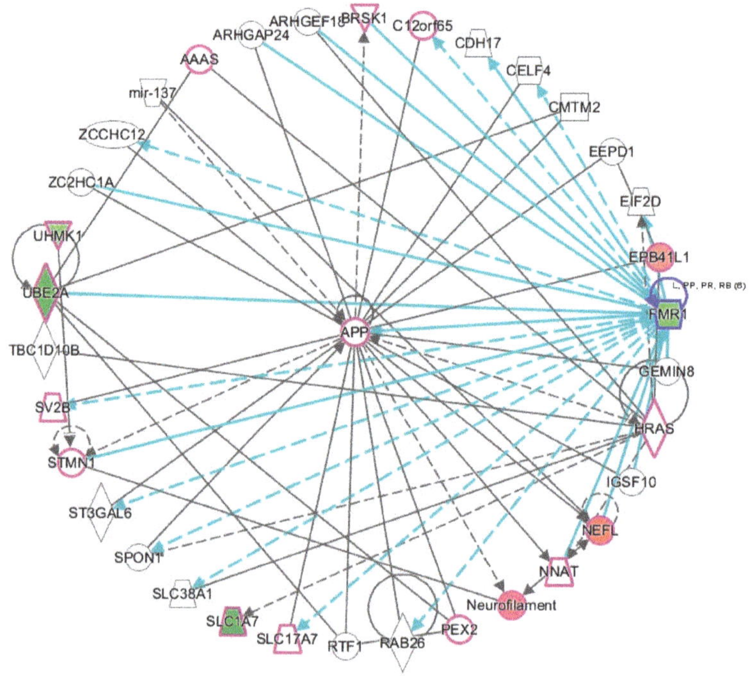

Figure 5. Gene network associated with DAGs enriched for ASD or intellectual disability. All genes involved in developmental disorder are outlined in purple. Genes colored red are hypermethylated while those colored green are hypomethylated. The turquoise colored lines indicate relationships between *FMR1* and other genes in the network. Solid lines denote direct interactions; dashed lines denote indirect interactions.

2.3. Proximity of Hypermethylated and Hypomethylated CpGs to the TSS of the DAGs

Aside from identifying DAGs in each subtype, we also separately investigated the genes associated with hypermethylated and hypomethylated CpGs that were less than 500 bp from the TSS. Interestingly, two of the top genes associated with ASD or intellectual disability in the severely language-impaired subtype, *FMR1* and *UBE2A*, were among the hypomethylated genes closest to the TSS in this subgroup (Table 3). Other ASD-relevant genes within 500 bp of the TSS are *PAX8* and *SHANK1* (both hypomethylated), and *CADM1* and *PAX6* (both hypermethylated). PAX6 and PAX8 are members of the paired box (PAX) family of transcription factors. While PAX 6 is involved in modulating the fate of neural progenitor cells [37], genetic variants in *PAX8* are associated with sleep disturbance [38,39], a frequent comorbidity of ASD. SHANK1 is a scaffolding protein at the postsynaptic density that has been found to be involved in ASD [40]. Mutations in *CADM1*, which codes for a synaptic adhesion molecule, are also associated with ASD [41].

Table 3. Neurological functions and diseases enriched among DAGs implicated by CpGs within 500 bp of the TSS in the severely language-impaired subgroup.

Nervous System Development & Function	*p*-Value *	DAGs (<500 bp from TSS)
Severely language-impaired subtype		*Hypermethylated*
Cell-cell adhesion of neurons	2.29×10^{-4}	CADM1, NINJ2
Induction of neural crest	2.37×10^{-3}	TFAP2A
Scaffolding of postsynaptic region	3.55×10^{-3}	CADM1
Corticogenesis	3.55×10^{-3}	PAX6
Quantity of neurons	7.25×10^{-3}	CADM1, NPTX2, PAX6, TFAP2A
Abnormal morphology of brain	7.37×10^{-3}	CRMP1, EPB41L1, PAX6, TFAP2A
Size of growth cone	1.65×10^{-2}	PAX6
Morphology of nervous system	3.71×10^{-2}	CADM1, CRMP1, EPB41L1, PAX6, TFAP2A
Memory consolidation	3.73×10^{-2}	PAX6
Quantity of nerve ending	3.73×10^{-2}	CADM1
Development of sensory neurons	3.95×10^{-2}	PAX6
Abnormal morphology of forebrain	4.58×10^{-2}	PAX6, TFAP2A
Severely language-impaired subtype		*Hypomethylated*
Abnormal morphology of sensory neurons	6.21×10^{-4}	ATP2B2, CETN2, KCNQ1, OPN4, PAX8
Delay in initiation of maturation of interneurons	5.93×10^{-3}	FMR1
Abnormal morphology of neurons	6.49×10^{-3}	ATP2B2, CABP4, CCL11, CETN2, CORT, FMR1, KCNQ1, NOS3, OPN4, PAX8, SHANK1
Long term synaptic depression of hippocampal cells	9.57×10^{-3}	FMR1, INS
Circadian phase shifting	1.18×10^{-2}	OPN4
Remodeling of dendrites	1.18×10^{-2}	FMR1
Density of GABAergic synapse	1.18×10^{-2}	FMR1
Neurological Diseases	***p*-Value ***	**DAGs (<500 bp from TSS)**
Severely language-impaired subtype		*Hypermethylated*
Autosomal dominant mental retardation type 11	1.19×10^{-3}	EPB41L1
Cognitive impairment	1.33×10^{-3}	CRMP1, EPB41L1, GSTM1, NPTX2, PAX6, TFAP2A
Epileptic seizure	3.70×10^{-2}	CCN1, NPTX2
Mental retardation	4.09×10^{-2}	EPB41L1, PAX6, TFAP2A
Abnormal morphology of forebrain	4.58×10^{-2}	PAX6, TFAP2A
Severely language impaired subtype		*Hypomethylated*
Syndromic X-linked mental retardation	2.20×10^{-5}	BCAP31, FMR1, PHF8, SLC1A7, SLC9A6, UBE2A
Cognitive impairment	1.65×10^{-3}	BCAP31, FMR1, GRM4, INS, KCNQ1, LRRN4, NOS3, PDZK1, PHF8, POLR3C, SHANK1, SLC1A7, SLC9A6, UBE2A, UHMK1
Fragile X-associated tremor ataxia syndrome	5.93×10^{-3}	FMR1
Fragile X syndrome with Prader-Willi-like phenotype	5.93×10^{-3}	FMR1
Movement Disorders	1.15×10^{-2}	ATP2B2, ATP2B3, BCAP31, C9, CCL11, CETN2, COL6A3, F8A1, FCGR3A/FCGR3B, FMR1, KCNQ1, MYH7, OPN4, SDC4, SGCG, SLC17A4, SLC1A7, SLC9A6, TGM6

* Fisher exact *p*-value indicating the probability that the function or disorder is not enriched among the DAGs for this subgroup.

Table 4. Neurological functions and diseases enriched among DAGs implicated by CpGs within 500 bp of the TSS in the intermediate subgroup.

Nervous System Development & Function	*p*-Value *	DAGs (<500 bp from TSS)
Intermediate subtype		*Hypermethylated*
Loss of neurites	4.64×10^{-4}	CORT, GJB1, NTF3, SERPINA3
Activation of neuroglia	1.11×10^{-3}	C1QA, CCL11, CCL22, FGF1, GJB1, NOS3, SMPD3
Abnormal morphology of neurons	1.22×10^{-3}	ATP2B2, C1QA, CABP4, CCL11, CORT, GJB1, KCNQ1, NOS3, NTF3, OPN4, PAX8, PLP1, RHO, SERPINA3, SORBS2
Abnormal morphology of nerve ending	1.66×10^{-3}	C1QA, NTF3
Abnormal morphology of sensory neurons	2.16×10^{-3}	ATP2B2, KCNQ1, NTF3, OPN4, PAX8
Loss of axons	2.38×10^{-3}	CORT, GJB1, NTF3
Activation of astrocytes	3.04×10^{-3}	C1QA, CCL11, FGF1, SMPD3
Formation of excitatory synapses	3.22×10^{-3}	NTF3, SORBS2
Abnormal morphology of neurites	5.98×10^{-3}	CORT, GJB1, NTF3, PLP1, SERPINA3, SORBS2
Evoked potential	6.24×10^{-3}	ATP2B2, KCNQ1, NTF3, PAX8
Abnormal morphology of nervous system	6.49×10^{-3}	ATP2B2, C1QA, CABP4, CCL11, CNGA2, CORT, FGF1, GJB1, KCNQ1, NOS3, NR5A1, NTF3, OPN4, PAX8, PLP1, RHO, SERPINA3, SMPD3, SORBS2
Intermediate subtype		*Hypomethylated*
Morphology of brain	8.83×10^{-4}	ARSA, CTNNB1, GBX2, GSX1, TFAP2A
Differentiation of sensory progenitor cells	9.40×10^{-4}	CTNNB1
Neurogenesis of dopaminergic neurons	1.88×10^{-3}	CTNNB1
Abnormal morphology of forebrain	2.42×10^{-3}	ARSA, GSX1, TFAP2A
Abnormal morphology of brain	3.12×10^{-3}	ARSA, GBX2, GSX1, TFAP2A
Auditory evoked potential	3.15×10^{-3}	ARSA, KCNQ1
Cell survival of dopaminergic neurons	3.76×10^{-3}	CTNNB1
Formation of forebrain	3.77×10^{-3}	CTNNB1, GBX2, GSX1
Accumulation of microglia	7.50×10^{-3}	CTNNB1
Lack of cerebellum	8.43×10^{-3}	GBX2
Neurological Diseases	***p*-Value ***	**DAGs (<500 bp from TSS)**
Intermediate subtype		*Hypermethylated*
Abnormal morphology of mechanosensory neurons	8.56×10^{-4}	ATP2B2, KCNQ1, NTF3, PAX8
Lack of muscle sensory neurons	7.85×10^{-3}	NTF3
Intermediate subtype		*Hypomethylated*
Early-onset neurological disorder	3.20×10^{-4}	ARSA, GABRA3, KCNQ1, PDZRN3
Cognitive impairment	3.54×10^{-4}	ARSA, CTNNB1, GABRA3, GSTM1, KCNQ1, TFAP2A
Autosomal dominant mental retardation type 19	9.40×10^{-4}	CTNNB1
Early-onset schizophrenia	1.13×10^{-3}	GABRA3, PDZRN3
Lack of cerebellum	8.43×10^{-3}	GBX2

* Fisher exact *p*-value indicating the probability that the function or disorder is not enriched among the DAGs for this subgroup.

Table 4 shows the neurological functions and disorders enriched among the hyper- and hypomethylated genes with CpGs closest (<500 bp) to the TSS in the intermediate subgroup. Notable among this set of genes are the hypermethylated genes, *CORT* (corticostatin) and *NTF3* (neurotrophin 3), which are both involved in the loss of neurites. CORT is a neuropeptide that is involved in the depression of neuronal activity and the induction of slow-wave sleep, while NTF3 is a protein that controls the survival and differentiation of mammalian neurons. Among the ASD-relevant hypomethylated genes in this subgroup are *CTNNB1* and *GABRA3*. CTNNB1 (catenin beta1) plays a role in seizure susceptibility and cortical malformation as demonstrated in a *Ctnnb1* knock-out mouse model [42], and GABRA3, a GABA receptor that mediates fast inhibitory effects of GABA in the brain, is reduced in the cerebellum of individuals with ASD [43].

Among the top hypermethylated genes that are enriched in neurological functions and disorders in the mild subgroup are *ARX* and *CNTNAP2* (Table 5; Table 6). *ARX* (Aristaless related homeobox gene) is involved in a number of neurological diseases, including mental retardation, autism, epilepsy, and dystonia [44]. Its function as a homeobox gene is responsible for the wide range of neurological disease phenotypes that result from its mutation or dysregulation. *CNTNAP2*, a member of the neurexin family of proteins that serves as a cell adhesion molecule, is one of the most well-studied ASD risk genes [45–49]. Like *ARX*, mutations in *CNTNAP2* can lead to multiple neurological disease phenotypes, including autism, epilepsy, intellectual disability, obsessive compulsive disorder, and schizophrenia [50]. Notable among the hypomethylated genes in this subgroup are a number of chemokine genes, including *CCL1*, *CCL11*, *CCL2*, *CCL22*, *CCL5*, and *CCL7*. Not surprisingly, these DAGs are enriched among genes that are involved in the activation of neuroglia and neuroinflammation that have been associated with ASD [51,52]. Interestingly, hypomethylated genes associated with schizophrenia include a number of neurotransmitter receptors (e.g., cholinergic, cannabinoid, dopamine, GABA, glutamate, and serotonin) as well as ion channels and ion transporter proteins. These schizophrenia-associated DAGs in the mild ASD subgroup are significantly enriched for GABA receptor signaling (Fisher's exact p-value = 1.98×10^{-6}), neuroinflammation pathway signaling ($p = 4.21 \times 10^{-5}$, serotonin receptor signaling (1.75×10^{-5}), calcium signaling (1.29×10^{-3}), G-protein coupled receptor signaling (2.56×10^{-3}), and glutamate receptor signaling (7.61×10^{-3}) pathways. Overall, the proximity of the differentially methylated CpGs to the TSS of the DAGs enriched for neurological functions and diseases (as shown in Tables 3–6) suggests that these sites may play a role in the transcriptional regulation of the associated genes.

Table 5. Neurological functions enriched among DAGs implicated by CpGs within 500 bp from the TSS in the mild subgroup.

Nervous System Development & Function	p-Value *	DAGs (<500 bp from TSS)
Mild subtype		*Hypermethylated*
Development of striatum	1.26×10^{-6}	ARX, CNTNAP2, GSX1, PAX6
Abnormal morphology of nervous system	3.61×10^{-6}	ARX, ATP8A2, CDH11, CNTNAP2, EDN3, FOXB1, FST, GSX1, OSTM1, PAX6, RBP1, SYN2, TFAP2A, TLX3, ZIC1
Abnormal morphology of glutamatergic neuron	4.96×10^{-5}	PAX6,TLX3
Migration of neurons	5.84×10^{-5}	ARX, CNTNAP2, ERRFI1, FLRT2, LRP12, PAX6, TLX3
Development of neurons	9.20×10^{-5}	ARX, ATP8A2, CADM1, CCN1, CDH1, CNTNAP2, FLRT2, ITGA1, LRP12, PAX6, SYN2, TLX3, TPBG
Quantity of neurons	1.19×10^{-4}	ARX, CADM1, CNTNAP2, ENTPD3, FST, PAX6, PTGER2, SYN2, TFAP2A
Abnormal morphology of brain	1.23×10^{-4}	ARX, CNTNAP2, FOXB1, GSX1, OSTM1, PAX6, SYN2, TFAP2A, ZIC1
Abnormal morphology of forebrain	1.94×10^{-4}	ARX, CNTNAP2, FOXB1, GSX1, PAX6, TFAP2A
Growth of cerebellum	2.30×10^{-4}	FOXB1, ZIC1
Cell cycle progression of neurons	9.71×10^{-4}	PAX6, ZIC1
Growth of brain	1.22×10^{-3}	ARX, FOXB1, PAX6, ZIC1
Developmental process of synapse	1.83×10^{-3}	CADM1, CDH1,FLRT2, SYN2, TPBG
Initiation of migration of neurons	2.90×10^{-3}	ARX
Formation of forebrain	3.02×10^{-3}	ARX, CNTNAP2, GSX1, PAX6, ZIC1
Synaptic transmission of hippocampal CA1 region	4.14×10^{-3}	CNTNAP2, SYN2
Development of sensory neurons	4.39×10^{-3}	PAX6, TLX3
Association of synaptic vesicles	5.80×10^{-3}	SYN2

Table 5. *Cont.*

Nervous System Development & Function	*p*-Value *	DAGs (<500 bp from TSS)
Mild subtype		*Hypomethylated*
Sensory system development	6.57×10^{-9}	ABCA4, ADCY1, AIPL1, AIRE, ALDH1A2, ALOX15, APOB, AQP1, ARSG, ASPA, ATP2B2, BBS1, BBS7, BCL9L, BFSP2, BMPR1B, BRD1, C5AR1, CABP4, CCL1, CDH5, CDK20, CNGA3, COL18A1, COL1A1, COL8A2, CPLX4, CRX, CRYAA/CRYAA2, CRYAB, CRYBA4, CRYBB2, CRYGA, CRYGB, CRYGC, CXCR3, DNMT3A, DPT, DSC1, EGFR, ELOVL4, EMX1, FABP7, FASLG, FEZF2, FGF1, FGF7, FGFR2, FYCO1, GDF3, GFRA1, GJA3, GNAT2, GRK1, GUCA1A, GUCY2F, HCN1, HGF, HK2, HRG, IL1R1, IRX3, KERA, KNG1, KRT12, KRT4, LCK, LCTL, LHX2, LRAT, LRP8, LYVE1, MARCKSL1, METRN, MFAP2, MFRP, MGAT5, MSX2, NEUROD2, NEUROD4, NOTCH3, NRTN, NTF3, NTF4, NXNL1, OLIG2, OPN4, PDCD1, PDE6B, PDE6C, PF4V1, PLA2G3, POR, POU4F2, POU4F3, PPT2, PRPH2, PTGS2, PTPRS, PYGO1, RB1, RBP3, RDH8, RHO, RPE65, RUNX3, S1PR3, SERPINF1, SIX3, SIX6, SLC17A8, SLC39A5, SOX10, SOX11, SPI1, TFB1M, TH, THBS1, TP63, TRPV4, TUB, TULP1, TYRP1, USH2A, VCAM1, VSX2, WNT2
Activation of neuroglia	1.35×10^{-8}	ABCA4, ADIPOQ, AGT, ALB, C1QA, C5AR1, CCL1, CCL11, CCL21, CCL22, CCL5, CCL7, CD40LG, CHGA, CNGA3, CSF3, DRD2, EGFR, F2, FASLG, FGA, FGF1, FGG, GFAP, GJB1, GJC2, GRK2, IL10, IL1R1, MC4R, MOG, MSTN, MYOD1, NOS3, NR4A1, NRG1, PDE6B, PDK4, PTGS2, RDH8, SERPINF2, SLC6A4, SST, TLR7, TLR9, TREM2, TRPM2, VTN

* Fisher exact *p*-value indicating the probability that the function is not enriched among the DAGs for this subgroup.

Table 6. Neurological diseases enriched among DAGs implicated by CpGs within 500 bp from the TSS in the mild subgroup.

Neurological Diseases	*p*-Value *	DAGs (<500 bp from TSS)
Mild subtype		*Hypermethylated*
Cerebellar ataxia with intellectual disability	2.95×10^{-4}	ATP8A2, PAX6
Movement Disorders	6.67×10^{-4}	ARX, ATP8A2, CDH11, DKK3, ERRFI1, FGF12, FLRT2, GABRE, GYPC, NKX6-2, PAX6, PDE4B, SYN2, ZIC1
Epilepsy	7.73×10^{-4}	ARX, CCN1, CNTNAP2, ERRFI1, FGF12, GABRE, SYN2
Epilepsy or neurodevelopmental disorder	1.08×10^{-3}	ARX, CCN1, CNTNAP2, EDN3, ERRFI1, FGF12, GABRE, SYN2
ARX-related X-linked mental retardation	2.90×10^{-3}	ARX
Moderate to severe stage mental retardation	2.90×10^{-3}	ARX
Severe hypotonia	2.90×10^{-3}	ARX
Susceptibility to autism type 15	2.90×10^{-3}	CNTNAP2
Cerebellar ataxia, mental retardation, and dysequilibrium syndrome type 4	2.90×10^{-3}	ATP8A2
Autism	3.95×10^{-3}	ARX, CNTNAP2, GABRE
Seizures	4.52×10^{-3}	ARX, CCN1, CNTNAP2, ERRFI1, FGF12, GABRE, SYN2
Familial pervasive developmental disorder	4.64×10^{-3}	ARX, CNTNAP2
Ataxia	5.23×10^{-3}	ARX, ATP8A2, NKX6-2, PAX6, ZIC1

Table 6. *Cont.*

Neurological Diseases	*p*-Value *	DAGs (<500 bp from TSS)
Mild subtype		*Hypomethylated*
Schizophrenia	9.17×10^{-11}	ACSBG1, ADRA2B, APOA4, APOB, ATP1A4, ATP2B2, ATP4A, ATP4B, BPIFC, CA1, CA5A, CA7, CA9, CAD, CALY, CAP2, CCDC60, CCK, CCKAR, CHI3L1, CHRM1, CHRNA1, CHRNA2, CHRNA9, CHRNB4, CNR1, COL3A1, CPLX2, CRHBP, CYP2D6, CYP2E1, CYP3A5, DAB1, DAO, DDR1, DLG2, DRD1, DRD2, DRD5, DRP2, EGFR, ERBB4, FABP7, FAM3D, FCGR2A, FCGR3A/FCGR3B, GABRA3, GABRA5, GABRA6, GABRG3, GABRP, GABRR1, GFAP, GPR37, GRIK1, GRIK5, GRIN1, GRIN3A, GRM4, GRM7, HIPK3, HRH1, HTR2B, HTR3A, HTR3B, HTR3C, HTR3D, HTR3E, HTR5A, HTR6, INS, LAMA1, LGALS1, MAGEC1, MC4R, MEST, MT2A, MTNR1B, NEFM, NELL1, NOTCH4, NPAS3, NRG1, NRXN1, NTF3, NTNG2, OFCC1, OXTR, PDZRN3, PLP1, PMP22, POMC, PRL, PTGS2, RCAN2, RIT2, RPP21, SCG2, SCG5, SCN2B, SCN3B, SCN4A, SCN9A, SLC14A1, SLC18A1, SLC18A2, SLC31A2, SLC5A7, SLC6A4, SLC7A11, SOX10, SST, STON1, SYN3, SYT3, SYT4, TAC1, TF, THBS1, TRAK1, TTR, UGT1A3, XDH

* Fisher exact *p*-value indicating the probability that the neurological disease is not enriched among the DAGs for this subgroup.

2.4. Shared DAGs among Case Groups Converge on Inflammatory Responses

We also used IPA to analyze the 67 DAGs (from Figure 4) shared by all three subgroups and the combined case group. Figure 6 shows the top network resulting from the network prediction analysis of the shared DAGs. This network is enriched in genes associated with inflammatory responses, suggesting that neuroinflammation may be a common theme underlying core features of ASD that are manifested in all subtypes. These results collectively demonstrate the value of reducing heterogeneity by subphenotyping individuals with ASD to maximize the ability to identify not only ASD-related DAGs but also ASD-associated functions, pathways, and disorders over-represented within each subgroup. Specifically, 1.62 times as many unique DAGs (4155) are identified among the three subphenotypes in comparison to that of the combined case group (2570).

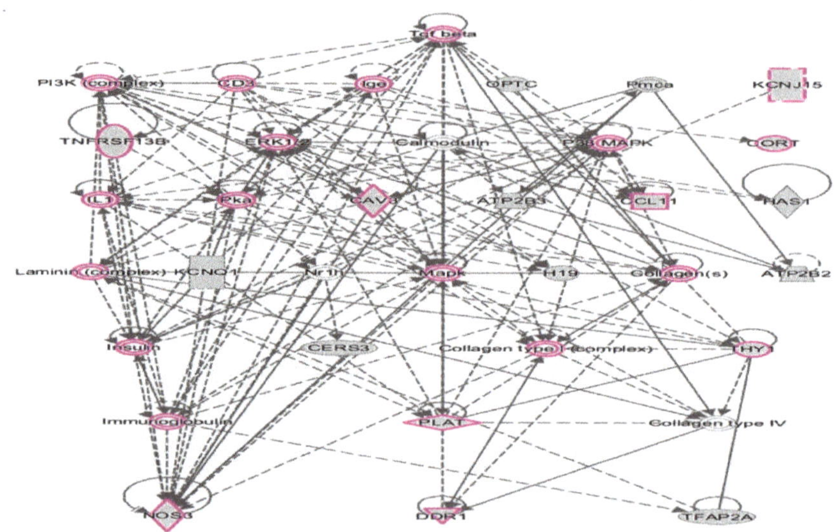

Figure 6. Hierarchical layout of top network of DAGs shared among 3 subphenotypes of ASD and the combined case group. Genes outlined in purple are involved in inflammatory responses.

2.5. Overlap of DAGs and Differentially Expressed Genes (DEGs) from Analogous Phenotypic Subgroups from the Simplex Population

The subgroup-associated DAGs from the present methylation study were compared with DEGs from a separate study investigating transcriptomic data on individuals from the SSC cohort who were divided into subphenotypes using cluster analyses of ADI-R scores (Hu, V.W. and Bi, C., unpublished data). The overlapping genes for each subgroup and the combined case group included 12 DEGs from the severely language-impaired subgroup (hypergeometric cumulative q-value = 0.30), 8 DEGs from the intermediate subgroup (q = 0.35), 76 DEGs from the mild subgroup (q = 7.14 × 10^{-4}, and 68 DEGs from the combined case group (q = 2.31 × 10^{-4}) (Table 7). Thus, there is a significant overlap between DEGs and DAGs from the mild subgroup and combined case group but not from the severely language-impaired subgroup or intermediate subgroup, suggesting at least partial functional validation with regard to regulation of expression for the overlapping genes. It is not expected that all of the DEGs would be regulated by methylation differences between cases and controls. It should also be noted that there were fewer individuals in the transcriptomic investigation, with 7 case-control sibling pairs in the severely language-impaired subgroup, 26 pairs in the intermediate subgroup, 41 pairs in the mild subgroup, and 74 pairs in the combined case group. Furthermore, although the cases from the transcriptomic analysis were phenotypically representative of those from the three subgroups in this methylation study, the samples were not the same as those included in the present study.

Table 7. Overlapping genes among DAGs and Differentially Expressed Genes (DEGs) from the three phenotypic subgroups of ASD and the combined case group.

Overlap between DAGs and DEGs in Language-Impaired Subgroup (hypergeom. q=0.30)	Overlap between DAGs and DEGs in Intermediate Subgroup (q = 0.35)	Overlap between DAGs and DEGs in Mild Subgroup (q = 7.14 × 10⁻⁴)		Overlap between DAGs and DEGs in Combined Case Group (q = 2.31 × 10⁻⁴)	
ALOX15B	AIM2	AADAC	LIMS2	AIM2	LCN2
CARD14	ARSA	AMPH	MATK	ASB10	LHX3
CAV3	ATP8B1	APOB	MEP1B	ASCL2	LYST
CCL11	KCNQ1	BNC1	MMP10	BGN	MAGEA11
COL6A3	LDHC	C15orf32	MS4A12	BMP10	MAGEA8
CTRB1	NEFL	C19orf18	MS4A6A	BMX	MEPE
FAM83A	RGS3	C8B	NKX6-2	BTNL2	MS4A12
HIPK4	SMPD3	CADPS	NNAT	C14orf39	MS4A6A
HSPB8		CCDC54	NR1I3	C15orf32	NR1I3
PSG4		CDH5	NR4A1	CARD14	NR5A1
SEMA3B		CEACAM3	NRXN1	CCR9	OR10A4
WFDC8		CHI3L1	NRXN3	CHRNA1	OR10H1
		COX4I2	OR10H1	CNKSR1	OR1N1
		CPA6	P4HA3	CYP2C9	OR3A3
		DCN	PCDHB7	CYP4F3	P4HA3
		DLK1	PHYHIP	DEFB126	PABPC5
		DNMT3L	RGS12	EGFL7	PLAT
		DOCK1	S100A3	FBLN1	PMCHL1
		EDNRB	SATB1	FLRT2	PNLIPRP1
		FMR1NB	SCARF1	GALR1	RASL12
		FRMPD2	SCN3B	GATA5	RGS13
		FXYD3	SLC13A5	GKN1	RHOJ
		GATA5	SLC35E4	GLIS1	SCGB1D1
		GIPR	SLC6A11	GRIK2	SLC6A11
		GLIS1	SPATA3	GUCA2B	SPATA21
		GUCA2B	SPINK4	GUCY2F	SPRR3
		HBE1	SPOCK3	HCRTR1	SPTB
		IFNA16	SPTB	IFNA17	TFAP2B
		IQCF1	ST6GAL2	IGSF11	TRPM5
		KLHDC7A	SYN3	IQCF1	TTLL2
		KLK3	SYNE2	KIF25	WFDC5
		KLK9	TMEM119	KLK9	WWP1
		KRTAP20-1	TMEM40	KRT1	ZBED2
		LAD1	TNNI1	LCE3C	ZDHHC11
		LCE3C	TRIM16		
		LCN2	USH2A		
		LHX3	ZDHHC11		
		LILRA5	ZPLD1		

2.6. Comparison with Other DNA Methylation Studies of ASD

DNA methylation has long been implicated as a contributor to the etiology of ASD-related disorders, such as Rett syndrome and Fragile X [53–56]. With respect to idiopathic ASD, we were the first to demonstrate that DNA methylation differences across multiple genes could be correlated to dysregulated expression of those genes in LCLs from discordantly diagnosed monozygotic twins and sibling pairs [7,57]. Since then, a number of other studies using blood-derived cells, buccal cells, and brain tissues have confirmed aberrant DNA methylation as a likely contributory factor to ASD [7–15]. However, there has been relatively low consistency with respect to the specific DAGs identified among the various studies, which is possibly due to the heterogeneity both within and among the cohorts used for the different analyses.

To our knowledge, this is the first study to undertake methylation analysis of ASD probands and unaffected siblings from the simplex population after dividing the cases into phenotypic subgroups to lessen the clinical heterogeneity inherent to ASD. A recent study that involved a meta-analysis of blood DNA methylation from two cohorts of individuals with ASD and controls did not find any DAGs that were significant after Bonferroni correction for multiple testing despite having 796 cases and 858 controls [58]. One of the cohorts included 343 probands and their respective sibling controls from the SSC. Among the 7 genes that were suggestively associated with ASD with p-value $< 1 \times 10^{-5}$, only one, *DIO3*, was found among DAGs from the mild subgroup tested here. Similarly, another recent methylation study using neonatal bloodspots from 1263 infants (of whom 50% were later diagnosed with ASD) concluded that ASD is not associated with robust differential methylation between the diagnosed children and the unaffected ones [59]. Another large methylome-wide association study (MWAS), which used cord blood from 701 8-year-olds and their respective scores on the Social and Communication Disorders Checklist as a measure of autistic traits, found no significant CpGs associated with the social traits [14]. Moreover, Massrali et al. [14] reported that a meta-analysis of the blood and blood spot data from the previous two MWAS studies [58,59] did not reveal any significant concordance in effect direction with their cord blood study; they therefore concluded that none of the MWAS studies identified any significant DAGs. It should be noted that all of these studies used methylation data collected on Illumina Infinium HumanMethylation450K BeadChip arrays, which offer greater potential for identifying differentially methylated CpG sites in comparison to the HumanMethylation27K array from which we derived the methylation data for our study. We therefore suggest that our ability to identify a large number of significant DAGs—some of which are replicated in different subgroups (or cohorts)—is due to the reduction in phenotypic or clinical heterogeneity among the cases in each subgroup. This interpretation is borne out by the smaller delta β values for DAGs when all the cases are combined into one group for methylation analysis. While we have used cluster analyses of ADI-R scores for phenotypic subgrouping in this study, heterogeneity reduction by genetic subgrouping (e.g., by *CHD8* mutations or by 16p11.2 deletions) has also resulted in enhanced ability to detect significant DAGs between ASD cases and controls [60]. In the same study, Siu et al. also reported no significant DAGs with a heterogeneous group of cases with idiopathic ASD, thereby reaffirming the value of heterogeneity reduction in genome-wide DNA methylation studies of ASD. Aside from the subgrouping methods discussed above, heterogeneity reduction in ASD can also be accomplished by subtyping individuals by associated comorbidities, such as intellectual disability, immune dysfunction, or gastrointestinal disease.

2.7. Advantages and Limitations of Study Design and Future Considerations

This study examines the impact of applying clinical subtyping to methylation analyses of males with ASD from the simplex population. While the inclusion of only males eliminates sex as a confounding factor, future studies should also include females to investigate the potential for sex-related differences in DNA methylation. The main limitation here is the relatively small number of cases studied, particularly in the severely language-impaired subgroup, which represents the smallest phenotypic subgroup identified by ADI-R cluster analyses of cases from simplex families. Despite this limitation, the severely language-impaired subgroup exhibited the largest differences in β values (and fold-change) between cases and controls relative to that of the other groups, perhaps reflecting the heightened clinical severity of this subgroup. Furthermore, network prediction analyses show that this subgroup was most enriched in neurological functions and comorbidities associated with ASD and was also the sole subgroup enriched for genes directly involved in autism and intellectual disability.

Another limitation is that we were not able to confirm the DAGs identified in each subgroup inasmuch as this bioinformatics study focused on a re-analysis of existing methylation data, and we did not have access to the samples for pyrosequencing analyses. Future studies should therefore address the confirmation of these results not only with regard to methylation analyses of specific DAGs, but also with respect to application of this subtyping method to methylation analyses of an additional cohort of individuals with ASD from the simplex population, preferably with more CpG sites interrogated. Nevertheless, the overlap of DAGs between and among the three phenotypic subgroups represents replication of at least these specific DAGs in different cohorts, as there is no overlap of individuals among the subgroups. In addition, the overlap of DAGs from this study and DEGs from a separate transcriptomic study involving analogous subgroups from the simplex population offers functional support for a fraction of the DAGs identified here. Finally, the Infinium HumanMethylation27K BeadChip array, which was used to generate the methylation data analyzed in this study, is also a limitation in terms of the relatively low number of CpGs interrogated. More recent BeadChip arrays currently probe over 800K CpG sites, and whole genome bisulfite sequencing can assess even more. Thus, in light of our study demonstrating increased discovery of significant DAGs as well as ASD-associated neurological functions and disorders as a result of phenotypic subgrouping, it will be of interest for future studies to analyze more comprehensive methylation data in the context of ASD subtypes to confirm the main findings reported here.

3. Materials and Methods

3.1. Acquisition of Methylation Data for Individuals with ASD from the Simplex Population

DNA methylation data from a study of individuals with ASD and their unaffected siblings who were included in the Simons Simplex Collection (SSC) (New York, NY, USA) were downloaded from the National Database for Autism Research (NDAR). NDAR is a repository of clinical, omics, and brain imaging data from autism studies that is maintained by the NIMH Data Archives (NDA) (Rockville, MD, USA). The original data were deposited by Dr. Stephen Warren (Emory University, Atlanta, GA, USA) for a methylation pilot study entitled "Epigenetic marks as peripheral biomarkers for autism" (Study ID: #287). For the pilot study, DNA methylation for over 300 simplex cases and their respective sibling controls was analyzed on Illumina Infinium HumanMethylation27K BeadChips covering 27,578 CpG dinucleotides, with the raw data deposited into NDAR.

3.2. Phenotypic Subtyping for ASD Individuals from Simplex Families

The Autism Diagnostic Interview-Revised (ADI-R), which is considered a gold-standard diagnostic tool for autism, is based on a series of questions posed to parents or primary caregivers that interrogate a subject's performance on a wide range of behaviors impacted by ASD [61]. These behaviors are scored for severity by a trained neuropsychologist according to the parent/caregiver's response. Raw ADI-R scoresheets for 1900 individuals with ASD (i.e., probands) were obtained from the SSC. As described previously for multiplex families [16], 123 severity scores on 63 ADI-R items (see Table S8) for each individual were subjected to K-means cluster (KMC) analyses, which showed that K = 3 (representing separation into 3 subgroups) resulted in an optimum separation of cases with distinguishable severity profiles. Based on these profiles, the three subgroups were described as mild, intermediate, and severely language impaired, which are similar to three of the four subgroups previously identified in multiplex families [16]. The fourth subgroup in the multiplex population, which exhibited a noticeably higher frequency of savant skills, was not clearly discernible within the simplex population.

The sample identification numbers (IDs) of the probands from the Warren pilot methylation study were then cross-referenced against the sample IDs associated with 1900 ADI-R scoresheets of individuals with ASD from the SSC. Based on the severity profiles that resulted from the ADI-R cluster analyses, 292 cases (all males) with available methylation data were stratified into three subphenotypes as follows: mild ($n = 149$), intermediate ($n = 121$), and severely language impaired ($n = 22$). Differences in the severity profiles of the 292 individuals selected for our study were verified by hierarchical clustering (HCL) and principal components analyses (PCA) using open-access Multiexperiment Viewer software [62]. The demographic information on individuals included in the current study is presented in Table S9.

3.3. Identification of Differentially Methylated Regions (DMR) and DMR-Associated Genes (DAG)

Raw signal intensities were extracted from idat files derived from the Illumina Infinium HumanMethylation27K BeadChip analyses using Illumina's GenomeStudio Methylation Module v1.8 (Illumina, San Diego, CA, USA). The DNA methylation level of each interrogated CpG site is reported in the GenomeStudio software as an average β value, ranging from 0 (completely unmethylated) to 1 (100% methylated). The β value is defined as the ratio of signal from the methylated probe (M) to the sum of the signals from the methylated probe (M) and unmethylated probe (U) plus 100, or $\beta = M/(M + U + 100)$. Analysis of differential methylation between ASD cases and sibling controls was performed in GenomeStudio using the Illumina Custom Model. This error model developed by Illumina assumes a normal distribution of the β values among biological replicates and results in a differential methylation score (DiffScore) for each interrogated CpG site. Using the absolute value of DiffScores reported by the GenomeStudio software, p-values were calculated with the following formula: $p = 10^{-(|\text{DiffScore}|/10)}$. $|\text{DiffScore}| > 13.0103$ is equivalent to a p-value < 0.05. Correction for multiple comparisons was accomplished by computing the false discovery rate (FDR), which is integrated into the GenomeStudio software. Interrogated CpG sites were annotated in GenomeStudio with respect to their corresponding genes. DAGs with FDR-adjusted $p < 0.05$ were classified as significant. The three ASD subgroups were analyzed separately as well as in combination (i.e., combined case group) for DNA methylation differences when compared to their respective sibling controls. Volcano plots showing the overall distribution of significant DAGs for each subgroup or the combined case group were generated by plotting $|\text{DiffScore}|$ against delta β, i.e., ($\beta_{case} - \beta_{control}$). The distance of the differentially methylated CpGs to the TSS of the nearest gene was obtained from Illumina's content file for the HumanMethylation27K BeadChip array, which provides the mapping information for each CpG as well as its location with respect to CpG islands. All of the CpG sites were within 1500 bp of a TSS, suggesting their potential involvement in the regulation of gene expression.

3.4. Network Prediction Analyses of DAGs

Ingenuity Pathway Analysis (IPA) network prediction software (Qiagen, Germantown, MD, USA) was used to identify enriched functions, pathways, and disorders associated with DAGs from the methylation analyses based on Fisher exact p-values of $p \leq 0.05$, using genes in IPA's Knowledgebase as the reference set of genes to determine enrichment in pathways or functions among the DAGs.

3.5. Hypergeometric Distribution Analyses

Hypergeometric distribution analyses were employed to identify the significance of overlap between DAGs and differentially expressed genes (DEGs) from analogous phenotypic subgroups of ASD from a separate study (Hu, V.W. and Bi, C., unpublished data), which involved re-analysis of transcriptomic data from a previously published study that used LCLs from the SSC [63]. Theoverlapping genes were identified using an open-access Venn diagram software program called Venny 2.1.0 (https://bioinfogp.cng.csic.es/tools/venny/) [64]. Significant overlap between the DAGs and DEGs was determined by hypergeometric distribution analyses using the open-access CASIO Keisan Online Calculator (http://keisan.casio.com/exec/system/1180573201), with significance determined by an upper cumulative *q*-value of ≤ 0.05. Venny 2.1.0 was also used to identify overlap among subgroup-associated DAGs and those from the combined case group.

4. Conclusions

This is the first study to investigate differential methylation in individuals with ASD from the simplex population who were divided into distinct phenotypic subgroups by cluster analyses of ADI-R scores. This study is important because it demonstrates a link between DNA methylation and the etiology of ASD in this population. We suggest that subphenotyping enables more efficient identification of statistically significant DAGs which, in turn, reveal subphenotype-dependent functions and comorbidities that are associated with each ASD subgroup. Such discrimination of the biological differences between ASD subphenotypes is essential to our understanding of the complex pathobiology of ASD as well as our ability to develop targeted ASD subtype-directed therapeutics.

Supplementary Materials: The following are available online at http://www.mdpi.com/1422-0067/21/18/6877/s1, Figure S1. |DiffScore| vs. log2 Fold-change values for all groups; Figure S2. Gene network associated with DAGs involved in neuritogenesis in the severely language-impaired subgroup; Figure S3. Gene network associated with DAGs involved in abnormal morphology of neurons in the intermediate subgroup; Figure S4. Gene network associated with DAGs involved in sensory system development in the mild subgroup; Figure S5. Gene network associated with DAGs involved in cognitive impairment in the severely language-impaired subgroup; Figure S6. Gene network associated with DAGs involved in motor dysfunction in the severely language-impaired subgroup; Figure S7. Gene network associated with DAGs involved in schizophrenia in the intermediate subgroup; Figure S8. Gene network associated with DAGs involved in schizophrenia in the mild subgroup; Figure S9. Hierarchical layout of a top gene network of DAGs associated with ASD and ID in the severely language-impaired subgroup; Table S1. Significant DAGs associated with the severely language-impaired subgroup; Table S2. Significant DAGs associated with the intermediate subgroup; Table S3. Significant DAGs associated with the mild subgroup; Table S4. Significant DAGs associated with the combined case group; Table S5. Map positions (distance from TSS) of the differentially methylated CpG sites in each subtype and the combined case group; Table S6. Over-represented neurological functions among DAGs in all subgroups and the combined case group; Table S7. Over-represented neurological and developmental disorders among DAGs in all subgroups and the combined case group; Table S8. List of ADI-R items with score adjustments used for cluster analyses, as described in [16]; Table S9. Demographic information for probands and siblings used in this study.

Author Contributions: Conceptualization, V.W.H.; Formal analysis, E.C.L. and V.W.H.; Supervision, V.W.H.; Visualization, V.W.H.; Writing—original draft, E.C.L. and V.W.H.; Writing—review & editing, E.C.L. and V.W.H. All authors have read and agreed to the published version of the manuscript.

Funding: This research received no external funding.

Acknowledgments: The methylation data used in the preparation of this manuscript were obtained from the National Institute of Mental Health (NIMH) Data Archive (NDA). NDA is a collaborative informatics system created by the National Institutes of Health to provide a national resource to support and accelerate research in mental health. Dataset identifier: [NIMH Data Archive Collection ID #287; DOI: 10.15154/1165651]. This manuscript reflects the views of the authors and may not reflect the opinions or views of the NIH or of the Submitters submitting original data to NDA. We also acknowledge Stephen Warren (Emory University, Atlanta, GA) as the submitter of the pilot methylation data deposited into the NDA. We thank the SSC for providing raw ADI-R scoresheets for probands in the SSC (to VWH) and the families of individuals with ASD for making these data as well as biological specimens available for research.

Conflicts of Interest: The authors declare no conflict of interest.

References

1. American Psychiatric Association. *Diagnostic and Statistical Manual of Mental Disorders: DSM-5*, 5th ed.; American Psychiatric Association: Arlington, VA, USA, 2013.

2. Bakulski, K.M.; Singer, A.B.; Fallin, M.D. Genes and environment in autism spectrum disorders: An integrated perspective. In *Frontiers in Autism Research: New Horizons for Diagnosis and Treatment*; Hu, V.W., Ed.; World Scientific Publishing Co.: Singapore, 2014; pp. 335–374.

3. Siu, M.T.; Weksberg, R. Epigenetics of Autism Spectrum Disorder. In *Neuroepigenomics in Aging and Disease*; Delgado-Morales, R., Ed.; Springer International Publishing: Cham, Switzerland, 2017; pp. 63–90.

4. Moosa, A.; Shu, H.; Sarachana, T.; Hu, V.W. Are Endocrine Disrupting Compounds Environmental Risk Factors for Autism Spectrum Disorder? *Horm. Behav.* **2018**, *101*, 13–21. [CrossRef] [PubMed]

5.   Ciernia, A.V.; LaSalle, J. The Landscape of DNA Methylation Amid a Perfect Storm of Autism Aetiologies. *Nat. Rev. Neurosci.* **2016**, *17*, 411–423. [CrossRef] [PubMed]

6.   Ladd-Acosta, C.; Fallin, M.D. DNA Methylation Signatures as Biomarkers of Prior Environmental Exposures. *Curr. Epidemiol. Rep.* **2019**, *6*, 1–13. [CrossRef] [PubMed]

7.   Nguyen, A.; Rauch, T.A.; Pfeifer, G.P.; Hu, V.W. Global Methylation Profiling of Lymphoblastoid Cell Lines Reveals Epigenetic Contributions to Autism Spectrum Disorders and a Novel Autism Candidate Gene, *RORA*, Whose Protein Product is Reduced in Autistic Brain. *FASEB J.* **2010**, *24*, 3036–3051. [CrossRef]

8.   Ginsberg, M.R.; Rubin, R.A.; Falcone, T.; Ting, A.H.; Natowicz, M.R. Brain Transcriptional and Epigenetic Associations with Autism. *PLoS ONE* **2012**, *7*, e44736. [CrossRef]

9.   Ladd-Acosta, C.; Hansen, K.D.; Briem, E.; Fallin, M.D.; Kaufmann, W.E.; Feinberg, A.P. Common DNA Methylation Alterations in Multiple Brain Regions in Autism. *Mol. Psychiatry* **2014**, *19*, 862–871. [CrossRef]

10.   Nardone, S.; Sharan Sams, D.; Reuveni, E.; Getselter, D.; Oron, O.; Karpuj, M.; Elliott, E. DNA Methylation Analysis of the Autistic Brain Reveals Multiple Dysregulated Biological Pathways. *Transl. Psychiatry* **2014**, *4*, e433. [CrossRef]

11.   Berko, E.R.; Suzuki, M.; Beren, F.; Lemetre, C.; Alaimo, C.M.; Calder, R.B.; Ballaban-Gil, K.; Gounder, B.; Kampf, K.; Kirschen, J.; et al. Mosaic Epigenetic Dysregulation of Ectodermal Cells in Autism Spectrum Disorder. *PLoS Genet.* **2014**, *10*, e1004402. [CrossRef]

12.   Wong, C.C.Y.; Meaburn, E.L.; Ronald, A.; Price, T.S.; Jeffries, A.R.; Schalkwyk, L.C.; Plomin, R.; Mill, J. Methylomic Analysis of Monozygotic Twins Discordant for Autism Spectrum Disorder and Related Behavioural Traits. *Mol. Psychiatry* **2014**, *19*, 495–503. [CrossRef]

13.   Feinberg, J.I.; Bakulski, K.M.; Jaffe, A.E.; Tryggvadottir, R.; Brown, S.C.; Goldman, L.R.; Croen, L.A.; Hertz-Picciotto, I.; Newschaffer, C.J.; Fallin, M.D.; et al. Paternal Sperm DNA Methylation Associated with Early Signs of Autism Risk in an Autism-Enriched Cohort. *Int. J. Epidemiol.* **2015**, *14*, 1–12. [CrossRef]

14.   Massrali, A.; Brunel, H.; Hannon, E.; Wong, C.; Baron-Cohen, S.; Warrier, V. Integrated Genetic and Methylomic Analyses Identify Shared Biology between Autism and Autistic Traits. *Mol. Autism* **2019**, *10*, 31. [CrossRef] [PubMed]

15.   Wong, C.C.Y.; Smith, R.G.; Hannon, E.; Ramaswami, G.; Parikshak, N.N.; Assary, E.; Troakes, C.; Poschmann, J.; Schalkwyk, L.C.; Sun, W.; et al. Genome-Wide DNA Methylation Profiling Identifies Convergent Molecular Signatures Associated with Idiopathic and Syndromic Autism in Post-Mortem Human Brain Tissue. *Hum. Mol. Genet.* **2019**, *28*, 2201–2211. [CrossRef] [PubMed]

16.   Hu, V.W.; Steinberg, M.E. Novel Clustering of Items from the Autism Diagnostic Interview-Revised to Define Phenotypes within Autism Spectrum Disorders. *Autism Res.* **2009**, *2*, 67–77. [CrossRef] [PubMed]

17.   Hu, V.W.; Sarachana, T.; Kim, K.S.; Nguyen, A.; Kulkarni, S.; Steinberg, M.E.; Luu, T.; Lai, Y.; Lee, N.H. Gene Expression Profiling Differentiates Autism Case-Controls and Phenotypic Variants of Autism Spectrum Disorders: Evidence for Circadian Rhythm Dysfunction in Severe Autism. *Autism Res.* **2009**, *2*, 78–97. [CrossRef]

18.   Hu, V.W.; Addington, A.; Hyman, A. Novel Autism Subtype-Dependent Genetic Variants are Revealed by Quantitative Trait and Subphenotype Association Analyses of Published GWAS Data. *PLoS ONE* **2011**, *6*, e19067. [CrossRef]

19.   Talebizadeh, Z.; Arking, D.E.; Hu, V.W. A Novel Stratification Method in Linkage Studies to Address Inter and Intra Family Heterogeneity in Autism. *PLoS ONE* **2013**, *8*, e67569. [CrossRef] [PubMed]

20.   Hu, V.W.; Devlin, C.A.; Debski, J.J. ASD Phenotype-genotype Associations in Concordant and Discordant Monozygotic and Dizygotic Twins Stratified by Severity of Autistic Traits. *Int. J. Mol. Sci.* **2019**, *20*, 3804. [CrossRef] [PubMed]

21.   Courchesne, E.; Pramparo, T.; Gazestani, V.H.; Lombardo, M.V.; Pierce, K.; Lewis, N.E. The ASD Living Biology: From Cell Proliferation to Clinical Phenotype. *Mol. Psychiatry* **2019**, *24*, 88–107. [CrossRef]

22.   Bakos, J.; Bacova, Z.; Grant, S.G.; Castejon, A.M.; Ostatnikova, D. Are Molecules Involved in Neuritogenesis and Axon Guidance Related to Autism Pathogenesis? *Neuromol. Med.* **2015**, *17*, 297–304. [CrossRef]

23.   Nguyen, H.T.N.; Kato, H.; Masuda, K.; Yamaza, H.; Hirofuji, Y.; Sato, H.; Pham, T.T.M.; Takayama, F.; Sakai, Y.; Ohga, S.; et al. Impaired Neurite Development Associated with Mitochondrial Dysfunction in Dopaminergic Neurons Differentiated from Exfoliated Deciduous Tooth-Derived Pulp Stem Cells of Children with Autism Spectrum Disorder. *Biochem. Biophys. Rep.* **2018**, *16*, 24–31. [CrossRef]

24. Phillips, M.; Pozzo-Miller, L. Dendritic Spine Dysgenesis in Autism Related Disorders. *Neurosci. Lett.* **2014**, *601*, 30–40. [CrossRef] [PubMed]

25. Guang, S.; Pang, N.; Deng, X.; Yang, L.; He, F.; Wu, L.; Chen, C.; Yin, F.; Peng, J. Synaptopathology Involved in Autism Spectrum Disorder. *Front. Cell. Neurosci.* **2018**, *12*, 470. [CrossRef] [PubMed]

26. Vargas, D.L.; Nascimbene, C.; Krishnan, C.; Zimmerman, A.W.; Pardo, C.A. Neuroglial Activation and Neuroinflammation in the Brain of Patients with Autism. *Ann. Neurol.* **2005**, *57*, 67–81. [CrossRef] [PubMed]

27. Prata, J.; Machado, A.S.; von Doellinger, O.; Almeida, M.I.; Barbosa, M.A.; Coelho, R.; Santos, S.G. The Contribution of Inflammation to Autism Spectrum Disorders: Recent Clinical Evidence. *Methods Mol. Biol.* **2019**, *2011*, 493–510. [PubMed]

28. Chang, M.C.; Parham, L.D.; Blanche, E.I.; Schell, A.; Chou, C.-P.; Dawson, M.; Clark, F. Autonomic and Behavioral Responses of Children with Autism to Auditory Stimuli. *Am. J. Occup. Ther.* **2012**, *66*, 567–576. [CrossRef] [PubMed]

29. Baum, S.H.; Stevenson, R.A.; Wallace, M.T. Behavioral, Perceptual, and Neural Alterations in Sensory and Multisensory Function in Autism Spectrum Disorder. *Prog. Neurobiol.* **2015**, *134*, 140–160. [CrossRef]

30. Wang, G.; Li, W.; Han, Y.; Gao, L.; Dai, W.; Su, Y.; Zhang, X. Sensory Processing Problems and Comorbidities in Chinese Preschool Children with Autism Spectrum Disorders. *J. Autism Dev. Disord.* **2019**, *49*, 4097–4108. [CrossRef]

31. Lai, M.-C.; Lombardo, M.V.; Baron-Cohen, S. Autism. *Lancet* **2014**, *383*, 896–910. [CrossRef]

32. McKeague, I.W.; Brown, A.S.; Bao, Y.; Hinkka-Yli-Salomäki, S.; Huttunen, J.; Sourander, A. Autism with Intellectual Disability Related to Dynamics of Head Circumference Growth during Early Infancy. *Biol. Psychiatry* **2015**, *77*, 833–840. [CrossRef]

33. Bryson, S.E.; Bradley, E.A.; Thompson, A.; Wainwright, A. Prevalence of Autism among Adolescents with Intellectual Disabilities. *Can. J. Psychiatry* **2008**, *53*, 449–459. [CrossRef]

34. McCarthy, J. Children with Autism Spectrum Disorders and Intellectual Disability. *Curr. Opin. Psychiatry* **2007**, *20*, 472–476. [CrossRef] [PubMed]

35. McCleery, J.P.; Elliott, N.A.; Sampanis, D.S.; Stefanidou, C.A. Motor Development and Motor Resonance Difficulties in Autism: Relevance to Early Intervention for Language and Communication Skills. *Front. Integr. Neurosci.* **2013**, *7*, 30. [CrossRef] [PubMed]

36. Whyatt, C.; Craig, C. Sensory-Motor Problems in Autism. Front. *Integr. Neurosci.* **2013**, *7*, 51.

37. Kikkawa, T.; Casingal, C.R.; Chun, S.H.; Shinohara, H.; Hiraoka, K.; Osumi, N. The Role of Pax6 in Brain Development and its Impact on Pathogenesis of Autism Spectrum Disorder. *Brain Res.* **2019**, *1705*, 95–103. [CrossRef] [PubMed]

38. Lane, J.M.; Liang, J.; Vlasac, I.; Anderson, S.G.; Bechtold, D.A.; Bowden, J.; Emsley, R.; Gill, S.; Little, M.A.; Luik, A.I.; et al. Genome-Wide Association Analyses of Sleep Disturbance Traits Identify New Loci and Highlight Shared Genetics with Neuropsychiatric and Metabolic Traits. *Nat. Genet.* **2017**, *49*, 274–281. [CrossRef]

39. Jones, S.E.; Tyrrell, J.; Wood, A.R.; Beaumont, R.N.; Ruth, K.S.; Tuke, M.A.; Yaghootkar, H.; Hu, Y.; Teder-Laving, M.; Hayward, C.; et al. Genome-Wide Association Analyses in 128,266 Individuals Identifies New Morningness and Sleep Duration Loci. *PLoS Genet.* **2016**, *12*, e1006125. [CrossRef]

40. Gong, X.H.; Wang, H.Y. SHANK1 and Autism Spectrum Disorders. *Sci. China Life Sci.* **2015**, *58*, 985–990. [CrossRef]

41. Kitagishi, Y.; Minami, A.; Nakanishi, A.; Ogura, Y.; Matsuda, S. Neuron Membrane Trafficking and Protein Kinases Involved in Autism and ADHD. *Int. J. Mol. Sci.* **2015**, *16*, 3095–3115. [CrossRef]

42. Campos, V.E.; Du, M.; Li, Y. Increased Seizure Susceptibility and Cortical Malformation in Beta-Catenin Mutant Mice. *Biochem. Biophys. Res. Commun.* **2004**, *320*, 606–614. [CrossRef]

43. Fatemi, S.H.; Reutiman, T.J.; Folsom, T.D.; Thuras, P.D. GABAA Receptor Downregulation in Brains of Subjects with Autism. *J. Autism Dev. Disord.* **2009**, *39*, 223–230. [CrossRef]

44. Sherr, E.H. The ARX Story (Epilepsy, Mental Retardation, Autism, and Cerebral Malformations): One Gene Leads to Many Phenotypes. *Curr. Opin. Pediatr.* **2003**, *15*, 567–571. [CrossRef] [PubMed]

45. Arking, D.E.; Cutler, D.J.; Brune, C.W.; Teslovich, T.M.; West, K.; Ikeda, M.; Rea, A.; Guy, M.; Lin, S.; Cook, E.H.; et al. A Common Genetic Variant in the Neurexin Superfamily Member CNTNAP2 Increases Familial Risk of Autism. *Am. J. Hum. Genet.* **2008**, *82*, 160–164. [CrossRef] [PubMed]

46. Alarcon, M.; Abrahams, B.S.; Stone, J.L.; Duvall, J.A.; Perederiy, J.V.; Bomar, J.M.; Sebat, J.; Wigler, M.; Martin, C.L.; Ledbetter, D.H.; et al. Linkage, Association, and Gene-Expression Analyses Identify CNTNAP2 as an Autism-Susceptibility Gene. *Am. J. Hum. Genet.* **2008**, *82*, 150–159. [CrossRef] [PubMed]

47. Bakkaloglu, B.; O'Roak, B.J.; Louvi, A.; Gupta, A.R.; Abelson, J.F.; Morgan, T.M.; Chawarska, K.; Klin, A.; Ercan-Sencicek, A.G.; Stillman, A.A.; et al. Molecular Cytogenetic Analysis and Resequencing of Contactin Associated Protein-Like 2 in Autism Spectrum Disorders. *Am. J. Hum. Genet.* **2008**, *82*, 165–173. [CrossRef] [PubMed]

48. Peñagarikano, O.; Abrahams, B.S.; Herman, E.I.; Winden, K.D.; Gdalyahu, A.; Dong, H.; Sonnenblick, L.I.; Gruver, R.; Almajano, J.; Bragin, A.; et al. Absence of CNTNAP2 Leads to Epilepsy, Neuronal Migration Abnormalities, and Core Autism-Related Deficits. *Cell* **2011**, *147*, 235–246. [CrossRef]

49. Canali, G.; Garcia, M.; Hivert, B.; Pinatel, D.; Goullancourt, A.; Oguievetskaia, K.; Saint-Martin, M.; Girault, J.-A.; Faivre-Sarrailh, C.; Goutebroze, L. Genetic Variants in Autism-Related CNTNAP2 Impair Axonal Growth of Cortical Neurons. *Hum. Mol. Genet.* **2018**, *27*, 1941–1954. [CrossRef]

50. Poot, M. Connecting the CNTNAP2 Networks with Neurodevelopmental Disorders. *Mol. Syndr.* **2015**, *6*, 7–22. [CrossRef]

51. Pardo, C.A.; Vargas, D.L.; Zimmerman, A.W. Immunity, Neuroglia and Neuroinflammation in Autism. *Int. Rev. Psychiatry* **2005**, *17*, 485–495. [CrossRef]

52. Matta, S.M.; Hill-Yardin, E.L.; Crack, P.J. The Influence of Neuroinflammation in Autism Spectrum Disorder. *Brain Behav. Immun.* **2019**, *79*, 75–90. [CrossRef]

53. Kraan, C.M.; Godler, D.E.; Amor, D.J. Epigenetics of Fragile X Syndrome and Fragile X-Related Disorders. *Dev. Med. Child Neurol.* **2019**, *61*, 121–127. [CrossRef]

54. Lavery, L.A.; Zoghbi, H.Y. The Distinct Methylation Landscape of Maturing Neurons and its Role in Rett Syndrome Pathogenesis. *Curr. Opin. Neurobiol.* **2019**, *59*, 180–188. [CrossRef] [PubMed]

55. Tremblay, M.W.; Jiang, Y. DNA Methylation and Susceptibility to Autism Spectrum Disorder. *Annu. Rev. Med.* **2019**, *70*, 151. [CrossRef] [PubMed]

56. Gabel, H.W.; Kinde, B.; Stroud, H.; Gilbert, C.S.; Harmin, D.A.; Kastan, N.R.; Hemberg, M.; Ebert, D.H.; Greenberg, M.E. Disruption of DNA-Methylation-Dependent Long Gene Repression in Rett Syndrome. *Nature* **2015**, *522*, 89–93. [CrossRef]

57. Hu, V.W.; Frank, B.C.; Heine, S.; Lee, N.H.; Quackenbush, J. Gene Expression Profiling of Lymphoblastoid Cell Lines from Monozygotic Twins Discordant in Severity of Autism Reveals Differential Regulation of Neurologically Relevant Genes. *BMC Genom.* **2006**, *7*, 118. [CrossRef]

58. Andrews, S.V.; Sheppard, B.; Windham, G.C.; Schieve, L.A.; Schendel, D.E.; Croen, L.A.; Chopra, P.; Alisch, R.S.; Newschaffer, C.J.; Warren, S.T.; et al. Case-Control Meta-Analysis of Blood DNA Methylation and Autism Spectrum Disorder. *Mol. Autism* **2018**, *9*, 40. [CrossRef] [PubMed]

59. Hannon, E.; Schendel, D.; Ladd-Acosta, C.; Grove, J.; Hansen, C.S.; Andrews, S.V.; Hougaard, D.M.; Bresnahan, M.; Mors, O.; Hollegaard, M.V.; et al. Elevated Polygenic Burden for Autism is Associated with Differential DNA Methylation at Birth. *Genome Med.* **2018**, *10*, 19. [CrossRef] [PubMed]

60. Siu, M.T.; Butcher, D.T.; Turinsky, A.L.; Cytrynbaum, C.; Stavropoulos, D.J.; Walker, S.; Caluseriu, O.; Carter, M.; Lou, Y.; Nicolson, R.; et al. Functional DNA Methylation Signatures for Autism Spectrum Disorder Genomic Risk Loci: 16p11.2 Deletions and CHD8 Variants. *Clin. Epigenetics* **2019**, *11*, 103. [CrossRef]

61. Lord, C.; Rutter, M.; Le Couteur, A. Autism Diagnostic Interview-Revised: A Revised Version of a Diagnostic Interview for Caregivers of Individuals with Possible Pervasive Developmental Disorders. *J. Autism Dev. Disord.* **1994**, *24*, 659–685. [CrossRef]

62. Saeed, A.I.; Sharov, V.; White, J.; Li, J.; Liang, W.; Bhagabati, N.; Braisted, J.; Klapa, M.; Currier, T.; Thiagarajan, M.; et al. TM4: A Free, Open-Source System for Microarray Data Management and Analysis. *BioTechniques* **2003**, *34*, 374–378. [CrossRef]

63. Luo, R.; Sanders, S.J.; Tian, Y.; Voineagu, I.; Huang, N.; Chu, S.H.; Klei, L.; Cai, C.; Ou, J.; Lowe, J.K.; et al. Genome-Wide Transcriptome Profiling Reveals the Functional Impact of Rare De Novo and Recurrent CNVs in Autism Spectrum Disorders. *Am. J. Hum. Genet.* **2012**, *91*, 38–55. [CrossRef]
64. Oliveros, J.C. Venny. An Interactive Tool for Comparing Lists with Venn's Diagrams. 2007. Available online: https://bioinfogp.cnb.csic.es/tools/venny/ (accessed on 18 September 2020).

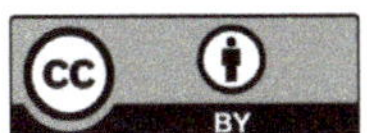

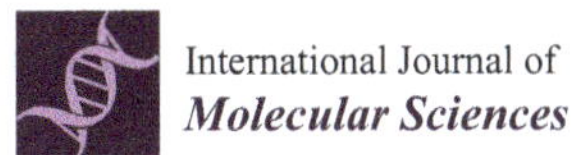 International Journal of
Molecular Sciences

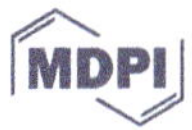

Article

Tracing Autism Traits in Large Multiplex Families to Identify Endophenotypes of the Broader Autism Phenotype

Krysta J. Trevis [1,2,†], Natasha J. Brown [3,4,†], Cherie C. Green [1,2,5], Paul J. Lockhart [6,7], Tarishi Desai [1,2], Tanya Vick [4], Vicki Anderson [2,8,9], Emmanuel P. K. Pua [1], Melanie Bahlo [10,11], Martin B. Delatycki [3,6,7], Ingrid E. Scheffer [1,3,9,12,‡] and Sarah J. Wilson [1,2,12,*,‡]

[1] Department of Medicine, Austin Health, The University of Melbourne, Heidelberg, VIC 3084, Australia; kjtrevis@gmail.com (K.J.T.); c.green@latrobe.edu.au (C.C.G.); tdesai@unimelb.edu.au (T.D.); pk.pua@unimelb.edu.au (E.P.K.P.); i.scheffer@unimelb.edu.au (I.E.S.)

[2] Melbourne School of Psychological Sciences, The University of Melbourne, Parkville, VIC 3010, Australia; vaa@unimelb.edu.au

[3] Victorian Clinical Genetics Services, Murdoch Children's Research Institute, Parkville, VIC 3052, Australia; natasha.brown@vcgs.org.au (N.J.B.); martin.delatycki@vcgs.org.au (M.B.D.)

[4] Barwon Health, Geelong, VIC 3220, Australia; cats-info@unimelb.edu.au

[5] Department of Psychology and Counselling, School of Psychology and Public Health, La Trobe University, Bundoora, VIC 3086, Australia

[6] Bruce Lefroy Centre for Genetic Health Research, Murdoch Children's Research Institute, Parkville, VIC 3052, Australia; paul.lockhart@mcri.edu.au

[7] Department of Paediatrics, The University of Melbourne, Parkville, VIC 3010, Australia

[8] Psychological Service, The Royal Children's Hospital, Parkville, VIC 3052, Australia

[9] Clinical Sciences Research, Murdoch Children's Research Institute, Parkville, VIC 3052, Australia

[10] Population Health and Immunity Division, The Walter and Eliza Hall Institute of Medical Research, Parkville, VIC 3052, Australia; bahlo@wehi.edu.au

[11] Department of Medical Biology, The University of Melbourne, Parkville, VIC 3010, Australia

[12] The Florey Institute of Neuroscience and Mental Health, Parkville, VIC 3052, Australia

* Correspondence: sarahw@unimelb.edu.au

† These authors contributed equally.

‡ These authors contributed equally.

Received: 21 September 2020; Accepted: 21 October 2020; Published: 27 October 2020

Abstract: Families comprising many individuals with Autism Spectrum Disorders (ASD) may carry a dominant predisposing mutation. We implemented rigorous phenotyping of the "Broader Autism Phenotype" (BAP) in large multiplex ASD families using a novel endophenotype approach for the identification and characterisation of distinct BAP endophenotypes. We evaluated ASD/BAP features using standardised tests and a semi-structured interview to assess social, intellectual, executive and adaptive functioning in 110 individuals, including two large multiplex families (Family A: 30; Family B: 35) and an independent sample of small families ($n = 45$). Our protocol identified four distinct psychological endophenotypes of the BAP that were evident across these independent samples, and showed high sensitivity (97%) and specificity (82%) for individuals classified with the BAP. Patterns of inheritance of identified endophenotypes varied between the two large multiplex families, supporting their utility for identifying genes in ASD.

Keywords: Broader Autism Phenotype; genetic; autism spectrum disorder; multiplex family

---

1. Introduction

Autism Spectrum Disorders (ASD) are a group of neurodevelopmental conditions characterised by deficits in social communication and social interaction, and restricted and repetitive patterns of behaviours, interests, or activities [1]. Recent estimates from the Centers for Disease Control and Prevention indicate a prevalence of 1 in 54 children aged 8 years for ASD [2]. There is strong evidence for the contribution of genetic factors to the aetiology of ASD [3]. Despite recent molecular advances, the cause remains unidentified in the majority of cases [4].

The recognition of milder phenotypes has facilitated an increased understanding and interest in the wide spectrum of clinical presentations in ASD. Family members of individuals with ASD have been observed to express milder forms, known as the Broader Autism Phenotype (BAP), that are not sufficient to meet diagnostic criteria for ASD [5,6]. The BAP includes a range of subtle behavioural and cognitive features that have qualitatively similar presentations to the core domains of ASD. While clinically significant impairment in these areas of functioning is seen in ASD [1,7], BAP traits are continuously distributed in the general population [8]. Several studies have reported the expression of at least one BAP trait in 20% of relatives of children with ASD, as well as a higher rate of BAP traits compared to controls across domains of pragmatic language [9,10], personality [11], social cognition [10,12,13] and executive function [14,15]. Monozygotic twins demonstrate 65–90% concordance for ASD [16,17] with a higher estimate when the BAP is considered [18,19], while dizygotic twin concordance is ~20% [20]. Together these findings suggest a strong genetic basis for ASD.

An estimated 25% of ASD cases can be identified clinically or molecularly with a predominant monogenic cause [21–23]. Although the aetiology for the majority of cases is still unknown, increasing evidence suggests a polygenic basis due to the interaction of multiple genetic risk variants following complex inheritance, with or without environmental factors [24–27]. Complementary techniques will be necessary to investigate the genetic aetiology of ASD in unsolved cases. Typically, family studies combine many small families (2–3 affected individuals), however, these are likely to be confounded by genetic heterogeneity. Very large multiplex families (> 8 affected) where ASD traits appear dominantly inherited are rare, but more genetically homogeneous. In other complex disorders, such as epilepsy, phenotypic characterisation of such families has proved powerful in gene discovery [28], however this approach has received limited attention in ASD. In multiplex ASD families, the identification of family members with BAP traits, or endophenotypes, may serve as markers of risk variants for ASD [29,30]. In turn, this may facilitate gene identification [31].

Endophenotypes are measurable features within a disorder that are proposed to reduce its complexity into more quantifiable elements [32]. These components can be represented at any level of analysis, including but not limited to biochemical, neuroanatomical, neurophysiological, cognitive or neuropsychological measurements. They have been hypothesised to reflect more aetiologically homogeneous subgroups within genetically heterogeneous conditions. Endophenotypes are also presumed to be located closer to aetiological mechanisms in the pathway between genotype and disease, compared to more overt phenotypes that are used to define clinical syndromes [33,34]. Clinically, the use of endophenotypes offers increased statistical power to localise and identify genes associated with disease [35]. Importantly, an endophenotype must indicate genetic susceptibility to disease independent of disease status, and by definition may serve as a marker of genetic liability in individuals without the disorder [34]. In individuals with the BAP, the mild expression of ASD-related traits is hypothesised to be due to an increased genetic liability for ASD. There are several BAP traits that may be considered "endophenotypes" from within the domains of language, executive function, and social cognition [31]. In the context of a single large family where numerous individuals demonstrate ASD or the BAP, recognition of BAP endophenotypes should allow granular identification of autism genes of dominant effect. This study is the first known to the authors to apply this approach in autism.

The aim of our study was to analyse ASD traits within large multiplex families to examine inheritance of ASD by identifying endophenotypes of the BAP. We achieved this aim through an iterative process of characterising, refining, and assessing BAP endophenotypes. This involved

(1) rigorous phenotyping of large multiplex families to identify BAP traits and potential endophenotypes, (2) validation of putative endophenotypes and their cut-off scores in an independent aggregated sample of 20 small families (each with at least one member with ASD), and (3) classification of BAP endophenotypes in large multiplex families (from step 1) based on optimal cut-off scores following validation analysis (from step 2) to assess their utility for examining inheritance patterns. We hypothesised that (1) multiple individuals in large families would demonstrate the BAP, (2) distinct BAP endophenotypes would be identified, and (3) BAP endophenotypes would vary in presentation between large multiplex families.

2. Results

2.1. Hypothesis 1: Multiple Individuals in Large Families Demonstrate the BAP

Based on our rigorous protocol for phenotyping the BAP in large multiplex families, we identified 32 members with the BAP across Family A and B. Of the 23 members in Family A who did not have an ASD diagnosis, we detected the BAP in 17 (74%) individuals, with 6 individuals unaffected. In Family B, we detected 15 (63%) individuals with the BAP, with 9 individuals unaffected (Table 1).

Table 1. Intellectual functioning in Family A and B by diagnostic classification.

	Participants (*n*) (Female)	Mean Age (Range)	Cognitive Data (*n*)	FSIQ Mean (SD)	VIQ Mean (SD)	PIQ Mean (SD)
Family A						
ASD	7 (1)	11.43 (4–34)	5	107 (16)	97 (15)	101 (30)
Unaffected	6 (5)	25.83 (2–50)	5	127 (17)	130 (17)	117 (15)
BAP	17 (8)	49.18 (13–79)	16 [a]	119 (13)	117 (13)	115 (12)
Total	30 (14)	35.7 (2–79)	26	118 (15)	116 (17)	113 (18)
Family B						
ASD	9 (3)	15.00 (8–20)	5	95 (20)	89 (28)	105 (16)
Unaffected	9 (7)	37.33 (10–73)	9	110 (14)	111 (14)	108 (11)
BAP	15 (10)	47.40 (15–73)	15	102 (17)	105 (18)	99 (17)
Total	33 (20)	35.06 (6–73)	29	103 (17)	104 (19)	102 (15)
Total	63 (34)	35.37 (2–79)	55 [a]	110 (18)	110 (19)	107 (17)

FSIQ = Full Scale Intelligence Quotient, VIQ = Verbal Intelligence Quotient, PIQ = Performance Intelligence Quotient. Note. Average FSIQ = 80–119; Superior FSIQ = ≥120. [a] One individual only completed VIQ and select executive functioning subtests.

Intellectual function was assessed in 54/63 (86%) individuals. Overall, participants were of average or greater intelligence. Average full scale intelligence quotient (FSIQ) was observed in 32/54 (59%) individuals, while 20/54 (37%) demonstrated superior or very superior FSIQ (Table 1). We performed group-level comparisons of cognitive, social and adaptive functions between family members with and without the BAP using non-parametric and parametric tests (Mann–Whitney U and *t*-tests, respectively), with the more conservative parametric tests reported here as there were no differences between these approaches. On average, individuals with the BAP demonstrated poorer pragmatic language, with significantly higher mean Pragmatic Rating Scale (PRS) scores ($M = 8.75$, $SD = 7.08$) compared to unaffected individuals ($M = 2.00$, $SD = 3.05$), t (40.99) $= -4.42$, $p < 0.001$. No significant differences were observed for general intellect, the Faux Pas Task (FPT), executive (D-KEFS) or adaptive function measures (ABAS-II, BRIEF; See Materials and Methods).

2.2. Hypothesis 2: Specific BAP Endophenotypes Exist Across BAP Domains

Based on our iterative characterisation process, four distinct endophenotypes of the BAP were reliably identified in the small families sample. From the natural grouping of traits, these reflected "socially unaware", "pedantic", "aloof", and "obsessive'" endophenotypes (Table 2). At the highest level of the dendrogram of the 33 BAP traits there was a clear split, whereby traits of the socially unaware and pedantic endophenotypes were more similar to each other and more dissimilar to the combination of traits of the aloof and obsessive endophenotypes. There was a significant difference between the mean proportional scores of the unaffected and BAP groups, with the BAP group demonstrating significantly higher scores on all four endophenotypes (all $p < 0.015$).

Table 2. Four endophenotypes of the BAP in the small families sample.

Mean Proportional Score (SD)		Cut-off Score	BAP Traits
Unaffected (*n* = 11)	BAP (*n* = 30)		
'Socially unaware': *Poor self-regulation and reciprocity in conversation*			
0.20 (0.18)	0.69 (0.06) **	>0.17	• Reduced capacity for clear narrative • Difficulty answering open ended questions • Making inappropriate or awkward comments either on history or during assessments • Tangential pragmatic style • Tendency to monologue rather than participate in reciprocal conversation • Tendency to anger easily • Reduced quantity of verbal output
'Pedantic': *Self-focused and technical in interactions*			
0.04 (0.05)	0.11 (0.12) *	>0.14	• An unusual or awkward greeting style • Unusual eye gaze • Speech has little variation in tone (i.e., monotonous) • Unusual speech volume • Precise articulation and language • Terse pragmatic style • Overly technical language • Narcissistic personality style • Focus on technicalities or minutiae • Fastidious regarding personal appearance • Self perception incongruent with views of others
'Aloof': *Difficulties relating to other's emotions and expressing own emotions*			
0.12 (0.07)	0.31 (0.16) ***	>0.20	• Aloof personality style • Difficult or limited interpersonal relationships • Reduced emotional empathy • A limited capacity to develop rapport with assessors • Reduced affection • Awkward social interactions • Opinionated in conversation • Reduced cognitive empathy • Little appreciation of humour (during the Cartoon task)

Table 2. *Cont.*

Mean Proportional Score (SD)		Cut-off Score	BAP Traits
Unaffected (*n* = 11)	BAP (*n* = 30)		
'Obsessive': *Regimented approach to life and tendency to ruminate*			
0.13 (0.10)	0.27 (0.18) ***	>0.25	• Hobby or interest of unusual intensity, or restricted range of interests relative to peers • Large collections or hoarding of items • Fastidious cleaning • Preference for structure in activities of daily living • Recurrent thoughts that are not distressing • Excessive worry

$* p < 0.05, ** p < 0.01, *** p < 0.001.$

Analysis of receiver operating characteristic (ROC) curves indicated relatively good discrimination within the small families for the socially unaware, aloof and obsessive endophenotypes (all AUC > 0.73, all $p < 0.025$), and acceptable discrimination for the pedantic endophenotype (AUC = 0.68, $p = 0.077$). Although we note that Box's M was violated in the discriminant function analysis (likely due to variation in the sample sizes), combined the four endophenotypes captured 93% of cases (Wilk's $\lambda = 0.47$, $\chi^2 = 27.83$, $p < 0.001$). In particular, the endophenotypes showed high sensitivity for the BAP group (97%) characterised by higher proportional scores, and good specificity for the unaffected group (82%) with lower proportional scores (Table 2).

2.3. Hypothesis 3: BAP Endophenotypes Vary in Large Multiplex Families

Applying the endophenotype thresholds to the proportional scores of the 33 BAP traits for members of Family A and B led to the identification of all individuals classified as having the BAP. Two additional BAP cases were identified in Family B based on the presence of above threshold endophenotype scores, indicating good utility of this approach (Figure 1). One individual was excluded from this analysis due to incomplete data. Across both families, the aloof endophenotype was most common (62%), followed by obsessive (60%), pedantic (55%) and socially unaware (48%). Approximately one quarter of family members met criteria for only one endophenotype, 15% met criteria for two, and the remainder met criteria for 3–4 (62%) (Figure 1). The dominant endophenotype across both families, as determined by the highest score, was aloof (47%), followed by obsessive (26%), socially unaware (18%) and pedantic (9%).

Family A appeared to have two endophenotype profiles, with one characterised by the presence of a single endophenotype (35%) seen in individuals who were mostly married-in (67%), contrasting with the second profile (41%) of all four endophenotypes, most evident in core family members (72%) (Figure 1). Overall, the obsessive endophenotype occurred most frequently (77%), followed equally by pedantic (65%) and aloof (65%), and then socially unaware (53%). The co-occurrence of the obsessive and pedantic endophenotypes was relatively common, seen in 29% of married-ins and core family members. Overall, there was a range of dominant endophenotypes across individuals, with aloof the most frequent (35%) particularly in core family members (83%).

Contrasting with Family A, Family B had more individuals (70%) with multiple endophenotypes, in both married-in and core family members (Figures 1 and 2). All four endophenotypes were again most frequently observed in core family members, indicative of a more severe BAP presentation. Unlike Family A, however, the aloof endophenotype occurred most frequently in Family B (88%), followed by obsessive (71%), pedantic (65%), and socially unaware (65%). The aloof endophenotype was also identified as dominant (59%), evident in 70% of core family members.

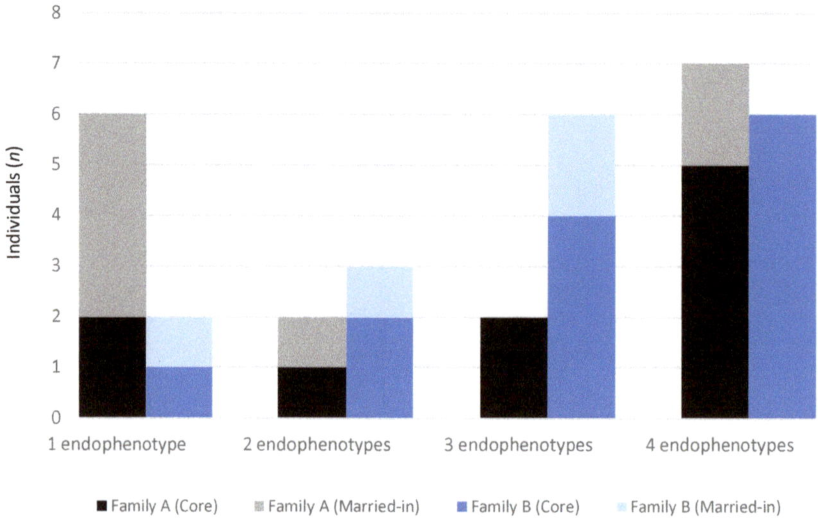

Figure 1. Number of BAP endophenotypes present in Family A and B. Individuals married-in to Family A tend to have a single endophenotype indicating a milder BAP presentation, in contrast with core family members who have multiple endophenotypes (obsessive most frequent). In Family B, married-in and core family members tend to have more than one endophenotype, with the aloof endophenotype the most frequent.

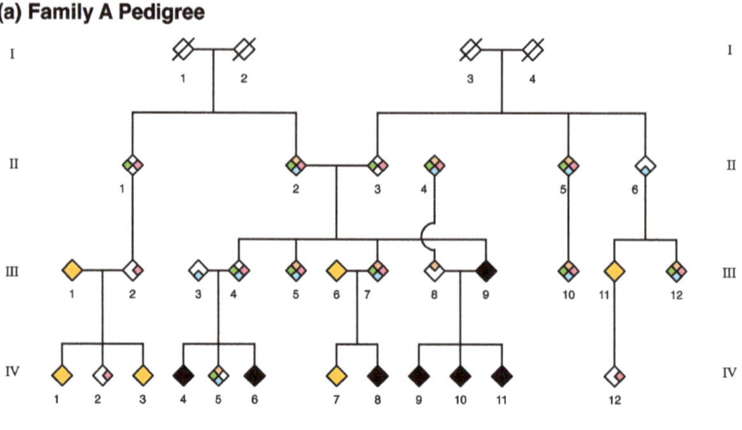

Figure 2. *Cont.*

(b) Family B Pedigree

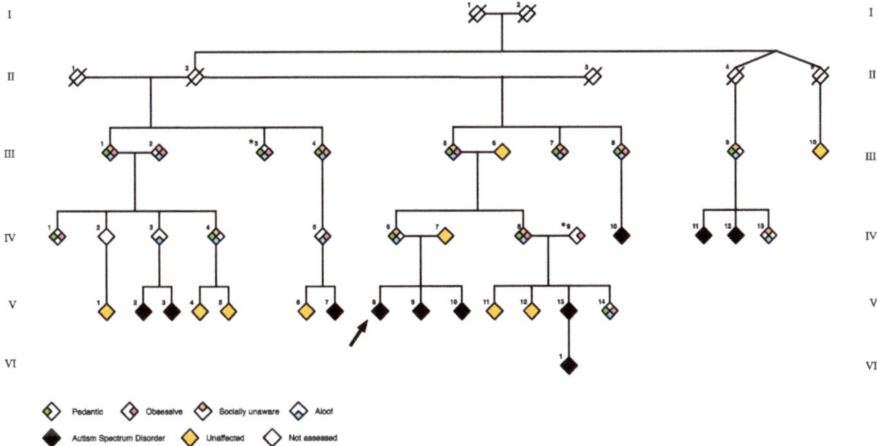

Figure 2. Scrambled pedigrees for Family A (panel **a**) and Family B (panel **b**) showing phenotypes and endophenotypes. All individuals with ≥1 endophenotype had the BAP, with the exception of two individuals from Family B (III-3 and IV-9) marked with an asterisk. These two individuals were clinically determined as unaffected but had above threshold endophenotype scores based on ROC curves. Some family members who were not phenotyped are not shown to preserve the anonymity of these families. The arrow indicates the proband shown in this pedigree. *: "All individuals with ≥1 endophenotype had the BAP, with the exception of two individuals from Family B (III-3 and IV-9) marked with an asterisk. These two individuals were clinically determined as unaffected but had above threshold endophenotype scores based on ROC curves.".

2.4. Correlates of the BAP Endophenotypes

Across both families, no sex or age differences were observed for any of the endophenotypes (all $p > 0.200$). Overall, a more severe BAP presentation (indicated by a greater number of endophenotypes) was associated with reduced social adaptive functioning on both self-report and objective measures of social communication (Table 3), demonstrating good convergent validity. In particular, a more severe BAP presentation showed a strong correlation with more severe pragmatic language difficulties, with scores for each endophenotype also significantly correlated. A similar relationship was evident for the ability to detect a faux pas in social discourse and self-reported social functioning, particularly for family members with the socially unaware endophenotype (Table 3).

For the cognitive measures, a more severe BAP presentation was associated with reduced executive functioning, particularly for nonverbal measures of cognitive flexibility (switching and fluency; Table 3). A pattern of weaker correlations was also evident for specific endophenotypes, including lower IQ in the socially unaware and aloof endophenotypes (Table 3).

Table 3. Correlations between endophenotypes and quantitative measures in Families A and B.

Domain	Task	Socially Unaware	Pedantic	Aloof	Obsessive	Total Number
				Endophenotypes		
Social communication	PRS	0.83 **	0.73 **	0.76 **	0.45 **	0.86 **
	FPT	−0.43 **	−0.28	−0.24	−0.18	−0.40 **
Intellect	FSIQ	−0.36 *	−0.10	−0.31 *	−0.02	−0.28
	VIQ	−0.29	−0.05	−0.31 *	−0.03	−0.28
	PIQ	−0.36 *	−0.13	−0.19	−0.02	−0.26
Executive functions	Trails (numbers) [a]	−0.32 *	−0.20	−0.29	0.17	−0.19
	Trails (switch) [a]	−0.24	−0.23	−0.27	−0.22	−0.34 *
	Design fluency (switch) [a]	−0.27	−0.25	−0.15	−0.09	−0.34 *
	Design fluency (composite) [a]	−0.27	−0.25	−0.25	−0.03	−0.32 *
	Tower task (achievement) [a]	−0.40 **	−0.19	−0.27	−0.22	−0.26
	Sorting (confirmed)	−0.33 *	−0.23	−0.32 *	−0.22	−0.33 *
	Sorting (free sort)	−0.31	−0.15	−0.24	−0.37*	−0.37 *
Adaptive function	Social index (self-report)	−0.46 *	−0.35	−0.19	−0.31	−0.43 *

$* \ p < 0.05$; $** \ p < 0.01$. PRS = Pragmatic Rating Scale, FPT = Faux Pas Test, FSIQ = Full Scale Intelligence Quotient, VIQ = Verbal Intelligence Quotient, PIQ = Performance Intelligence Quotient. [a] Nonverbal executive function subtests.

3. Discussion

We investigated the BAP to capture phenotypic variation within and between high-risk ASD families, with the aim of improving characterisation and identification of individuals for accurate molecular genetic analysis. We identified multiple individuals with the BAP in large multiplex families using rigorous phenotyping and a novel reliable endophenotyping approach, validated in an independent sample of small ASD families and with objective measures of cognitive, social and adaptive functioning. This deep phenotyping showed that specific BAP endophenotypes exist beyond the conventional BAP domains of social relationships, communication, and circumscribed interests and behaviour, allowing for more granular detection of subtle features of the BAP. Distinct patterns of inheritance were identified by applying the endophenotype approach in two large multiplex families, highlighting the utility of such a framework to identify putative ASD genes of dominant effect.

The research model employed here to phenotype rare large multiplex families reveals a pattern consistent with autosomal dominant inheritance of ASD/BAP traits that would not have been captured without deep phenotyping. Fifteen individuals (23%) met criteria for ASD and 33 (51%) the BAP, including some married-in individuals. Our promising endophenotype analysis provides further insight into specific profiles of the BAP and its varied presentation. Traditionally, ASD family studies include 2–3 affected individuals [36,37]. For example, four candidate ASD genes were identified in seven ASD/BAP pedigrees with ≥ 3 affected individuals [38]. Larger multiplex families remain scarce in the literature [30,39]. Here, we identified more subtle indicators of carrier status in two large families, using a robust endophenotyping method with good sensitivity and specificity to detect the BAP in two independent samples.

The BAP is strongly associated with ASD and may be considered a marker of genes that contribute to ASD risk [31,40]. Here we delineated the BAP into distinct endophenotypes that fulfil Gottesman and Gould's criteria for a true endophenotype (Supplementary Table S1) [41]. This includes recent proposed revisions to account for the strong overlap in the complex aetiology and genetic liability underlying the spectrum of trait expression across many neuropdevelopmental and psychiatric conditions, with the expectation that putative endophenotypes may not be strictly disorder-specific [34]. Each endophenotype cluster was characterised by a combination of communication, personality and behavioural indicators showing how specific traits across the traditional BAP domains may group together to form distinct endophenotypes or 'profiles' that capture phenotypic variation within and between families. As summarised in Table 4, these profiles capture identifiable 'personas' that have core characteristics with high face validity. These profiles also vary with functional correlates in distinct ways, supporting their construct validity. For example, the aloof endophenotype was characterised by a lack of innate social motivation or ability to meaningfully connect and empathise with others, associated with decreased theory of mind, and lower executive and intellectual functioning. One individual dominant for the aloof endophenotype described social interactions as "a means to an end". In contrast, the pedantic endophenotype was primarily characterised by detail-oriented traits, showing no associations with intellectual, executive or adaptive functions. Unsurprisingly, given the importance of social communication deficits in ASD and the BAP, all endophenotypes were associated with poor social communication, with the socially unaware endophenotype most broadly affected across social, intellectual, executive and adaptive functions (Table 4).

Table 4. Summary of the BAP endophenotypes and their functional correlates.

Endophenotype	Core Characteristic	Associated Functional Domains			
		Social	Intellect	Executive	Adaptive
Socially unaware	Poor self-regulation and reciprocity in conversation	✓	✓	✓	✓
Pedantic	Self-focused and technical in interactions	✓			
Aloof	Difficulties expressing and relating to other's emotions	✓	✓	✓	
Obsessive	Regimented approach to life and tendency to ruminate	✓		✓	

In contrast to conventional approaches that commonly rely on broad and non-specific classification of the BAP, the endophenotype framework implemented in the present study reliably identifies individuals that meet threshold criteria for a specific endophenotype profile potentially linked to susceptibility genes that confer risk for ASD. Clustering traits across conventional BAP domains to achieve granular characterisation of endophenotype profiles may thus improve detection of the BAP to facilitate gene discovery. We propose that such a framework is necessary to increase the efficacy of assessment protocols. It may also allow for a more sophisticated mapping of psychological and neural correlates to delineate the neurobiology of ASD, which has been characterised by inconsistencies in the literature to date [42–46].

Phenotypic heterogeneity was evident in both families at the endophenotype level suggesting that a single familial mutation may produce a phenotypic spectrum, with other genetic, epigenetic and environmental factors potentially influencing expression. With the advancement of high-throughput next generation sequencing technologies, meticulous phenotypic characterisation of both affected and apparently unaffected individuals remains essential for accurate data interpretation. In other words, identification of subtle endophenotypes, such as the four identified here, are crucial for advancing gene discovery programs. Importantly, these proposed BAP endophenotypes should be replicated and validated in subsequent research and further endophenotypes sought through a deep phenotyping approach.

Although multiplex families with ASD are genetically homogeneous, our phenotyping analysis suggests possible bi-lineal inheritance of the BAP in both families. Therefore, multiple risk alleles may contribute to ASD/BAP in later generations, consistent with recent genetic and phenotyping evidence [47,48]. The importance of unique de novo genetic changes in both sporadic (or 'simplex') ASD [25], and small multiplex ASD families [39] has become increasingly apparent. However, with at least seven individuals with ASD and many more with the BAP in our families, there is less likelihood of de novo changes contributing to each phenotype. It is much more likely that there is a single genetic variant of major phenotypic effect in each family, with the possibility that there are additional de novo genetic changes in some individuals that contribute to phenotypic severity.

The intensive nature of the study meant that clinicians were not blinded to family relationships, potentially leading to investigator bias. However, our diagnostic method of using the independent assessments of experienced clinicians and subsequent consensus agreement aligns with current best practice for ASD/BAP diagnosis. This method was further strengthened by objective cognitive and behavioural testing using quantitative measures. We selected a relatively low threshold for BAP classification, leading to the identification of many affected individuals. However, this approach is justified in a family with a clear genetic liability for ASD and was validated by the finding of consistent data-driven endophenotypes in the small families. Successful gene identification in future work requires capture of all individuals who may carry the putative variant, with the approach outlined here designed to enable more robust gene identification work. Future genetic investigations are required to test the reproducibility of the four identified endophenotypes over time and in additional independent samples, as well as determine their rate of occurrence in affected families compared to the general population (see Supplementary Materials for materials and guidelines on assessment and scoring of the four endophenotypes).

4. Materials and Methods

4.1. Large Multiplex Families

Large multiplex families were primarily ascertained from the Barwon Autism Database as part of a broader Collaborative Autism Study [49]. For inclusion as a multiplex family, >8 individuals with a diagnosis or suspected diagnosis of ASD or the BAP were required. The two fully characterised large multiplex families used to examine inheritance patterns using BAP endophenotypes are referred to as 'Family A', ascertained from the Barwon Autism Database, and 'Family B', who were self-referred. All available relatives were recruited, including those with and without reported BAP traits. The study was approved by the appropriate institutional review boards including the Human Research Ethics Committees of Barwon Health (HREC 02/34 and 04/57; reviewed 9 August 2017) and The Royal Children's Hospital (HREC 25043Y; reviewed 26 September 2017), Australia. Informed consent was obtained from all participants or a parent/guardian, and all study methods were carried out in accordance with relevant guidelines and regulations.

4.2. Protocol for Diagnosing ASD in Large Multiplex Families

ASD diagnoses were confirmed using the Autism Diagnostic Observation Schedule—Generic [50] (ADOS-G), or the Autism Diagnostic Interview—Revised [51] (ADI-R), based on Diagnostic and Statistical Manual of Mental Disorders, Fourth Edition, Text Revision (DSM-IV-TR) criteria [52]. For adults, the structured Family History Interview [5] (FHI) was administered by NJB, while for adolescents, a detailed developmental and medical history was obtained. Quantitative measures of intellect, executive functioning, adaptive behaviour and social functioning were also completed (Table 5). Testing was undertaken over a number of days to minimise fatigue effects. A physical examination was conducted for dysmorphic and neurocutaneous features and growth parameters. Standard genetic testing (karyotype, fragile X testing) and metabolic investigations were performed on probands.

Table 5. Protocol for diagnosing ASD and phenotyping the Broader Autism Phenotype (BAP) in large multiplex families.

	Participants with ASD		Participants without ASD		
Protocol Item	Child or Adolescent ≥ 4.5–17 yr	Adult ≥ 18 yr	Child < 13 yr	Adolescent ≥ 13–17 yr	Adult ≥ 18 yr
ADI-R + ADOS-G *or* DSM-IV interview + ADOS-G	+	±	−	−	−
Detailed developmental, medical, psychiatric and behavioural history	+	+	+	+	+
Family History Interview	−	+	−	−	±
Standardised testing of cognition and executive function [a]	±	+	+	+	±
Questionnaires of adaptive behaviour [b]	+	+	+	+	±
Broader Autism Phenotype Interview, the Faux Pas Task, Cartoon Task and Pragmatic Rating Scale	−	±	−	+	+
Physical Examination	+	+	+	+	+
High resolution molecular karyotype, Fragile X testing, metabolic investigations	+	−	−	−	−

ASD = Autism Spectrum Disorder, ADI-R = Autism Diagnostic Interview-Revised, ADOS-G = Autism Diagnostic Observation Schedule-Generic, DSM-IV = Diagnostic and Statistical Manual of Mental Disorders (4th edition). + all individuals completed this assessment, ± only some individuals completed this assessment, − no individuals completed this assessment. [a] Wechsler Abbreviated Scale of Intelligence and subtests of the Delis–Kaplan Executive Function System. [b] The Adaptive Behavioural Assessment System (2nd edition) and The Behavioural Rating Inventory of Executive Function.

Across Family A and B, 65 individuals were recruited: 16 children (2–12 years), 9 adolescents (13–17 years) and 40 adults (18–79 years) spanning 4 generations. Of these, 16/65 met criteria for a diagnosis of ASD. Family B also reported a deceased family member who had a diagnosis of ASD (not shown on the pedigree to preserve anonymity), an additional family member with ASD who was not recruited, and a child who had been diagnosed with ASD but was not assessed. Scrambled pedigrees of affected status are presented to preserve participant anonymity (Figure 3). In each family, individuals directly related to a matriarch are classified as 'core family'; others are referred to as 'married-in'. Family A comprised 30 individuals, including 7 diagnosed with ASD (6/9 children, 1/6 adults; Figure 3a). Nineteen were core family; 11 were married-in. In Family B, the matriarch (II-2) was elderly and too unwell to be behaviourally assessed and subsequently passed away during the study. Three children and three adolescents participated in a limited range of phenotyping activities and as such, these individuals were excluded from final analyses. Nine participants had ASD (5/7 children, 1/5 adolescents, 3/22 adults; Figure 3b); 31 were core family, and four were married-in.

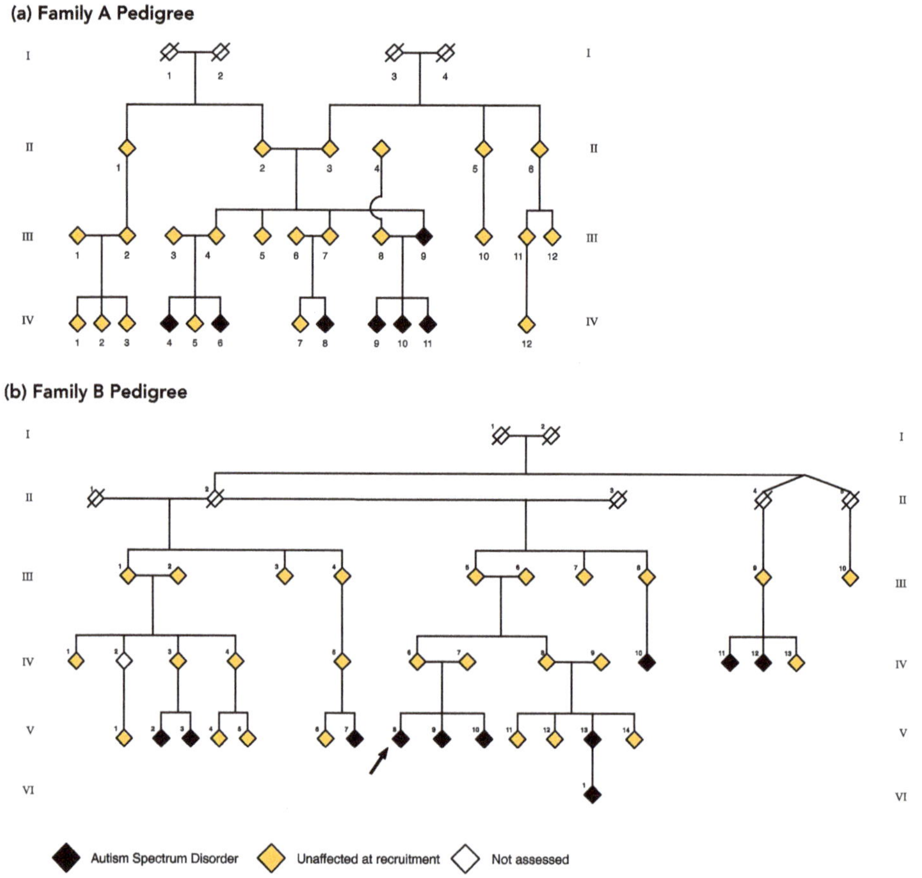

(a) Family A Pedigree

(b) Family B Pedigree

Figure 3. Scrambled pedigrees for Family A (Panel **a**) and Family B (Panel **b**) at recruitment. Individuals with a diagnosis of ASD are marked in black, and individuals recruited from the broader families are marked in yellow. White diamonds are individuals who were not assessed but are represented here to preserve the pedigree lines. One individual in Family B with a diagnosis of ASD was deceased (not shown to preserve anonymity) and one was too young to be assessed. The arrow indicates the proband shown in this pedigree.

4.3. Protocol for Phenotyping the BAP in Large Multiplex Families

We employed a mixed methods approach to rigorously assess the BAP, including an evaluation of general intellect, executive functions, adaptive behaviour, social cognition and language pragmatics (Table 5). A purpose developed semi-structured interview, the Broader Autism Phenotype Interview (BAPI), was also administered by three clinicians with expertise in neurobehavioural disorders (NJB, SJW, IES) to all individuals ≥ 13 years to characterise the presence, nature and extent of BAP traits. Interview responses were independently rated by the clinicians on all traits, with consensus agreement used to determine the presence of the BAP. Questions focused on the participant's life story, personal qualities, relationships, social functioning, and developmental, medical, psychiatric and vocational history. During the interview we included one or two "intentional errors" to elicit pragmatic elements of the BAP, such as terse speech [10]. Quantitative measures of social cognition and language pragmatics were also included within the interview. Social cognition was assessed using an adapted Faux Pas Task [53,54] (FPT), involving the standardised administration of four faux pas stories and four control stories [55] (maximum score = 40, M = 37, SD = 4). Pragmatic language was assessed with the Goldman-Eisler Cartoon task [56], which has previously been used to assess overly detailed speech and longer pauses between words in the BAP [10]. This task measures discourse production by eliciting a description of an eight frame captionless cartoon, "The Cowboy Story", over three successive trials [57]. Control individuals show increased verbal fluency with successive trials compared with decreased fluency in individuals with communication deficits [56]. Following the interview, the Pragmatic Rating Scale (PRS) [10] was independently completed by the three clinicians and consensus ratings reached. A score $\geq$ 4 defined pragmatic impairment [11] (Table 5).

Other cognitive domains and adaptive behaviour were assessed by a member of the team trained in psychometric assessment (TV) on a separate testing occasion. This included estimating full scale (FSIQ), verbal (VIQ) and performance (PIQ) intelligence quotients, derived with the four subtest Weschler Abbreviated Scale of Intelligence [58] (WASI; M = 100, SD = 15). Executive functions were measured with seven subtests of the Delis–Kaplan Executive Function System [59] (D-KEFS; M = 10, SD = 3). The second edition of the Adaptive Behavioural Assessment System [60] (ABAS-II) and the Behavioural Rating Inventory of Executive Function [61] (BRIEF) were used to assess adaptive functioning. The quantitative assessment provided a measure of convergent validity for the BAPI. At the completion of testing, final review of all qualitative and quantitative data by the three clinicians was used to confirm BAP status based on consensus agreement.

4.4. Small Families

We recruited an independent sample of 45 individuals from 20 small families with at least one member diagnosed with ASD, through advertisements and from the Barwon Autism Database. All participants provided written informed consent, as described above. Inclusion criteria were: (i) no diagnosis of ASD (based on DSM-IV or DSM-V criteria), (ii) $\geq$1 family member with ASD (based on DSM-IV or DSM-V criteria), and (iii) >12 years of age. Individuals were classified as having the BAP if they met $\geq$2 criteria for a BAP diagnosis on the Broader Autism Phenotype Rating Scale [5] (BAPRS) administered by an independent ASD expert (CG). Individuals were classified as unaffected if they did not meet criteria for any BAP traits or a diagnosis of ASD. This identified 30 individuals with the BAP (4 adolescents, 26 adults) in the 20 families, ranging in age from 14–71 years, and 11 unaffected adult family members ranging in age from 18–53 years. Four adult individuals showed only one BAP trait on the BAPRS and thus, were excluded from analyses based on the above criteria. All 45 individuals were also administered the BAPI by the independent ASD expert (CG) to characterise and rate their BAP traits. To ensure inter-rater agreement, video recordings of the interviews of a subset of these individuals were independently rated by two of the three clinicians (SJW, IES), with ratings confirmed by consensus agreement.

In 31/45 individuals, the WASI-II [62] was administered to measure Verbal Comprehension (VCI) and Perceptual Reasoning (PRI) and to estimate FSIQ. All individuals were within the normal range based on FSIQ (Table 6), with no significant differences between unaffected and BAP individuals for age or intellect (all p > 0.250). For 27 individuals, average total scores were available for the Broader Autism Phenotype Questionnaire (BAPQ) collected as part of a separate study. Consistent with expectations, there was a trend for higher scores on the BAPQ in the BAP group, with a medium effect size (t (24.56) = −1.96, p = 0.062, d = 0.70).

Table 6. Demographics of the small families sample.

	Unaffected	BAP
Number of participants (female)	11 (6)	30 (19)
Mean age (range)	41.09 (18–53)	39.50 (14–53)
Mean BAPQ (SD) [a]	2.43 (0.38)	2.92 (0.92)
Mean FSIQ (SD) [b]	108 (14)	111 (13)
Mean VCI (SD) [b]	106 (18)	109 (15)
Mean PRI (SD) [b]	109 (7)	110 (15)

BAPQ = Broader Autism Phenotype Questionnaire, FSIQ = Full Scale Intelligence Quotient, VCI = Verbal Comprehension Index, PRI = Perceptual Reasoning Index. [a] Data available for unaffected ($n = 9$) and BAP ($n = 18$). [b] Data available for unaffected ($n = 10$) and BAP ($n = 21$).

4.5. Endophenotyping Procedure

We used an iterative process to characterise, refine and assess endophenotypes of the BAP in the two independent samples, as summarised in Figure 4.

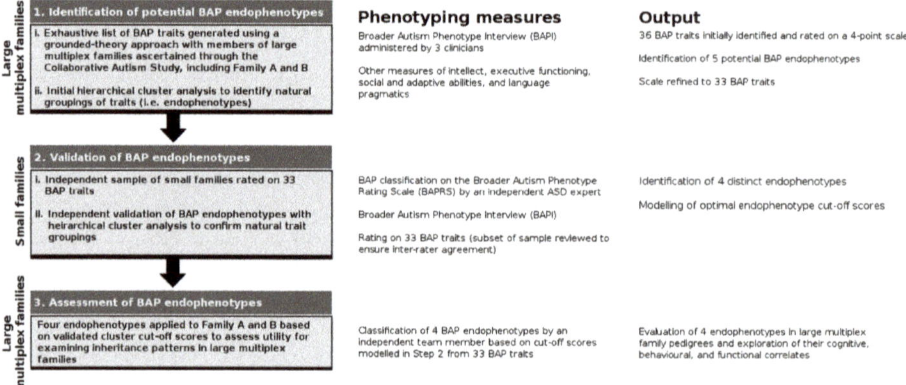

Figure 4. Iterative process used to identify and assess BAP endophenotypes. Step 1: An exhaustive list of BAP traits was generated through detailed clinical assessment of a number of large multiplex families, resulting in the identification of a final set of 33 BAP traits. Step 2. Validation analyses in an independent and aggregated sample of small families resulted in a 4-cluster solution representing distinct BAP endophenotypes. Step 3. Cut-off scores modelled in Step 2 were independently applied to large multiplex Family A and B for endophenotype classification and assessment of inheritance patterns.

4.5.1. Step 1: Identification of Potential BAP Endophenotypes in Large Multiplex Families

Using a grounded theory approach, BAP traits were initially identified from a detailed literature review targeting the theoretical domains described in the seminal work of Bolton (1994), on which the conceptualisation of the BAP is largely based. The domains included speech, literacy, pragmatics, relationships, and circumscribed interests, which were explored in-depth using our BAP phenotyping protocol (described above) in members of a number of unrelated large multiplex families primarily ascertained through the Collaborative Autism Study [55]. This in-depth characterisation was phenomenologically based [63], whereby the number of traits within each domain was fully expanded through administration of the semi-structured interview (BAPI) with separate family members until no further traits were identified (saturation) to capture the entire range of BAP traits (Supplementary Table S2).

This deep phenotyping produced an exhaustive list of 36 BAP traits. Ordinal ratings of these traits were then assigned to capture subtle variations in their presentation, with severity rated on a scale of 0 = absent, 1 = mild, 2 = moderate, and 3 = severe. The presence of traits through each individual's developmental history was also evaluated where available. Exploratory hierarchical cluster analysis was then performed to identify potential BAP endophenotypes. We used Ward's method with Euclidean squared distances based on z-scores to progressively group traits by minimising the variability within clusters and maximising the variance between clusters [64]. Interpretation of cluster groupings was informed by the relative similarity and dissimilarity in the linkage output combined with clinical judgement, leading to the initial identification of five endophenotypes. Inspection of these endophenotypes revealed a consistent rating of 0 for two of the 36 traits across all interviews, leading to their removal. One further trait reflecting inflexibility to intentional errors was removed due to challenges in reliably assessing the trait across interviewers, resulting in a final set of 33 BAP traits (Supplementary Figure S1).

4.5.2. Step 2: Validation of BAP Endophenotypes in Small Families

In the small families sample, an independent expert in ASD assessment (CG) interviewed and rated 45 participants on the 33 BAP traits based on all qualitative and quantitative data, with a subset (9%) rated via consensus between CG, IES and SJW to ensure consistency in ratings across both samples and to clarify borderline cases. As above, Ward's hierarchical cluster analysis was used to examine natural trait groupings. This led to the identification of four endophenotypes that showed a high degree of similarity to the initial five cluster solution (Spearman's r range = 0.710–0.976, $p < 0.001$).

To account for a varying number of traits in each cluster we computed proportional scores, whereby scores on each trait (range 0–3) were summed and divided by the maximum total score for that cluster, to produce four cluster scores for each individual. An ROC curve was plotted for each cluster in the small families sample to identify optimum cut-off scores for determining endophenotypic status using Youden's Index to allow mildly affected individuals to be included [65,66]. The highest score was used to represent the most prominent endophenotype for each individual, calculated as the difference between the observed endophenotype (i.e., cluster) score and the threshold score for the endophenotype (i.e., cut-off score).

4.5.3. Step 3: Assessment of BAP Endophenotypes in Family A and B

A team member who had not been involved in the phenotyping of Family A and B (Step 1) performed the endophenotype analysis (KT). Proportional scores for the four endophenotypes were calculated, and family members classified as having the endophenotype if their proportional score was greater than or equal to the cut-off scores identified in the small families analysis (Step 2). As above, the highest score (observed endophenotype score—threshold endophenotype score) for any endophenotype was used to represent an individual's most prominent endophenotype. A discriminant function analysis was then used to determine the sensitivity and specificity of the endophenotype approach to identifying the presence of the BAP in these families. In addition, endophenotype results were correlated with measures of intellect, executive, social and adaptive functions using conservative non-parametric Spearman's correlations (r_s). Materials used for assessment and scoring of endophenotypes are available in Supplementary Materials.

5. Conclusions

Despite significant advances towards unravelling the genetic heterogeneity of ASD, the underlying genetic aetiology remains unsolved for the majority of cases, in part due to significant challenges in identifying endophenotypes and potential carriers. We used a rigorous phenotyping approach to characterise the BAP in two large multiplex families with dominant inheritance of ASD and the BAP. Deep phenotyping identified four endophenotypes, showing differentiation of BAP features beyond traditional domain approaches. The proposed endophenotype approach advances current understanding and characterisation of the phenotypic spectrum for improved detection of the BAP that may facilitate gene discovery.

Supplementary Materials: The following are available online at http://www.mdpi.com/1422-0067/21/21/7965/s1.

Author Contributions: K.J.T. contributed to data analysis and draft manuscript; N.J.B. contributed phenotyping, data analysis and the draft manuscript; C.C.G. contributed to phenotyping and data analysis; P.J.L. and M.B. contributed to project conception; T.D., T.V. and V.A. contributed to phenotyping; E.P.K.P. contributed to data interpretation, data curation, visualisation, the draft manuscript; M.B.D. contributed to project coordination and data analysis; I.E.S. contributed to project conception and co-ordination, phenotyping and the draft manuscript; S.J.W. contributed to project co-ordination, phenotyping, data analysis and the draft manuscript. All authors have read and agreed to the published version of the manuscript.

Funding: This project received financial support from the National Health and Medical Research Council of Australia (Grant Numbers: 490037, 566759, 1044175, 1098255), the Australian Research Council (Grant Number: FT100100764), the Jack Brockhoff Foundation, Pfizer Australia, the Percy Baxter Charitable Trust, Perpetual Trustees, the Murdoch Children's Research Institute, and The University of Melbourne. PJL is supported by an NHMRC Career Development Fellowship (GNT1032364). This work was made possible through Victorian State Government Operational Infrastructure Support and Australian Government NHMRC IRIISS. The funding bodies played no role in the study design, or data collection, analysis or interpretation nor in writing of this manuscript.

Acknowledgments: We wish to acknowledge the late Peter Hewson, who was the founding father of the project.

Conflicts of Interest: The authors declare no conflict of interest.

Data Availability: All data is available within the manuscript and its Supporting Information, although scrambled pedigrees have been used to preserve participant anonymity.

References

1. American Psychiatric Association. *Diagnostic and Statistical Manual of Mental Disorders*, 5th ed.; American Psychiatric Association: Washington, DC, USA, 2013.

2. Maenner, M.J.; Shaw, K.A.; Baio, J. Prevalence of autism spectrum disorder among children aged 8 years—Autism and developmental disabilities monitoring network, 11 sites, United States, 2016. *Mmwr Surveill. Summ.* **2020**, *69*, 1. [CrossRef] [PubMed]

3. Yuen, R.K.; Merico, D.; Bookman, M.; Howe, J.L.; Thiruvahindrapuram, B.; Patel, R.V.; Whitney, J.; Deflaux, N.; Bingham, J.; Wang, Z. Whole genome sequencing resource identifies 18 new candidate genes for autism spectrum disorder. *Nat. Neurosci.* **2017**, *20*, 602–611. [CrossRef] [PubMed]

4. Trost, B.; Engchuan, W.; Nguyen, C.M.; Thiruvahindrapuram, B.; Dolzhenko, E.; Backstrom, I.; Mirceta, M.; Mojarad, B.A.; Yin, Y.; Dov, A. Genome-wide detection of tandem DNA repeats that are expanded in autism. *Nature* **2020**, *586*, 80–86. [CrossRef] [PubMed]

5. Bolton, P.; Macdonald, H.; Pickles, A.; Rios, P.; Goode, S.; Crowson, M.; Bailey, A.; Rutter, M. A case-control family history study of autism. *J. Child Psychol. Psychiatry* **1994**, *35*, 877–900. [CrossRef] [PubMed]

6. Kanner, L. Autistic Disturbances of Affective Contact. *Nerv. Child* **1943**, *2*, 34.

7. Barak, B.; Feng, G. Neurobiology of social behavior abnormalities in autism and Williams syndrome. *Nat. Neurosci.* **2016**, *19*, 647–655. [CrossRef] [PubMed]

8. Constantino, J.N.; Todd, R.D. Intergenerational transmission of subthreshold autistic traits in the general population. *Biol. Psychiatry* **2005**, *57*, 655–660. [CrossRef]

9. Piven, J.; Palmer, P.; Jacobi, D.; Childress, D.; Arndt, S. Broader autism phenotype: Evidence from a family history study of multiple-incidence autism families. *Am. J. Psychiatry* **1997**, *154*, 185–190. [CrossRef]

10. Landa, R.; Piven, J.; Wzorek, M.M.; Gayle, J.O.; Chase, G.A.; Folstein, S.E. Social language use in parents of autistic individuals. *Psychol. Med.* **1992**, *22*, 245–254. [CrossRef]

11. Piven, J.; Wzorek, M.; Landa, R.; Lainhart, J.; Bolton, P.; Chase, G.A.; Folstein, S. Personality characteristics of the parents of autistic individuals. *Psychol. Med.* **1994**, *24*, 783–795. [CrossRef]

12. Eyuboglu, M.; Baykara, B.; Eyuboglu, D. Broad autism phenotype: Theory of mind and empathy skills in unaffected siblings of children with autism spectrum disorder. *Psychiatry Clin. Psychopharmacol.* **2018**, *28*, 36–42. [CrossRef]

13. Folstein, S.E.; Santangelo, S.L.; Gilman, S.E.; Piven, J.; Landa, R.; Lainhart, J.; Hein, J.; Wzorek, M. Predictors of cognitive test patterns in autism families. *J. Child Psychol. Psychiatry* **1999**, *40*, 1117–1128. [CrossRef] [PubMed]

14. Hughes, C.; Russell, J.; Robbins, T.W. Evidence for executive dysfunction in autism. *Neuropsychologia* **1994**, *32*, 477–492. [CrossRef]

15. Hughes, C.; Plumet, M.H.; Leboyer, M. Towards a cognitive phenotype for autism: Increased prevalence of executive dysfunction and superior spatial span amongst siblings of children with autism. *J. Child Psychol. Psychiatry* **1999**, *40*, 705–718. [CrossRef] [PubMed]

16. Ronald, A.; Hoekstra, R.A. Autism spectrum disorders and autistic traits: A decade of new twin studies. *Am. J. Med. Genet. Part B Neuropsychiatr. Genet.* **2011**, *156*, 255–274. [CrossRef] [PubMed]

17. Constantino, J.N. Recurrence rates in autism spectrum disorders. *JAMA* **2014**, *312*, 1154–1155. [CrossRef] [PubMed]

18. Castelbaum, L.; Sylvester, C.M.; Zhang, Y.; Yu, Q.; Constantino, J.N. On the nature of monozygotic twin concordance and discordance for autistic trait severity: A quantitative analysis. *Behav. Genet.* **2019**, *50*, 263–272. [CrossRef]

19. Colvert, E.; Tick, B.; McEwen, F.; Stewart, C.; Curran, S.R.; Woodhouse, E.; Gillan, N.; Hallett, V.; Lietz, S.; Garnett, T. Heritability of autism spectrum disorder in a UK population-based twin sample. *JAMA Psychiatry* **2015**, *72*, 415–423. [CrossRef]

20. Frazier, T.W.; Thompson, L.; Youngstrom, E.A.; Law, P.; Hardan, A.Y.; Eng, C.; Morris, N. A twin study of heritable and shared environmental contributions to autism. *J. Autism Dev. Disord.* **2014**, *44*, 2013–2025. [CrossRef]

21. Codina-Sola, M.; Rodriguez-Santiago, B.; Homs, A.; Santoyo, J.; Rigau, M.; Aznar-Lain, G.; Del Campo, M.; Gener, B.; Gabau, E.; Botella, M.P.; et al. Integrated analysis of whole-exome sequencing and transcriptome profiling in males with autism spectrum disorders. *Mol. Autism* **2015**, *6*, 21. [CrossRef]

22. Tammimies, K.; Marshall, C.R.; Walker, S.; Kaur, G.; Thiruvahindrapuram, B.; Lionel, A.C.; Yuen, R.K.; Uddin, M.; Roberts, W.; Weksberg, R.; et al. Molecular Diagnostic Yield of Chromosomal Microarray Analysis and Whole-Exome Sequencing in Children With Autism Spectrum Disorder. *JAMA* **2015**, *314*, 895–903. [CrossRef]

23. Fernandez, B.A.; Scherer, S.W. Syndromic autism spectrum disorders: Moving from a clinically defined to a molecularly defined approach. *Dialogues Clin. Neurosci.* **2017**, *19*, 353. [PubMed]

24. Waye, M.M.; Cheng, H.Y. Genetics and epigenetics of autism: A Review. *Psychiatry Clin. Neurosci.* **2018**, *72*, 228–244. [CrossRef]

25. O'Roak, B.J.; Vives, L.; Girirajan, S.; Karakoc, E.; Krumm, N.; Coe, B.P.; Levy, R.; Ko, A.; Lee, C.; Smith, J.D. Sporadic autism exomes reveal a highly interconnected protein network of de novo mutations. *Nature* **2012**, *485*, 246–250. [CrossRef] [PubMed]

26. Berg, J.M.; Geschwind, D.H. Autism genetics: Searching for specificity and convergence. *Genome Biol.* **2012**, *13*, 247. [CrossRef] [PubMed]

27. Gaugler, T.; Klei, L.; Sanders, S.J.; Bodea, C.A.; Goldberg, A.P.; Lee, A.B.; Mahajan, M.; Manaa, D.; Pawitan, Y.; Reichert, J. Most genetic risk for autism resides with common variation. *Nat. Genet.* **2014**, *46*, 881–885. [CrossRef]

28. Helbig, I.; Scheffer, I.E.; Mulley, J.C.; Berkovic, S.F. Navigating the channels and beyond: Unravelling the genetics of the epilepsies. *Lancet Neurol.* **2008**, *7*, 231–245. [CrossRef]

29. Bora, E.; Aydin, A.; Sarac, T.; Kadak, M.T.; Kose, S. Heterogeneity of subclinical autistic traits among parents of children with autism spectrum disorder: Identifying the broader autism phenotype with a data-driven method. *Autism Res.* **2017**, *10*, 321–326. [CrossRef]

30. Woodbury-Smith, M.; Paterson, A.D.; Thiruvahindrapduram, B.; Lionel, A.C.; Marshall, C.R.; Merico, D.; Fernandez, B.A.; Duku, E.; Sutcliffe, J.S.; O'Conner, I.; et al. Using extended pedigrees to identify novel autism spectrum disorder (ASD) candidate genes. *Hum. Genet.* **2015**, *134*, 191–201. [CrossRef]

31. Dawson, G.; Webb, S.; Schellenberg, G.D.; Dager, S.; Friedman, S.; Aylward, E.; Richards, T. Defining the broader phenotype of autism: Genetic, brain, and behavioral perspectives. *Dev. Psychopathol.* **2002**, *14*, 581–611. [CrossRef]

32. Gould, T.D.; Gottesman, I.I. Psychiatric endophenotypes and the development of valid animal models. *Genes Brain Behav.* **2006**, *5*, 113–119. [CrossRef] [PubMed]

33. Lenzenweger, M.F. Endophenotype, intermediate phenotype, biomarker: Definitions, concept comparisons, clarifications. *Depress. Anxiety* **2013**, *30*, 185–189. [CrossRef]

34. Beauchaine, T.P.; Constantino, J.N. Redefining the endophenotype concept to accommodate transdiagnostic vulnerabilities and etiological complexity. *Biomark. Med.* **2017**, *11*, 769–780. [CrossRef] [PubMed]

35. Glahn, D.C.; Knowles, E.E.; McKay, D.R.; Sprooten, E.; Raventós, H.; Blangero, J.; Gottesman, I.I.; Almasy, L. Arguments for the sake of endophenotypes: Examining common misconceptions about the use of endophenotypes in psychiatric genetics. *Am. J. Med. Genet. Part B Neuropsychiatr. Genet.* **2014**, *165*, 122–130. [CrossRef] [PubMed]

36. Duong, L.; Klitten, L.L.; Moller, R.S.; Ingason, A.; Jakobsen, K.D.; Skjodt, C.; Didriksen, M.; Hjalgrim, H.; Werge, T.; Tommerup, N. Mutations in NRXN1 in a family multiply affected with brain disorders: NRXN1 mutations and brain disorders. *Am. J. Med. Genet B Neuropsychiatr. Genet.* **2012**, *159*, 354–358. [CrossRef] [PubMed]

37. Shi, L.; Zhang, X.; Golhar, R.; Otieno, F.G.; He, M.; Hou, C.; Kim, C.; Keating, B.; Lyon, G.J.; Wang, K.; et al. Whole-genome sequencing in an autism multiplex family. *Mol. Autism* **2013**, *4*, 8. [CrossRef] [PubMed]

38. Chapman, N.H.; Nato, A.Q., Jr.; Bernier, R.; Ankenman, K.; Sohi, H.; Munson, J.; Patowary, A.; Archer, M.; Blue, E.M.; Webb, S.J.; et al. Whole exome sequencing in extended families with autism spectrum disorder implicates four candidate genes. *Hum. Genet.* **2015**, *134*, 1055–1068. [CrossRef]

39. Salyakina, D.; Cukier, H.N.; Lee, J.M.; Sacharow, S.; Nations, L.D.; Ma, D.; Jaworski, J.M.; Konidari, I.; Whitehead, P.L.; Wright, H.H.; et al. Copy number variants in extended autism spectrum disorder families reveal candidates potentially involved in autism risk. *PLoS ONE* **2011**, *6*, e26049. [CrossRef]

40. Losh, M.; Adolphs, R.; Poe, M.D.; Couture, S.; Penn, D.; Baranek, G.T.; Piven, J. Neuropsychological profile of autism and the broad autism phenotype. *Arch. Gen. Psychiatry* **2009**, *66*, 518–526. [CrossRef]

41. Gottesman, I.I.; Gould, T.D. The endophenotype concept in psychiatry: Etymology and strategic intentions. *Am. J. Psychiatry* **2003**, *160*, 636–645. [CrossRef]

42. Billeci, L.; Calderoni, S.; Conti, E.; Gesi, C.; Carmassi, C.; Dell'Osso, L.; Cioni, G.; Muratori, F.; Guzzetta, A. The Broad Autism (Endo)Phenotype: Neurostructural and Neurofunctional Correlates in Parents of Individuals with Autism Spectrum Disorders. *Front. Neurosci.* **2016**, *10*, 346. [CrossRef] [PubMed]

43. Pua, E.P.K.; Bowden, S.C.; Seal, M.L. Autism spectrum disorders: Neuroimaging findings from systematic reviews. *Res. Autism Spectr. Disord.* **2017**, *34*, 28–33. [CrossRef]

44. Pua, E.P.K.; Ball, G.; Adamson, C.; Bowden, S.; Seal, M.L. Quantifying individual differences in brain morphometry underlying symptom severity in Autism Spectrum Disorders. *Sci. Rep.* **2019**, *9*, 9898. [CrossRef] [PubMed]

45. Pua, E.P.K.; Malpas, C.B.; Bowden, S.C.; Seal, M.L. Different brain networks underlying intelligence in autism spectrum disorders. *Hum. Brain Mapp.* **2018**, *39*, 3253–3262. [CrossRef] [PubMed]

46. Pua, E.P.K.; Thomson, P.; Yang, J.Y.-M.; Craig, J.M.; Ball, G.; Seal, M. Individual Differences in Intrinsic Brain Networks Predict Symptom Severity in Autism Spectrum Disorders. *Cereb. Cortex* **2020**. [CrossRef] [PubMed]

47. Geschwind, D.H.; State, M.W. Gene hunting in autism spectrum disorder: On the path to precision medicine. *Lancet Neurol.* **2015**, *14*, 1109–1120. [CrossRef]

48. Leppa, V.M.; Kravitz, S.N.; Martin, C.L.; Andrieux, J.; Le Caignec, C.; Martin-Coignard, D.; DyBuncio, C.; Sanders, S.J.; Lowe, J.K.; Cantor, R.M.; et al. Rare Inherited and De Novo CNVs Reveal Complex Contributions to ASD Risk in Multiplex Families. *Am. J. Hum. Genet.* **2016**, *99*, 540–554. [CrossRef]

49. Icasiano, F.; Hewson, P.; Machet, P.; Cooper, C.; Marshall, A. Childhood autism spectrum disorder in the Barwon region: A community based study. *J. Paediatr. Child Health* **2004**, *40*, 696–701. [CrossRef]

50. Lord, C.; Risi, S.; Lambrecht, L.; Cook, E.H., Jr.; Leventhal, B.L.; DiLavore, P.C.; Pickles, A.; Rutter, M. The autism diagnostic observation schedule-generic: A standard measure of social and communication deficits associated with the spectrum of autism. *J. Autism Dev. Disord.* **2000**, *30*, 205–223. [CrossRef]

51. Lord, C.; Pickles, A.; McLennan, J.; Rutter, M.; Bregman, J.; Folstein, S.; Fombonne, E.; Leboyer, M.; Minshew, N. Diagnosing autism: Analyses of data from the Autism Diagnostic Interview. *J. Autism Dev. Disord.* **1997**, *27*, 501–517. [CrossRef]

52. American Psychiatric Association. *Diagnostic and Statistical Manual of Mental Disorders*, 4th ed.; Text Revision (DSM-IV-TR); American Psychiatric Association: Washington, DC, USA, 2000.

53. Stone, V.E.; Baron-Cohen, S.; Knight, R.T. Frontal lobe contributions to theory of mind. *J. Cogn. Neurosci.* **1998**, *10*, 640–656. [CrossRef]

54. Baron-Cohen, S.; O'Riordan, M.; Stone, V.; Jones, R.; Plaisted, K. Recognition of faux pas by normally developing children and children with Asperger syndrome or high-functioning autism. *J. Autism Dev. Disord.* **1999**, *29*, 407–418. [CrossRef]

55. Brown, N.J. *Family and Community Study of the Genetics of Autism Spectrum Disorder*; University of Melbourne: Melbourne, Australia, 2014.

56. Goldman Eisler, F. *Psycholinguistics: Experiments in Spontaneous Speech*; Academic Press Inc: London, UK, 1968.

57. Joanette, Y.; Goulet, P. Narrative Discourse in Right-Brain-Damaged Right-Handers. In *Discourse Ability and Brain Damage*; Joanette, Y., Brownell, H.H., Eds.; Springer: New York, NY, USA, 1990.

58. Wechsler, D. *Wechsler Abbreviated Scale of Intelligence*; Harcourt Assessment Inc: San Antonio, TX, USA, 1999.

59. Delis, D.C.; Kaplan, E.; Kramer, J.H. *Delis-Kaplan Executive Function System (D-KEFS)*; Pearson Psychological Corporation: San Antonio, TX, USA, 2018. [CrossRef]

60. Harrison, P.L.; Oakland, T. *Adaptive Behavior Assessment System—Second Edition (ABAS-II)*, 2nd ed.; The Psychological Corporation: San Antonio, TX, USA, 2003.

61. Roth, R.M.; Gioia, G.A.; Guy, S.C.; Kenworthy, L.; Isquith, P.K. *Behavior Rating Inventory of Executive Function: BRIEF*; Psychological Assessment Resources: Odessa, FL, USA, 2000.

62. Wechsler, D. *Wechsler Abbreviated Scale of Intelligence-II*; Harcourt Assessment Inc: San Antonio, TX, USA, 2011.

63. Smith, J.A. Reflecting on the development of interpretative phenomenological analysis and its contribution to qualitative research in psychology. *Qual. Res. Psychol.* **2004**, *1*, 39–54. [CrossRef]

64. Ward, J.H. Hierarchical Grouping to Optimize an Objective Function. *J. Am. Stat. Assoc.* **1963**, *58*, 236–244. [CrossRef]

65. Luo, J.; Xiong, C. Youden index and Associated Cut-points for Three Ordinal Diagnostic Groups. *Commun. Stat. Simul. Comput.* **2013**, *42*, 1213–1234. [CrossRef] [PubMed]

66. Youden, W.J. Index for rating diagnostic tests. *Cancer* **1950**, *3*, 32–35. [CrossRef]

Publisher's Note: MDPI stays neutral with regard to jurisdictional claims in published maps and institutional affiliations.

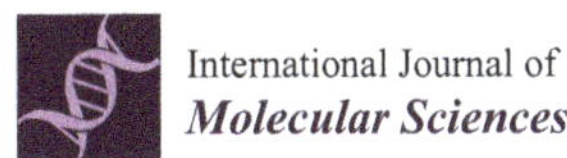
International Journal of
Molecular Sciences

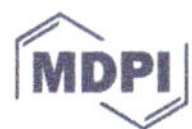

Review

An Overview of the Main Genetic, Epigenetic and Environmental Factors Involved in Autism Spectrum Disorder Focusing on Synaptic Activity

Elena Masini [1,†], **Eleonora Loi** [1,†], **Ana Florencia Vega-Benedetti** [1], **Marinella Carta** [2], **Giuseppe Doneddu** [3], **Roberta Fadda** [4] **and Patrizia Zavattari** [1,*]

[1] Department of Biomedical Sciences, Unit of Biology and Genetics, University of Cagliari, 09042 Cagliari, Italy; elena.masini97@gmail.com (E.M.); eleonora.loi@unica.it (E.L.); anaf.vegab@unica.it (A.F.V.-B.)

[2] Center for Pervasive Developmental Disorders, Azienda Ospedaliera Brotzu, 09121 Cagliari, Italy; marinellacarta@aob.it

[3] Centro per l'Autismo e Disturbi correlati (CADc), Nuovo Centro Fisioterapico Sardo, 09131 Cagliari, Italy; io.donez@gmail.com

[4] Department of Pedagogy, Psychology, Philosophy, University of Cagliari, 09123 Cagliari, Italy; robfadda@unica.it

* Correspondence: pzavattari@unica.it

† The authors contributed equally to this work.

Received: 30 September 2020; Accepted: 30 October 2020; Published: 5 November 2020

Abstract: Autism spectrum disorder (ASD) is a neurodevelopmental disorder that affects social interaction and communication, with restricted interests, activity and behaviors. ASD is highly familial, indicating that genetic background strongly contributes to the development of this condition. However, only a fraction of the total number of genes thought to be associated with the condition have been discovered. Moreover, other factors may play an important role in ASD onset. In fact, it has been shown that parental conditions and in utero and perinatal factors may contribute to ASD etiology. More recently, epigenetic changes, including DNA methylation and micro RNA alterations, have been associated with ASD and proposed as potential biomarkers. This review aims to provide a summary of the literature regarding ASD candidate genes, mainly focusing on synapse formation and functionality and relevant epigenetic and environmental aspects acting in concert to determine ASD onset.

Keywords: autism spectrum disorder; ASD; genetic factors; epigenetic factors; environmental factors; pervasive developmental disorder; post-synaptic density; CNV; SNP; gene fusion

---

1. Introduction

Autism is a complex syndrome characterized by a range of conditions and symptoms that frame it as a spectrum of disorders (autism spectrum disorder, ASD), including relevant physiological and biochemical ones, whose core symptoms includes social deficits and restrictive/repetitive behaviors. In the 1960s, thanks to the studies of Bernard Rimland, it was understood that ASD is a psychiatric disorder which might be grounded on a combination of genetic and environmental factors. To cope with ASD, it is necessary to achieve positive results through multidisciplinary, biomedical and behavioral therapies. Early diagnosis and intensive therapeutic interventions greatly improve the disease outcomes. In this context, the discovery of new diagnostic methods to detect ASD-related genetic alterations and biomarkers becomes fundamental in order to make an early diagnosis of the disorder.

In this review, we provide an overview of the genetic, epigenetic and environmental factors contributing to ASD pathogenesis.

2. Autism

2.1. Clinical Characteristics of ASD

ASD can be considered as a group of early-onset neuroevolutionary disorders which seem to be at the basis of alterations in brain connectivity, with cascading effects on many neuropsychological functions [1,2]. The The Diagnostic and Statistical Manual of Mental Disorders (DSM-5) (The American Psychiatric Association, APA, Philadelphia, PA, USA, 2013) gives the condition of autism the attribute of "spectrum" and uses criteria derived from diagnostic research assessment tools.

As indicated in the DSM-5 (APA, Philadelphia, PA, USA, 2013), individuals with ASD are characterized by persistent deficits in social communication and social interaction across multiple contexts and by restricted, repetitive patterns of behaviour, interests or activities. Deficiency in social communication and social interaction might appear in the form of deficits in social-emotional reciprocity, in nonverbal communicative behaviours used for social interaction and deficit in developing, maintaining and understanding age-appropriate relationships. As reported in the DSM-5, symptoms could be masked during early development and fully manifest only when social demands exceed limited capacities or may be hidden by learned strategies in later life. The impairments should cause clinically significant damage in social, occupational or other important areas of current functioning.

ASD symptoms should not be better explained by a diagnosis of intellectual disability (ID) or global developmental delay. Intellectual disability and ASD might co-occur.

The DSM-5 proposes differentiations based on commorbidity with intellectual impairment, language impairment, another neurodevelopmental, mental, or behavioral disorder, genetic or medical condition or environmental factors. Furthermore, it is possible to differentiate between different levels of severity according to the level of support required to function in daily contexts. According to this description, it is clear that different clinical variants of ASD exist and should be taken into account for diagnosis and intervention (APA, 2013). A distinction is made between a congenital form of ASD, representing a small percentage of cases in which the symptoms occur shortly after birth and in which the genetic fingerprint is prevalent, and a regressive or acquired form, in which the disorder appears after a period of typical development and it is not characterised by typical and constant genetic abnormalities, although several single nucleotide polymorphisms (SNPs) have been associated with the disease [3,4]. SNPs constitute variations of a single nucleotide in certain DNA traits. SNPs associated with ASD have been identified in genes encoding for proteins involved in different processes, including: cellular detoxification, some neuronal receptors and metabolism of several neurotransmitters and metabolites, in particular those of the metabolic circuits of methylation and transulfuration [5,6].

2.2. Epidemiology

Autism has been considered relatively rare for many years, with a prevalence of less than 1 in 1000 children, while today, the estimated rate is 1 in 160, and it seems likely to increase in the coming years (World Health Organization, Geneva, Switzerland, 2019). In the last decade, the study of ASD genetics has proved to be crucial not only to interpret and explain its phenotypic heterogeneity but also to discover new diagnostic procedures and therapies. It is estimated to-date that hundreds of genes are involved in ASD, resulting in a unified spectrum of different phenotypes, including different language and social deficits with various associated sub-phenotypes [7].

ASD show an unequal distribution based on gender: males have a four times higher risk of developing the disorder than females. A number of hypotheses have been made to interpret this unequal prevalence: in females, a higher dose of genetic "defect" is required than in males, consistent with the hypothesis of the contribution of protective genetic factors in females, because in males, there is only one X chromosome, so when alterations appear, it cannot be compensated by the normality of a second X chromosome. An association between testosterone levels and ASD risk has also been described: males have more frequent inflammatory reactions and use the brain in a more focal way and therefore suffer more from alterations in neuronal development that affect the connection systems between the different areas [8].

Genetic, environmental and developmental factors play a key role in the onset of autism spectrum disorders, as highlighted from many epidemiological studies [9,10]. It is unlikely that a single condition or event plays a major role in the causality of ASD; based on research to date, rather, none of the risk factors identified is a necessary and sufficient condition for ASD. Even for syndromic or secondary autism, which refers to autism with a single defined cause, such as fragile X syndrome and tuberous sclerosis, none of these etiologies are specific to autism because each of them encompasses a variable proportion of individuals with and without autism [11]. At present, ASD appears to have a multifactorial etiology to which developmental (in utero and early childhood), environmental and genetic aspects contribute, in as-yet unknown and different ways. Emerging methodologies in genomics and epigenomics research could be the key to elucidate the mysteries underlying the epidemiology of autism spectrum disorder.

3. Genetic and Epigenetic Factors

The involvement of genetic etiology in ASD was first suggested by a study on twins reported in the 1970s. The genetic heritability of a trait can be estimated by comparing the phenotypic concordance between monozygotic twins (MZ), which have 100% genetic similarity, and dizygotic twins (DZ), who have approximately 50% genetic similarity. The greater the difference between the concordance of MZ twins and DZ twins, the higher the genetic heritability and the contribution of genetics to that trait. The genetic fingerprint was confirmed by the high concordance of autism in monozygotic twins (60–90%) compared to dizygotic twins (5–40%) [12,13].

One of the largest studies to date, involving more than two million children born between 1982 and 2006 in Sweden, concluded that ASD has an inheritability of 45–56% [14]. A study of all twins born in the UK between 1994 and 1996 estimated an inheritability of more than 56% using concordance in MZ (0.77–0.99) compared to DZ (0.22–0.65) twins [13].

Considering all lines of evidence, the genetic heritability of ASD is estimated to play a fundamental role in ASD onset, together with environmental and epigenetic factors. However, despite most of the studies aimed at understanding the etiological basis of ASD having been focused on the genetic component, it has been possible to associate genetic variants to only a relatively small fraction of ASD patients. The problem, known as the "missing heritability issue", is common to most complex genetic diseases. Several hypotheses have been put forward to justify the missing heritability, such as the existence of poorly characterised variants, genotype/genotype interactions, incomplete penetrance, epigenetic factors and genotype/environment interactions [15–17].

In the 1990s, most of the research consisted of candidate gene studies, focusing on a particular gene that might be involved in ASD. From 2005, technologies such as whole-exome sequencing (WES), but also microarrays, have allowed genome-wide studies, leading to the identification of different variations in copy number (CNVs), DNA segments larger than 1 kilobase present in a variable copy number compared to a reference genome and single nucleotide variations (SNVs) in autistic patients, suggesting a highly heterogeneous genetic architecture. CNVs would contribute at about 15% and SNVs at 7% to the causes of ASD. Only a few of these genetic alterations have such complete penetrance that they are associated with ASD in almost every person who carries that variant [18]. On the contrary, genetic alterations with incomplete penetrance, variable expressivity or both are more frequently observed. However, the cause in most ASDs (>75%) remains elusive [18]. Genome-wide association studies (GWAS) have identified several SNPs associated with ASD. The first GWAS study allowed the identification of six polymorphisms, including some localized in *CDH10* and *CDH9*, genes encoding for cadherins, proteins that are important in cell adhesion, as common genetic variants in ASD [19].

However, the fact that several GWASs failed to identify some relevant loci despite the use of genetic data from more than 1000 families affected by autism suggests that the effect of individual common variants is relatively small [20].

On the other hand, WES analysis of affected and unaffected individuals has proven to be a powerful approach that offers new opportunities of sporadic cases studies and has the ability to detect mutations and de novo variants with incomplete penetrance [21]. WES has already led to the identification of over 150 new candidate genes for ASD.

In addition to SNPs, evidence is accumulating that CNVs play an important role in human neuropsychiatric diseases. ASD patients have three to five times more de novo CNVs than other family members and unaffected controls [22,23].

CNVs can influence gene expression, thus contributing to the pathogenesis of the disease through various mechanisms, including gene dosage, gene interruption, position effects, gene fusion and unmasking of recessive alleles or polymorphisms [24].

Screening for CNVs has proven to be a method of choice for identifying genes associated with ASD susceptibility [25]. Although CNVs associated with the disease are usually unique and show a low frequency in the population, they are identified in 8–21% of individuals with ASD and are most likely related to a severe clinical picture [26,27]. In addition, previous studies have indicated that individuals with syndromic ASD and intellectual disability have more pathogenic CNVs than individuals with non-syndromic ASD or ID [26,28].

CNVs may also lead to the generation of chimeric genes. Several studies have investigated whether fusion transcripts may lead to an increased ASD susceptibility. Holt and colleagues identified a fusion transcript involving *MAPKAPK5* and *ACAD10* genes in two ASD probands. However, the fusion transcript was detected at similar rates in both ASD patients and controls and had a premature stop codon, suggesting that it may be degraded by nonsense-mediated decay [29]. Similarly, Pagnamenta et al. identified a *DOCK4-IMMP2L* fusion transcript, likely to be subjected to nonsense-mediated decay in ASD individuals and their unaffected family members [30]. A study conducted on a multiplex family identified a *BST1-CD38* fusion transcript in one ASD proband with asthma, suggesting that it may be related to the more severe phenotype of this patient compared to the other ASD sibling [31]. qRT-PCR analysis showed that the fusion transcript was less expressed compared to the wild-type *BST1* transcript in the lymphoblastoid cell line derived from the proband, while the aberrant protein was not detected in a preliminary Western blot analysis [31]. Recently, our research group identified a microdeletion leading to the formation of an *ELMOD3-SH2D6* chimeric transcript in a multiplex ASD family [32]. *SH2D6* is expressed at extremely low levels in blood cells. On the other hand, the fusion transcript was highly expressed in PMBCs from the two ASD siblings and their unaffected mother carrying the deletion, suggesting that it was not subjected to nonsense-mediated decay. Bioinformatic analysis has shown that the fusion transcript would encode for a chimeric protein with an interrupted domain of ELMOD3 and would not contain the canonical SH2D6 sequence, suggesting an impaired function of the protein [32]. These results suggest a possible contribution of fusion transcripts in the complex ASD phenotype. Therefore, in case of copy number loss, the possible transcript fusion and chimeric protein product should be deeply investigated.

Recent studies have shown that epigenetic factors, including DNA methylation, hystone modifications and microRNAs (miRNAs), could play an important role in predisposition to autism.

We herein provide an overview of the main candidate genes (extensively reviewed in [33]) and epigenetic mechanisms involved in ASD etiology. Figure 1 summarizes some ASD candidate genes and epigenetic factors, belonging to the pathways mainly associated with ASD described in this review.

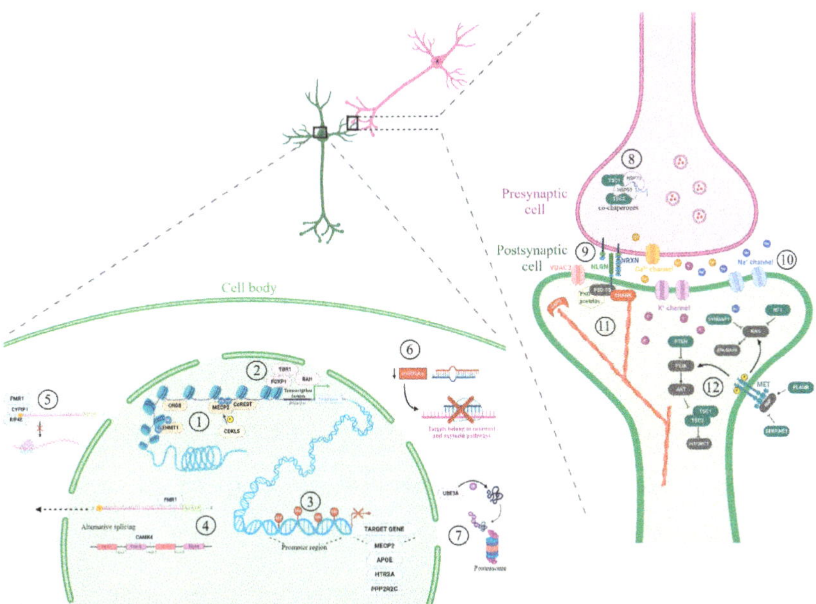

Figure 1. Candidate genes and epigenetic factors representative of the main processes involved in autism spectrum disorder (ASD) development. The illustration shows a synapse between neurons (presynaptic cell in violet and postsynaptic cell in green). On the bottom-left, a cell body of a neuron including different nuclear and cytoplasmic mechanisms involved in ASD. In the nucleus, several processes implicated in gene expression regulation are shown: **(1)** chromatin packaging and factors involved in chromatin remodeling; **(2)** gene transcription regulated by transcription factors; **(3)** DNA methylation at promoter region associated with transcription inhibition of target genes; **(4)** alternative splicing and mRNA export to the cytoplasm. In the cytoplasm, the following mechanisms are shown: **(5)** regulation of protein translation by the CYFIP1-EIF4E-FMR1 complex; **(6)** post-transcriptional regulation by miRNA; **(7)** protein ubiquitination and degradation by proteasome. On the right, the synapse architecture and functionality mechanisms associated with ASD. In the presynaptic cell, **(8)** TSC proteins and co-chaperons. **(9)** The neurexin/neuroligin transsynaptic complex and **(10)** the voltage-gated ion channels are represented. In the postsynaptic cell, **(11)** actin filaments, capping proteins and scaffold proteins; **(12)** some members of PI3K/AKT pathway, RAS signal transduction pathway and MET receptor tyrosine kinase pathway. Chromatin remodelers are indicated in beige, transcription factors in pink, proteins involved in RNA binding and export in light blue, protein ubiquitination in purple, scaffold proteins in red, cell growth and proliferation proteins in green and their related pathway members in grey. A more comprehensive list of ASD candidate genes can be found in Table 1 and along the text. Figure created using BioRender.com images.

3.1. Relevant Candidate Genes

Case-control studies on population and animal models have pointed out more than 800 genes associated with autism. The most affected genes in ASD encode for proteins involved in chromatin remodeling and transcriptional regulation, cell proliferation and mostly synaptic architecture and functionality. In this review, we will focus on this last category since our recent studies have also pointed out alterations in these genes fundamental for a proper synaptic function. Table 1 provides a summary of several genes clearly implicated in ASD, included in the SFARI Gene database as high confidence ASD genes (release 26 October 2020, gene.sfari.org) belonging to the other categories. Most of these genes were indicated in the largest exome sequencing study of ASD to date [34], as well as in the list narrowing down the number of amygdala-expressed genes associated to the social pathophysiology of ASD [35].

Table 1. Several relevant ASD candidate genes.

Category	Gene Symbol	Gene Name	Alterations	Associated Syndromes
Chromatin regulators	ANKRD11	Ankyrin repeat domain 11	Mutations; copy number loss	KBG syndrome; Cornelia de Lange syndrome
	ARID1B	AT-rich interaction domain 1B	Mutations; copy number loss; copy number gain; translocation	Coffin–Siris syndrome
	ASXL3	ASXL Transcriptional Regulator 3	Mutations	Bainbridge-Ropers syndrome
	ATRX	ATRX Chromatin Remodeler	Mutations; copy number loss	
	AUTS2	Autism susceptibility candidate 2	Mutations; copy number loss; copy number gain; inversion; translocation	
	CHD2	Chromodomain helicase DNA binding protein 2	Mutations; copy number loss	Tourette syndrome
	CHD7	Chromodomain helicase DNA binding protein 7	Mutations; copy number loss; translocation	CHARGE syndrome
	CHD8	Chromodomain helicase DNA binding protein 8	Mutations; copy number loss; copy number gain; translocation	
	CREBBP	CREB-binding protein	Mutations; copy number loss	Rubinstein–Taybi syndrome, Menke-Hennekam syndrome 1, Tourette syndrome
	EHMT1	Euchromatic histone-lysine N-methyltransferase 1	Mutations; copy number loss; copy number gain; translocation	Kleefstra syndrome
	MBD5	Methyl-CpG binding domain protein 5	Mutations; copy number loss; copy number gain; inversion; translocation	2q23.1 microdeletion syndrome, Kleefstra syndrome
	MECP2	Methyl CpG binding protein 2	Mutations; copy number loss; copy number gain; promoter methylation	Rett syndrome, X-linked intellectual disability, MECP2 duplication syndrome
	SETD5	SET domain containing 5	Mutations; copy number loss	
Transcription factors/regulators	ADNP	Activity-dependent neuroprotector homeobox	Mutations; copy number loss	Helsmoortel-Van der Aa syndrome
	FOXG1	Forkhead box G1	Mutations; copy number loss; copy number gain; translocation	Rett syndrome, FOXG1 syndrome, West syndrome,
	FOXP1	Forkhead box P1	Mutations; copy number loss; inversion; translocation	
	FOXP2	Forkhead box P2	Mutations; copy number loss; translocation	FOXP2-related speech and language disorder
	MED13L	Mediator complex subunit 13-like	Mutations; copy number loss; copy number gain	
	POGZ	Pogo transposable element with ZNF domain	Mutations; copy number loss; copy number gain	White–Sutton syndrome
	RAI1	Retinoic Acid Induced 1	Mutations; copy number loss; copy number gain	Smith–Magenis syndrome, Potocki–Lupski syndrome
	TBR1	T-box, brain, 1	Mutations; copy number loss	
	TCF4	Transcription factor 4	Mutations; copy number loss; translocation	Pitt–Hopkins syndrome
	ZBTB20	Zinc finger and BTB domain containing 20	Mutations; copy number loss; translocation	3q13.31 microdeletion syndrome, Primrose syndrome,
mRNA binding and trafficking regulator	FMR1 and its pathways	Fragile X mental retardation 1	Mutations; copy number loss	Fragile X syndrome, Fragile X-associated tremor/ataxia syndrome
Protein degradation	UBE3A	Ubiquitin protein ligase E3A	Mutations; copy number gain	Angelman syndrome
Cell growth/proliferation	DYRK1A	Dual-specificity tyrosine-(Y)-phosphorylation regulated kinase 1A	Mutations; copy number loss; inversion; translocation	
	NF1	Neurofibromin 1	Mutations; copy number loss	Cowden syndrome, Macrocephaly/autism syndrome, PTEN hamartoma tumor syndrome
	PTEN and its pathways	Phosphatase and tensin homolog	Mutations; copy number loss	
	SYNGAP1	Synaptic Ras GTPase activating protein 1	Mutations; copy number loss; translocation	
	TSC1/TSC2	Tuberous sclerosis 1/2	Mutations	
Protein modification	CDKL5	Cyclin-dependent kinase-like 5	Mutations; copy number loss; copy number gain translocation	Rett syndrome, Angelman syndrome

Prepared by the authors with data from gene.sfari.org (release 26 October 2020).

Synaptic Architecture and Functionality

It is not surprising that many candidate ASD genes are involved in synaptic architecture and function, which allows the transmission of information between neurons and between neurons and other cells, such as muscle, sensory and other cells. Many ASD candidate genes are involved in dendritic spine formation. Dendritic spines are small actin-rich protrusions that form the postsynaptic part of most excitatory synapses. Remodeling of actin cytoskeleton is responsible for the changes in the shape and size of dendritic spines and, consequently, to the synaptic functions [36]. Actin regulation mechanisms regulate the formation, maturation and plasticity of dendritic spines and of neuronal processes, such as learning and memory [36]. Abnormalities in the number and shape of dendritic spines have been observed in several neurological disorders, including autism, and contribute to brain dysfunction [37].

Post-synaptic density proteins (PSD), including cell adhesion molecules, scaffold proteins, receptors and cytoskeleton proteins, are fundamental for synaptic transmission and plasticity. Alterations of these proteins have been associated with many neurological disorders, including ASD [38].

- Cell adhesion molecules

Neurexins (NRXN) and neuroligins (NLGN) are transmembrane synaptic proteins that form the neurexin/neuroligin transsynaptic complex, crucial for synaptic function [39]. NLGNs bind to SHANK3 through PSD-95 and other synaptic proteins.

Loss of function NRX1 variants in ASD individuals have been identified in multiple studies [23,40,41]. Studies conducted in animal models knockout (KO) for *NLGN* and *NRXN* family members showed that mice develop ASD-like symptoms and have confirmed their role in synaptic function [42–44].

CNTNAP2, also known as *CASPR2*, encodes for a member of the NRXN family that serves as an adhesion protein, primarily between neuronal and glial cells. CNVs encompassing *CNTNAP2* and resulting in its decreased expression have been described in subjects with ASD [45–47]. The suppression of CNTNAP2 in murine models causes autistic behaviors, such as repetitive behaviors and reduced socialization and communication [48].

- Scaffold proteins

SHANK gene family, including *SHANK1*, *SHANK2* and *SHANK3*, has been suggested as a strong candidate for ASD. SHANK proteins are multi-domain post synaptic density scaffold proteins that connect neurotransmitter receptors, ion channels and other membrane proteins to cytoskeleton actin and signaling proteins. These proteins are important for synapse formation and dendritic spine maturation [49]. Rare deletions of *SHANK2* and de novo variants causing loss of protein function have been identified in individuals with ASD [50]. A microdeletion encompassing *SHANK3* determines Phelan–McDermid syndrome, characterized by intellectual disability, ASD, severe speech disorders and epilepsy [51]. A meta-analysis of SHANK mutations found low frequency of *SHANK1* and *SHANK2* deleterious mutations in contrast to the high frequency of loss of function *SHANK3* mutations in cases with ASD [52].

Our studies led to the identification of another promising ASD candidate gene, *CAPG*. This gene encodes for a member of the gelsolin family of actin-regulatory proteins, important for the remodeling of actin architecture. A microdeletion encompassing the entire *CAPG* gene has been recently described in three completely independent families in the heterozygous [53,54] and homozygous state [55]. Importantly, a reduced CAPG expression, both at transcriptional and protein levels, has been detected in the Sardinian family members carrying the deletion, and reduced *CAPG* mRNA levels have been also observed in an independent cohort of 13 non-Sardinian ASD cases compared to age-matched healthy controls [54].

Several studies have demonstrated the importance of CAPG for the formation of functional synapses. In fact, experiments conducted on cultured hippocampal neurons have demonstrated that capping proteins are present at the branched actin filament network of dendritic spine heads and they are fundamental for dendritic spine development [56,57]. In fact, *CAPG* knock-down led to a decline in spine density and to an increased number of filopodia-like protrusions [56].

- Voltage-gated ion channels

The role of genetic defects of different ion channels in the pathogenesis of ASD is well established. In fact, GWAS, WES and WGS have identified several polymorphisms and rare variants in calcium, sodium and potassium channels in ASD subjects (reviewed in [58]).

Point mutations in *CACNA1C* gene, which encode for L-type voltage-gated Ca^{2+} channel Cav1.2, lead to Timothy syndrome (TS), a disorder affecting multiple organs and characterized by an autistic phenotype [59,60]. L-type channels are mainly expressed in neuronal dendrites and cell bodies and are crucial for the activation of Ca^{2+}-signaling pathways and for neuronal excitability [61]. Defects in CACNA1C prevent the inactivation of the channel and lead to its prolonged opening and consequent increase in Ca^{2+} flux [60,62].

Mutations in other genes encoding for L-type and T-type Ca^{2+} channels, such as *CACNA1D*, *CACNA1E*, *CACNA1F* and *CACNA1H*, have been described in ASD [63–67]. Moreover, mutations of *CACNB2*, the gene encoding for the regulatory β2 subunit of CACNA1C, have been found in ASD families [68].

Genetic defects in genes encoding for sodium channels, such as *SCN1A*, *SCN2A*, *SCN3A*, *SCN7A* and *SNC8A*, have been also associated with ASD [69–73]. Voltage-dependent sodium channels are mainly expressed in neurons and glial cells and are fundamental for the initiation and propagation of action potentials. Mutations of SCN1A cause Dravet syndrome, characterized by seizures and frequently manifesting, also, autistic symptoms. A study has shown that *Scn1a+/−* heterozygous KO mice display stereotypical and anxious behaviors other than seizures [74].

Several studies have also shown that mutations in genes encoding for K^+ channels, including *KCNMA1*, *KCND2*, *KCNJ10*, *KCNQ3* and *KCNQ5*, may play a central role in ASD etiology [75–78]. It has been shown that KO of *Fmr1* in mice results in K^+ channel dysregulation and consequent dysregulation of synaptic transmission [79].

Some evidence has shown that voltage-dependent anion channel (VDAC) genes, a class of postsynaptic density genes highly expressed in several brain regions, could be implicated in ASD. In fact, autoantibodies against VDAC proteins have been detected in autistic individuals, suggesting a possible causal role in ASD pathogenesis [80]. Moreover, the beneficial effects observed in ASD patients treated with coenzyme Q, or other agents influencing the transport of electrons, have been attributed to the control of such molecules on the porin channels [81]. Recently, a study conducted by our research group identified a 2-bp frameshift deletion of *VDAC3* in an ASD family [54].

3.2. Epigenetic Factors

There is increasing evidence supporting the possible role of epigenetic aberrations, including DNA methylation alterations and microRNAs, in ASD etiology.

- DNA methylation

Several studies have conducted global methylation analyses in peripheral tissues as well as post-mortem brain tissues from ASD subjects and controls.

Studies conducted on lymphoblastoid cell lines and whole-blood DNA from monozygotic twins discordant for ASD diagnosis and controls identified several differentially methylated regions (DMRs) between discordant MZ twins and between ASD patients and control samples [82,83].

Zhu et al. identified 400 DMRs, enriched at promoters of genes involved in neuronal development, between placentas from children later diagnosed with ASD and those from typically developing controls. Methylation levels of two DMRs, mapping on *CYP2E1* and *IRS2*, were respectively associated with genotype within the DMR and prenatal vitamin use [84].

Conversely, a large epigenome-wide association study, performed on blood-DNA from 796 ASD cases and 858 controls, did not detect any differentially methylated CpG site after correction for multiple testing [85].

Similarly, Siu et al. did not detect any DNA methylation patterns clearly distinguishing heterogenous ASD cases from controls. However, they identified unique DNA methylation signatures for ASD individuals with 16p11.2 deletions or pathogenic variants of *CHD8* [86].

On the other hand, Kimura et al. identified a potential biomarker for adult ASD. The identified CpG site was hypermethylated in whole-blood DNA from ASD patients compared to controls and mapped on the *PPP2R2C* gene, which resulted down-regulated in ASD subjects [87].

Alterations in Alu methylation patterns have been observed in ASD cases sub-grouped based on Autism Diagnostic Interview-Revised scores compared with matched controls [88].

More recently, a genome-wide methylation study was performed on post-mortem tissue samples from different brain regions dissected from ASD subjects and controls. Wide-spread methylation differences, with more pronounced effects in cortical regions compared to cerebellum, were detected between idiopathic ASD cases and controls and in individuals carrying 15q11–13 duplication [89].

Another global methylation study has recently reported that differentially methylated CpG sites identified in ASD cases compared to controls are enriched in pathways converging on mitochondrial metabolism and protein ubiquitination, suggesting a possible role of DNA methylation and mitochondrial dysfunction in ASD [90].

Other studies measuring methylation levels of candidate genes using targeted approaches detected hypermethylation of genes including *APOE* [91] and *HTR2A* [92] and hypomethylation of genes such as *HTR4* [93] in ASD subjects compared to controls.

The functional impact of locus-specific *Mecp2* methylation on ASD onset has been recently demonstrated in vitro and in vivo. *MECP2* is known to be hypermethylated and down-regulated in ASD subjects. The authors of this study employed the CRISPR-dCas9 methylation editing system to induce methylation of the *Mecp2* transcription start site in Neuro-2a cells and in mouse models, resulting in *Mecp2* down-regulation and the acquisition of behavioral changes attributable to an ASD phenotype in mice [94].

- miRNA

Several studies have found that miRNA expression profiles are dysregulated in different matrices, including saliva, blood and brain tissues, from ASD individuals [95].

A study conducted on saliva samples from individuals with and without ASD has identified a panel of four microRNAs differentially expressed between ASD patients and controls [96]. A panel of five salivary miRNAs has shown an accuracy of about 90% in the detection of developmental disorders, including ASD [97].

Down-regulation of miR-6126 has been detected in peripheral blood samples from adult individuals with ASD. The predicted targets of this miRNA belong to neuronal and oxytocin pathways [98]. Similarly, Ozkul et al. identified a consistent decrease and a slight reduction in six microRNAs (miR-19a-3p, miR-361-5p, miR-3613-3p, miR-150-5p, miR-126-3p and miR-499a-5p) in serum samples from ASD children and their unaffected family members compared to healthy controls. This result was replicated in the blood, hypothalamus and sperm of two ASD mouse models [99]. Another study conducted on serum samples identified a panel of three miRNAs (miR-130-3p, miR-181b-5p and miR-320a) showing an area under the curve >0.85 in distinguishing ASD subjects from controls [100].

Studies conducted on knockout (KO) mouse models for some ASD candidate genes, including *Fmr1*, *Mecp2* and *Ube3A*, have observed dysregulation of different miRNAs and evaluated their regulatory role in neuronal context [101–103].

4. Environmental Factors

As mentioned above, several studies investigated the possible role of environmental factors in the etiology of ASD. According to recent studies, up to 40–50% of variance in ASD liability could be determined by environmental factors, such as drugs, toxic exposures, parental age, nutrition, fetal environment and many others [104–106]. However, while for some potential risk factors, there is strong evidence, supported by association studies but also by in vitro and in vivo studies, only weak associations have been described for many others.

Below is reported an overview of the most-studied environmental factors that have been found to potentially contribute to cause ASD (recently reviewed in [107]) (Figure 2).

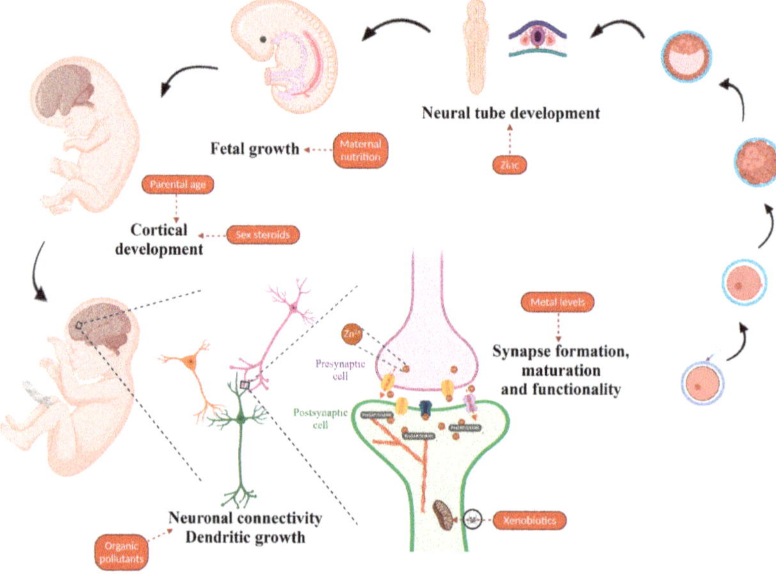

Figure 2. Environmental factors associated with ASD. The illustration indicates the putative impact of environmental factors on embryonic and fetal development with a particular focus on neuronal development and synaptic function. Figure created using BioRender.com images.

Parental age is one of the most established environmental ASD risk factors. In fact, much evidence has correlated advanced paternal age (APA) with the development of bipolar disorder, schizophrenia, ADHD and ASD [108]. A meta-analysis of 27 studies on the association between advanced parental age and ASD showed that a 10-year increase in maternal and paternal age is associated with a 20% higher risk of ASD in children [109]. A study has shown that age-related methylation changes observed in sperm could be related to an increased ASD risk in the offspring [110]. APA has been associated with reduced cortical thickness of the right posterior ventral cingulate cortex in ASD offspring [111]. Experiments conducted in mouse models have confirmed that APA is associated with the development of autism-like symptoms in the offspring [112,113] and with altered cortical morphology in male APA mice [112]. Moreover, behaviors related to ASD have also been observed in the second generation of mice with older grandfathers, suggesting that genetic and epigenetic alterations associated with APA are heritable [113].

Perinatal risk factors are also among the most-studied ASD risk factors and among the most difficult to determine and predict in advance. Two comprehensive meta-analyses examined 60 obstetric factors and found statistically significant associations between ASD risk and umbilical cord complications, injury or trauma at birth, multiple births, maternal hemorrhage, low birth weight, neonatal anemia, genital malformation, ABO or Rh blood group incompatibility and hyperbilirubinemia [114,115]. Another study has described an association between increased risk of autism and different factors, including caesarean section delivery, induced labor, management age less than 36 weeks and fetal distress [116].

Fetal exposure to sex steroids represents a potential risk factor for ASD. In fact, the fetal testosterone theory has been proposed to explain the higher ASD prevalence in males [8]. However, this hypothesis is controversial. In fact, while higher testosterone levels have been reported in ASD women, ASD males display testosterone levels similar to controls [117]. Baron-Cohen and colleagues have supposed that testosterone has effects on brain development during the prenatal masculinization window. The authors detected higher levels of sex steroids and cortisol in the amniotic fluid samples from male autistic patients compared with matched typically developing controls [118]. Recently, the same authors reported an association between fetal estrogen levels, important in synaptogenesis and corticogenesis, and autism risk [119]. Similarly, a study conducted on post-mortem brains detected reduced levels of estrogen receptor beta, aromatase and estrogen coactivators in the frontal gyrus of subjects with ASD compared to controls [120]. Moreover, several SNPs in genes encoding for proteins involved in sex steroid synthesis/transport have been associated with autistic traits [121].

The health condition of the mother has a major impact on the risk of ASD. It appears that maternal nutrition in pregnancy is of fundamental importance as it determines the nutrients available to support fetal growth [122]. Therefore, diets lacking specific nutrients can have adverse effects on fetal development. It has been shown that even short intervals between pregnancies can be harmful, since the body needs time, up to one year after childbirth, to recover acceptable levels of several essential substances [123].

Deficiencies of micronutrients, including vitamins and trace elements, have been associated with an increased risk of ASD. For instance, a Swedish study found that maternal vitamin D deficiency is associated with the risk of ASD with ID in the offspring [124]. Unbalanced levels of vitamins have also been detected in ASD children. Moreover, beneficial effects of vitamin supplementation have been observed in ASD patients [125]. Similarly, altered hair and/or blood concentrations of several trace elements, including chromium, magnesium and zinc, have been found in ASD patients compared with controls [126]. Association between maternal deficiency of microelements and ASD risk has also been reported. For example, iron deficiency, common in pregnant women, was associated with a five-fold increased risk of ASD, especially in the presence of other risk factors [127].

The involvement of altered trace elements concentrations on ASD phenotype is also supported by in vitro and animal studies. The effects on unbalanced metal levels on synapse formation and functionality have been evaluated on hippocampal cultured cells from rat brains, finding that the metal profile of autistic children led to down-regulation of crucial synaptic components, including Shank proteins and NMDA receptor subunits, and reduction of synaptic density. Interestingly, it was observed that zinc supplementation was able to revert the observed alterations [128]. The importance of zinc in ASD is supported by multiple pieces of evidence, including a strong association between low levels of this metal and ASD risk as well as a causative role of zinc deficiency in neuronal defects and development of ASD-related symptoms and "therapeutic" effects of zinc supplementation. In fact, low hair and serum levels of zinc and/or altered Zn/Cu ratio have been detected in children with ASD [129–131]. The effects of zinc deficiency on ASD have been observed in animal models. It has been shown that prenatal zinc deficiency alters social behavior in mice [132]. In vitro and in vivo studies have shown that zinc deficiency at the synaptic level leads to a decrease in ProSAP/Shank family members, a reduction in synaptic density and the development of ASD-related symptoms in mice [133]. In fact, other studies have shown that Zn^{2+} ions, highly abundant at PSD level, influence the recruitment of ProSAP1/Shank2 or ProSAP2/Shank3 for a correct formation and maturation of synapses [134]. The mechanism regulating the abundance of Zn at PSD levels has been hypothesized: Zn is released from pre-synaptic terminals and can translocate into post-synaptic neurons through Zn-permeable channels, including NMDA, and voltage-gated Ca^{2+} and AMPA channels [135]. Notably, a recent study has shown maternal zinc supplementation can prevent ASD-associated deficits in *Shank3* KO mouse models [136]. Recently, Shih et al. have elegantly demonstrated the impact of the crosstalk between genetic and environmental factors in the development of ASD. The authors have shown that KO of *Cttnbp2*, an actin cytoskeleton regulator, leads to a reduction in Zn concentration and expression levels of different synaptic proteins, consequently affecting dendritic spine formation and leading to the development of autism-like behaviors rescued by zinc supplementation [137].

The beneficial effects of zinc supplementation have been also observed in pregnant women, where an increase in zinc intake has been shown to reduce the risk of neural tube defects in the offspring [138].

The association between maternal obesity and risk of ASD in offspring is controversial. A Swedish study described a relationship between maternal BMI and ASD at population level; however, sibling analysis did not reveal any association between elevated maternal BMI and ASD risk [139]. On the other hand, a meta-analysis has shown a 28% and 36% increased risk of ASD in offspring born from overweight and obese mothers, respectively [140], even though there were relatively small numbers of ASD cases within the category of maternal underweight. However, it has also been shown that children born from underweight mothers are also at high risk of ASD [141]. Another study has shown that the combination of maternal obesity and maternal diabetes was associated with an increased risk of ASD and ID [142].

Maternal consumption of substances such as smoke, alcohol and medicines during pregnancy might be a potential risk factor as well. However, the association between smoking and alcohol-use with ASD is rather weak; in fact, two meta-analyses showed no evidence that smoking is a risk factor for ASD [143,144]. Moreover, cohort studies or case-control studies have examined the risk of ASD due to maternal alcohol consumption, indicating that mild to moderate consumption does not pose any risk [145–148].

The safety of medicines during pregnancy is very difficult to establish. In the ASD literature, antidepressant and anticonvulsant drugs have emerged as drugs of potential interest. An example is valproic acid, a drug that has been used to treat epilepsy or as a mood stabilizer in bipolar disorder. Its use during pregnancy leads to congenital malformations, developmental delay and cognitive malfunction [149,150]. Maternal use of selective serotonin uptake inhibitors has been associated with a 50% increase in ASD risk, although maternal psychiatric condition is a confounding factor [151].

An association between maternal diseases and ASD risk has been shown. A meta-analysis limited to case-control studies identified a 62% increased ASD risk among diabetic mothers compared to non-diabetic mothers [152], while a second study found a 74% increase in ASD risk for pregestational diabetes and 43% for gestational diabetes [153].

It has also been shown that maternal viral and bacterial infections are associated with ASD risk [154–156]. Two meta-analyses found that maternal autoimmune diseases are associated with an increased risk of ASD in offspring [157,158]. However, it is not the presence of viruses and bacteria per se to be associated with ASD development, but the immune response they cause, a conclusion supported by research identifying elevated inflammatory markers and antibodies in pregnant women with autistic children [159,160]. This hypothesis is supported by animal studies where maternal immune activation, induced by different immunogens, has been shown to induce post-natal brain dysfunction observable in a phenotype characteristic of ASD and other neurological disorders [161].

It is interesting to note that, although from different perspectives, much evidence points out the importance of maternal immune system condition during fetal development. Several studies have also reported an association between family history of autoimmune diseases and ASD [158,162,163]. It could be speculated that this link could be supported by maternal levels of zinc. In fact, our recent meta-analysis has shown that Zn concentrations in both serum and plasma levels of patients with autoimmunity are significantly lower compared to controls [164]. It is known that Zn plays an important role in the regulation of the immune system and, according to the studies provided above, it plays also an important role in neuronal tube formation.

Finally, exposure to toxic xenobiotics could represent another potential environmental risk factor. Substances such as brominated flame retardants could cause mitochondrial toxicity through a variety of mechanisms, leading to an altered energy balance in the brain [165], an important association with autism since mitochondrial dysfunction has been documented in patients with ASD [166]. Heavy metals can have a negative impact on many body functions by inducing neurological and behavioral damage. A meta-analysis of three case-control studies found a 60% increase in the risk of ASD due to exposure to high levels of inorganic mercury [167]. A recent case-control study found that exposure to organophosphates during pregnancy is associated with a 60% increase in the risk of ASD [168]. This category includes non-persistent organic pollutants, including phthalates and bisphenol A, and persistent organic pollutants, including DDT, PCB and PBDE. A research group found that three out of five studies on phthalate exposure showed a significant association between phthalate exposure and ASD risk [169]. Exposure to PCBs and PBDEs appears to alter calcium-related signal pathways, leading to alterations in dendritic growth and consequent abnormalities in neuronal connectivity, a key feature of ASD [170,171].

Table 2 summarizes several environmental factors associated with ASD described above.

Table 2. Several environmental factors associated with ASD.

Factor	Evidence	References
Parental age	Association studies; meta-analyses; animal studies	[108–113]
Perinatal factors	Meta-analyses	[114–116]
Sex steroids	Association studies	[117–121]
Maternal nutrition	Association studies; meta-analyses; in vitro studies, animal studies	[123–134,136–142]
Fetal exposure to drugs, smoke, alcohol	Association studies; meta-analyses	[143–151]
Maternal diseases	Meta-analyses	[152,153]
Maternal infections	Association studies; meta-analyses; animal studies	[154–161]
Fetal exposure to toxic xenobiotics	Association studies; meta-analyses; in vitro studies; animal studies	[166–171]

5. Conclusions

Given the complexity of the etiology of autism and the increasing prevalence of new confirmed cases of ASD worldwide, there is an urgent need to find effective diagnostic methods and study as many risk factors as possible—not only genetic but also epigenetic and environmental ones—without neglecting also genetic/environmental interactions, where risk factors influence each other.

Author Contributions: Conceptualization, E.L. and P.Z.; bibliographic search, E.M. and E.L.; writing—original draft preparation, E.M., E.L., R.F. and P.Z.; writing—review and editing, all authors; visualization, A.F.V.-B.; supervision, E.L. and P.Z.; funding acquisition, P.Z., M.C., G.D. All authors have read and agreed to the published version of the manuscript.

Funding: This research was funded by the Fondazione di Sardegna, grant number BSPROG21/2017.

References

1. Kana, R.K.; Uddin, L.Q.; Ekenet, T.; Echugani, D.; Müller, R.-A. Brain connectivity in autism. *Front. Hum. Neurosci.* **2014**, *8*, 349. [CrossRef] [PubMed]
2. Narzisi, A.; Muratori, F.; Calderoni, S.; Fabbro, F.; Urgesi, C. Neuropsychological Profile in High Functioning Autism Spectrum Disorders. *J. Autism Dev. Disord.* **2012**, *43*, 1895–1909. [CrossRef] [PubMed]
3. Goin-Kochel, R.P.; Myers, B.J. Congenital Versus Regressive Onset of Autism Spectrum Disorders. *Focus Autism Other Dev. Disabil.* **2005**, *20*, 169–179. [CrossRef]
4. Tamouza, R.; Fernell, E.; Eriksson, M.A.; Anderlid, B.; Manier, C.; Mariaselvam, C.M.; Boukouaci, W.; Leboyer, M.; Gillberg, C. HLA Polymorphism in Regressive and Non-Regressive Autism: A Preliminary Study. *Autism Res.* **2019**, *13*, 182–186. [CrossRef]
5. Cohen, J.; Eyu, S.; Efu, Y.; Eli, X. Synaptic proteins and receptors defects in autism spectrum disorders. *Front. Cell. Neurosci.* **2014**, *8*, 276. [CrossRef]

6.   James, S.J.; Melnyk, S.; Jernigan, S.; Cleves, M.A.; Halsted, C.H.; Wong, D.H.; Cutler, P.; Bock, K.; Boris, M.; Bradstreet, J.J.; et al. Metabolic endophenotype and related genotypes are associated with oxidative stress in children with autism. *Am. J. Med. Genet. Part B Neuropsychiatr. Genet.* **2006**, *141*, 947–956. [CrossRef] [PubMed]

7.   Iossifov, I.; O'Roak, B.J.; Sanders, S.J.; Ronemus, M.; Krumm, N.; Levy, D.; Stessman, H.A.; Witherspoon, K.T.; Vives, L.; Patterson, K.E.; et al. The contribution of de novo coding mutations to autism spectrum disorder. *Nature* **2014**, *515*, 216–221. [CrossRef] [PubMed]

8.   Werling, D.M. The role of sex-differential biology in risk for autism spectrum disorder. *Biol. Sex Differ.* **2016**, *7*, 1–18. [CrossRef]

9.   Newschaffer, C.J.; Croen, L.A.; Daniels, J.; Giarelli, E.; Grether, J.K.; Levy, S.E.; Mandell, D.S.; Miller, L.A.; Pinto-Martin, J.; Reaven, J.; et al. The Epidemiology of Autism Spectrum Disorders. *Annu. Rev. Public Health* **2007**, *28*, 235–258. [CrossRef] [PubMed]

10. Elsabbagh, M.; Mercure, E.; Hudry, K.; Chandler, S.; Pasco, G.; Charman, T.; Pickles, A.; Baron-Cohen, S.; Bolton, P.; Johnson, M.H. Infant Neural Sensitivity to Dynamic Eye Gaze Is Associated with Later Emerging Autism. *Curr. Biol.* **2012**, *22*, 338–342. [CrossRef] [PubMed]

11. Benvenuto, A.; Moavero, R.; Alessandrelli, R.; Manzi, B.; Curatolo, P. Syndromic autism: Causes and pathogenetic pathways. *World J. Pediatr.* **2009**, *5*, 169–176. [CrossRef] [PubMed]

12. Hu, V.W.; Devlin, C.A.; Debski, J.J. ASD Phenotype—Genotype Associations in Concordant and Discordant Monozygotic and Dizygotic Twins Stratified by Severity of Autistic Traits. *Int. J. Mol. Sci.* **2019**, *20*, 3804. [CrossRef]

13. Colvert, E.; Tick, B.; McEwen, F.; Stewart, C.; Curran, S.R.; Woodhouse, E.; Gillan, N.; Hallett, V.; Lietz, S.; Garnett, T.; et al. Heritability of Autism Spectrum Disorder in a UK Population-Based Twin Sample. *JAMA Psychiatry* **2015**, *72*, 415–423. [CrossRef] [PubMed]

14. Sandin, S.; Lichtenstein, P.; Kuja-Halkola, R.; Larsson, H.; Hultman, C.M.; Reichenberg, A. The Familial Risk of Autism. *JAMA* **2014**, *311*, 1770–1777. [CrossRef]

15. Eichler, E.E.; Flint, J.; Gibson, G.; Kong, A.; Leal, S.M.; Moore, J.H.; Nadeau, J.H. Missing heritability and strategies for finding the underlying causes of complex disease. *Nat. Rev. Genet.* **2010**, *11*, 446–450. [CrossRef]

16. Génin, E. Missing heritability of complex diseases: Case solved? *Hum. Genet.* **2020**, *139*, 103–113. [CrossRef]

17. Wiśniowiecka-Kowalnik, B.; Nowakowska, B.A. Genetics and epigenetics of autism spectrum disorder—Current evidence in the field. *J. Appl. Genet.* **2019**, *60*, 37–47. [CrossRef] [PubMed]

18. Fatemi, S.H. *The Molecular Basis of Autism*; Springer: New York, NY, USA, 2015; ISBN 9781493921904.

19. Wang, K.; Zhang, H.; Ma, D.; Bucan, M.; Glessner, J.T.; Abrahams, B.S.; Salyakina, D.; Imielinski, M.; Bradfield, J.P.; Sleiman, P.M.A.; et al. Common genetic variants on 5p14.1 associate with autism spectrum disorders. *Nature* **2009**, *459*, 528–533. [CrossRef]

20. Anney, R.; Klei, L.; Pinto, D.; Almeida, J.; Bacchelli, E.; Baird, G.; Bolshakova, N.; Bölte, S.; Bolton, P.F.; Bourgeron, T.; et al. Individual common variants exert weak effects on the risk for autism spectrum disorders. *Hum. Mol. Genet.* **2012**, *21*, 4781–4792. [CrossRef]

21. Sener, E.F.; Canatan, H.; Ozkul, Y. Recent Advances in Autism Spectrum Disorders: Applications of Whole Exome Sequencing Technology. *Psychiatry Investig.* **2016**, *13*, 255–264. [CrossRef]

22. Pinto, D.; Pagnamenta, A.T.; Klei, L.; Anney, R.; Merico, D.; Regan, R.; Conroy, J.; Magalhaes, T.R.; Correia, C.; Abrahams, B.S.; et al. Functional impact of global rare copy number variation in autism spectrum disorders. *Nature* **2010**, *466*, 368–372. [CrossRef]

23. Marshall, C.R.; Noor, A.; Vincent, J.B.; Lionel, A.C.; Feuk, L.; Skaug, J.; Shago, M.; Moessner, R.; Pinto, D.; Ren, Y.; et al. Structural Variation of Chromosomes in Autism Spectrum Disorder. *Am. J. Hum. Genet.* **2008**, *82*, 477–488. [CrossRef]

24. Lupski, J.R.; Stankiewicz, P. Genomic Disorders: Molecular Mechanisms for Rearrangements and Conveyed Phenotypes. *PLoS Genet.* **2005**, *1*, e49. [CrossRef] [PubMed]

25. Devlin, B.; Scherer, S.W. Genetic architecture in autism spectrum disorder. *Curr. Opin. Genet. Dev.* **2012**, *22*, 229–237. [CrossRef]

26. Napoli, E.; Russo, S.; Casula, L.; Alesi, V.; Amendola, F.A.; Angioni, A.; Novelli, A.; Valeri, G.; Menghini, D.; Vicari, S. Array-CGH Analysis in a Cohort of Phenotypically Well-Characterized Individuals with "Essential" Autism Spectrum Disorders. *J. Autism Dev. Disord.* **2018**, *48*, 442–449. [CrossRef]

27. Beaudet, A.L. The utility of chromosomal microarray analysis in developmental and behavioral pediatrics. *Child Dev.* **2013**, *84*, 121–132. [CrossRef] [PubMed]

28. Jacquemont, M.-L.; Sanlaville, D.; Redon, R.; Raoul, O.; Cormier-Daire, V.; Lyonnet, S.; Amiel, J.; Le Merrer, M.; Heron, D.; De Blois, M.-C.; et al. Array-based comparative genomic hybridisation identifies high frequency of cryptic chromosomal rearrangements in patients with syndromic autism spectrum disorders. *J. Med. Genet.* **2006**, *43*, 843–849. [CrossRef]

29. Holt, R.; Sykes, N.H.; Conceição, I.; Cazier, J.-B.; Anney, R.J.; Oliveira, G.G.; Gallagher, L.; Vicente, A.M.; Monaco, A.P.; Pagnamenta, A.T. CNVs leading to fusion transcripts in individuals with autism spectrum disorder. *Eur. J. Hum. Genet.* **2012**, *20*, 1141–1147. [CrossRef]

30. Pagnamenta, A.T.; Bacchelli, E.; De Jonge, M.V.; Mirza, G.; Scerri, T.S.; Minopoli, F.; Chiocchetti, A.; Ludwig, K.U.; Hoffmann, P.; Paracchini, S.; et al. Characterization of a Family with Rare Deletions in CNTNAP5 and DOCK4 Suggests Novel Risk Loci for Autism and Dyslexia. *Biol. Psychiatry* **2010**, *68*, 320–328. [CrossRef]

31. Ceroni, F.; Sagar, A.; Simpson, N.H.; Gawthrope, A.J.; Newbury, D.F.; Pinto, D.; Francis, S.M.; Tessman, D.C.; Cook, E.H.; Monaco, A.P.; et al. A Deletion Involving CD 38 and BST 1 Results in a Fusion Transcript in a Patient With Autism and Asthma. *Autism Res.* **2014**, *7*, 254–263. [CrossRef]

32. Loi, E.; Moi, L.; Blois, S.; Bacchelli, E.; Benedetti, A.F.V.; Cameli, C.; Fadda, R.; Maestrini, E.; Carta, M.; Doneddu, G.; et al. ELMOD3—SH2D6 gene fusion as a possible co-star actor in autism spectrum disorder scenario. *J. Cell. Mol. Med.* **2019**, *24*, 2064–2069. [CrossRef] [PubMed]

33. Yin, J.; Schaaf, C.P. Autism genetics—An overview. *Prenat. Diagn.* **2016**, *37*, 14–30. [CrossRef]

34. Satterstrom, F.K.; Kosmicki, J.A.; Wang, J.; Breen, M.S.; De Rubeis, S.; An, J.-Y.; Peng, M.; Collins, R.; Grove, J.; Klei, L.; et al. Large-Scale Exome Sequencing Study Implicates Both Developmental and Functional Changes in the Neurobiology of Autism. *Cell* **2020**, *180*, 568–584.e23. [CrossRef]

35. Herrero, M.J.; Velmeshev, D.; Hernandez-Pineda, D.; Sethi, S.; Sorrells, S.; Banerjee, P.; Sullivan, C.; Gupta, A.R.; Kriegstein, A.R.; Corbin, J.G. Identification of amygdala-expressed genes associated with autism spectrum disorder. *Mol. Autism* **2020**, *11*, 1–14. [CrossRef] [PubMed]

36. Hotulainen, P.; Hoogenraad, C. Actin in dendritic spines: Connecting dynamics to function. *J. Cell Biol.* **2010**, *189*, 619–629. [CrossRef]

37. Van Spronsen, M.; Hoogenraad, C.C. Synapse Pathology in Psychiatric and Neurologic Disease. *Curr. Neurol. Neurosci. Rep.* **2010**, *10*, 207–214. [CrossRef]

38. Kaizuka, T.; Takumi, T. Postsynaptic density proteins and their involvement in neurodevelopmental disorders. *J. Biochem.* **2018**, *163*, 447–455. [CrossRef]

39. Südhof, T.C. Neuroligins and neurexins link synaptic function to cognitive disease. *Nature* **2008**, *455*, 903–911. [CrossRef] [PubMed]

40. Kim, H.-G.; Kishikawa, S.; Higgins, A.W.; Seong, I.-S.; Donovan, D.J.; Shen, Y.; Lally, E.; Weiss, L.A.; Najm, J.; Kutsche, K.; et al. Disruption of Neurexin 1 Associated with Autism Spectrum Disorder. *Am. J. Hum. Genet.* **2008**, *82*, 199–207. [CrossRef]

41. Schaaf, C.P.; Boone, P.M.; Sampath, S.; Williams, C.; Bader, P.I.; Mueller, J.M.; Shchelochkov, O.A.; Brown, C.W.; Crawford, H.P.; Phalen, J.A.; et al. Phenotypic spectrum and genotype–phenotype correlations of NRXN1 exon deletions. *Eur. J. Hum. Genet.* **2012**, *20*, 1240–1247. [CrossRef]

42. Radyushkin, K.; Hammerschmidt, K.; Boretius, S.; Varoqueaux, F.; El-Kordi, A.; Ronnenberg, A.; Winter, D.; Frahm, J.; Fischer, J.; Brose, N.; et al. Neuroligin-3-deficient mice: Model of a monogenic heritable form of autism with an olfactory deficit. *Genes Brain Behav.* **2009**, *8*, 416–425. [CrossRef]

43. Liang, J.; Xu, W.; Hsu, Y.-T.; Yee, A.X.; Chen, L.; Südhof, T.C. Conditional neuroligin-2 knockout in adult medial prefrontal cortex links chronic changes in synaptic inhibition to cognitive impairments. *Mol. Psychiatry* **2015**, *20*, 850–859. [CrossRef] [PubMed]

44. Pak, C.; Danko, T.; Zhang, Y.; Aoto, J.; Anderson, G.R.; Maxeiner, S.; Yi, F.; Wernig, M.; Südhof, T.C. Human Neuropsychiatric Disease Modeling using Conditional Deletion Reveals Synaptic Transmission Defects Caused by Heterozygous Mutations in NRXN1. *Cell Stem Cell* **2015**, *17*, 316–328. [CrossRef]

45. Arking, D.E.; Cutler, D.J.; Brune, C.W.; Teslovich, T.M.; West, K.; Ikeda, M.; Rea, A.; Guy, M.; Lin, S.; Cook, E.H.; et al. A Common Genetic Variant in the Neurexin Superfamily Member CNTNAP2 Increases Familial Risk of Autism. *Am. J. Hum. Genet.* **2008**, *82*, 160–164. [CrossRef] [PubMed]

46. Alarcón, M.; Abrahams, B.S.; Stone, J.L.; Duvall, J.A.; Perederiy, J.V.; Bomar, J.M.; Sebat, J.; Wigler, M.; Martin, C.L.; Ledbetter, D.H.; et al. Linkage, Association, and Gene-Expression Analyses Identify CNTNAP2 as an Autism-Susceptibility Gene. *Am. J. Hum. Genet.* **2008**, *82*, 150–159. [CrossRef] [PubMed]

47. Nord, A.S.; Network, S.P.; Roeb, W.; Dickel, D.E.; Walsh, T.; Kusenda, M.; O'Connor, K.L.; Malhotra, D.; McCarthy, S.E.; Stray, S.M.; et al. Reduced transcript expression of genes affected by inherited and de novo CNVs in autism. *Eur. J. Hum. Genet.* **2011**, *19*, 727–731. [CrossRef]

48. Peñagarikano, O.; Abrahams, B.S.; Herman, E.I.; Winden, K.D.; Gdalyahu, A.; Dong, H.; Sonnenblick, L.I.; Gruver, R.; Almajano, J.; Bragin, A.; et al. Absence of CNTNAP2 Leads to Epilepsy, Neuronal Migration Abnormalities, and Core Autism-Related Deficits. *Cell* **2011**, *147*, 235–246. [CrossRef]

49. Kreienkamp, H.-J. Scaffolding Proteins at the Postsynaptic Density: Shank as the Architectural Framework. In *Protein-Protein Interactions as New Drug Targets*; Springer: Berlin, Germany, 2008; Volume 186, pp. 365–380.

50. Berkel, S.; Marshall, C.; Weiss, B.; Howe, J.; Roeth, R.; Moog, U.; Endris, V.; Roberts, W.; Szatmari, P.; Pinto, D.; et al. Mutations in the SHANK2 synaptic scaffolding gene in autism spectrum disorder and mental retardation. *Nat. Genet.* **2010**, *42*, 489–491. [CrossRef]

51. Jiang, Y.-H.; Ehlers, M.D. Modeling Autism by SHANK Gene Mutations in Mice. *Neuron* **2013**, *78*, 8–27. [CrossRef]

52. Leblond, C.S.; Nava, C.; Polge, A.; Gauthier, J.; Huguet, G.; Lumbroso, S.; Giuliano, F.; Stordeur, C.; Depienne, C.; Mouzat, K.; et al. Meta-analysis of SHANK Mutations in Autism Spectrum Disorders: A Gradient of Severity in Cognitive Impairments. *PLoS Genet.* **2014**, *10*, e1004580. [CrossRef]

53. Pinto, D.; Delaby, E.; Merico, D.; Barbosa, M.; Merikangas, A.; Klei, L.; Thiruvahindrapuram, B.; Xu, X.; Ziman, R.; Wang, Z.; et al. Convergence of Genes and Cellular Pathways Dysregulated in Autism Spectrum Disorders. *Am. J. Hum. Genet.* **2014**, *94*, 677–694. [CrossRef]

54. Bacchelli, E.; Loi, E.; Cameli, C.; Moi, L.; Vega-Benedetti, A.F.; Blois, S.; Fadda, A.; Bonora, E.; Mattu, S.; Fadda, R.; et al. Analysis of a Sardinian Multiplex Family with Autism Spectrum Disorder Points to Post-Synaptic Density Gene Variants and Identifies CAPG as a Functionally Relevant Candidate Gene. *J. Clin. Med.* **2019**, *8*, 212. [CrossRef]

55. Lahbib, S.; Leblond, C.S.; Hamza, M.; Regnault, B.; Lemée, L.; Mathieu, A.; Jaouadi, H.; Mkaouar, R.; Ben Youssef-Turki, I.; Belhadj, A.; et al. Homozygous 2p11.2 deletion supports the implication of ELMOD3 in hearing loss and reveals the potential association of CAPG with ASD/ID etiology. *J. Appl. Genet.* **2018**, *60*, 49–56. [CrossRef]

56. Fan, Y.; Tang, X.; Vitriol, E.A.; Chen, G.; Zheng, J.Q. Actin capping protein is required for dendritic spine development and synapse formation. *J. Neurosci.* **2011**, *31*, 10228–11033. [CrossRef] [PubMed]

57. Korobova, F.; Svitkina, T.M. Molecular Architecture of Synaptic Actin Cytoskeleton in Hippocampal Neurons Reveals a Mechanism of Dendritic Spine Morphogenesis. *Mol. Biol. Cell* **2010**, *21*, 165–176. [CrossRef]

58. Schmunk, G.; Gargus, J.J. Channelopathy pathogenesis in autism spectrum disorders. *Front. Genet.* **2013**, *4*, 222. [CrossRef]

59. Despang, P.; Salamon, S.; Breitenkamp, A.F.; Kuzmenkina, E.; Herzig, S.; Matthes, J. Autism-associated mutations in the CaVβ2 calcium-channel subunit increase Ba2+-currents and lead to differential modulation by the RGK-protein Gem. *Neurobiol. Dis.* **2020**, *136*, 104721. [CrossRef]

60. Splawski, I.; Timothy, K.W.; Sharpe, L.M.; Decher, N.; Kumar, P.; Bloise, R.; Napolitano, C.; Schwartz, P.J.; Joseph, R.M.; Condouris, K.; et al. CaV1.2 Calcium Channel Dysfunction Causes a Multisystem Disorder Including Arrhythmia and Autism. *Cell* **2004**, *119*, 19–31. [CrossRef]

61. Catterall, W.A.; Perez-Reyes, E.; Snutch, T.P.; Striessnig, J. International Union of Pharmacology. XLVIII. Nomenclature and Structure-Function Relationships of Voltage-Gated Calcium Channels. *Pharmacol. Rev.* **2005**, *57*, 411–425. [CrossRef]

62. Barrett, C.F.; Tsien, R.W. The Timothy syndrome mutation differentially affects voltage- and calcium-dependent inactivation of CaV1.2 L-type calcium channels. *Proc. Natl. Acad. Sci. USA* **2008**, *105*, 2157–2162. [CrossRef]

63. Hemara-Wahanui, A.; Berjukow, S.; Hope, C.I.; Dearden, P.K.; Wu, S.-B.; Wilson-Wheeler, J.; Sharp, D.M.; Lundon-Treweek, P.; Clover, G.M.; Hoda, J.-C.; et al. A CACNA1F mutation identified in an X-linked retinal disorder shifts the voltage dependence of Cav1.4 channel activation. *Proc. Natl. Acad. Sci. USA* **2005**, *102*, 7553–7558. [CrossRef]

64. Pinggera, A.; Lieb, A.; Benedetti, B.; Lampert, M.; Monteleone, S.; Liedl, K.R.; Tuluc, P.; Striessnig, J. CACNA1D De Novo Mutations in Autism Spectrum Disorders Activate Cav1.3 L-Type Calcium Channels. *Biol. Psychiatry* **2015**, *77*, 816–822. [CrossRef]

65. Pinggera, A.; Mackenroth, L.; Rump, A.; Schallner, J.; Beleggia, F.; Wollnik, B.; Striessnig, J. New gain-of-function mutation shows CACNA1D as recurrently mutated gene in autism spectrum disorders and epilepsy. *Hum. Mol. Genet.* **2017**, *26*, 2923–2932. [CrossRef]

66. Boczek, N.J.; Miller, E.M.; Ye, D.; Nesterenko, V.V.; Tester, D.J.; Antzelevitch, C.; Czosek, R.J.; Ackerman, M.J.; Ware, S.M. Novel Timothy syndrome mutation leading to increase in CACNA1C window current. *Heart Rhythm* **2015**, *12*, 211–219. [CrossRef]

67. Splawski, I.; Yoo, D.S.; Stotz, S.C.; Cherry, A.; Clapham, D.E.; Keating, M.T. CACNA1H Mutations in Autism Spectrum Disorders. *J. Biol. Chem.* **2006**, *281*, 22085–22091. [CrossRef]

68. Breitenkamp, A.F.S.; Matthes, J.; Nass, R.D.; Sinzig, J.; Lehmkuhl, G.; Nürnberg, P.; Herzig, S. Rare Mutations of CACNB2 Found in Autism Spectrum Disease-Affected Families Alter Calcium Channel Function. *PLoS ONE* **2014**, *9*, e95579. [CrossRef]

69. Morrow, E.M.; Yoo, S.-Y.; Flavell, S.W.; Kim, T.-K.; Lin, Y.; Hill, R.S.; Mukaddes, N.M.; Balkhy, S.; Gascon, G.; Hashmi, A.; et al. Identifying Autism Loci and Genes by Tracing Recent Shared Ancestry. *Science* **2008**, *321*, 218–223. [CrossRef]

70. Veeramah, K.R.; O'Brien, J.E.; Meisler, M.H.; Cheng, X.; Dib-Hajj, S.D.; Waxman, S.G.; Talwar, D.; Girirajan, S.; Eichler, E.E.; Restifo, L.L.; et al. De Novo Pathogenic SCN8A Mutation Identified by Whole-Genome Sequencing of a Family Quartet Affected by Infantile Epileptic Encephalopathy and SUDEP. *Am. J. Hum. Genet.* **2012**, *90*, 502–510. [CrossRef]

71. Chen, C.-P.; Lin, S.-P.; Chern, S.-R.; Chen, Y.-J.; Tsai, F.-J.; Wu, P.-C.; Wang, W. Array-CGH detection of a de novo 2.8 Mb deletion in 2q24.2→q24.3 in a girl with autistic features and developmental delay. *Eur. J. Med. Genet.* **2010**, *53*, 217–220. [CrossRef]

72. Sanders, S.J.; Murtha, M.T.; Gupta, A.R.; Murdoch, J.D.; Raubeson, M.J.; Willsey, A.J.; Ercan-Sencicek, A.G.; DiLullo, N.M.; Parikshak, N.N.; Stein, J.L.; et al. De novo mutations revealed by whole-exome sequencing are strongly associated with autism. *Nature* **2012**, *485*, 237–241. [CrossRef] [PubMed]

73. Weiss, L.A.; Escayg, A.; Kearney, J.A.; Trudeau, M.; Macdonald, B.T.; Mori, M.; Reichert, J.; Buxbaum, J.D.; Meisler, M.H. Sodium channels SCN1A, SCN2A and SCN3A in familial autism. *Mol. Psychiatry* **2003**, *8*, 186–194. [CrossRef]

74. Han, S.; Tai, C.; Westenbroek, R.E.; Yu, F.H.; Cheah, C.S.; Potter, G.B.; Rubenstein, J.L.; Scheuer, T.; De La Iglesia, H.O.; Catterall, W.A. Autistic-like behaviour in Scn1a+/− mice and rescue by enhanced GABA-mediated neurotransmission. *Nature* **2012**, *489*, 385–390. [CrossRef]

75. Gilling, M.; Rasmussen, H.B.; Calloe, K.; Sequeira, A.F.; Baretto, M.; Oliveira, G.; Almeida, J.; Lauritsen, M.B.; Ullmann, R.; Boonen, S.E.; et al. Dysfunction of the Heteromeric KV7.3/KV7.5 Potassium Channel is Associated with Autism Spectrum Disorders. *Front. Genet.* **2013**, *4*, 54. [CrossRef]

76. Gross, C.; Yao, X.; Pong, D.L.; Jeromin, A.; Bassell, G.J. Fragile X Mental Retardation Protein Regulates Protein Expression and mRNA Translation of the Potassium Channel Kv4.2. *J. Neurosci.* **2011**, *31*, 5693–5698. [CrossRef]

77. Sicca, F.; Imbrici, P.; D'Adamo, M.C.; Moro, F.; Bonatti, F.; Brovedani, P.; Grottesi, A.; Guerrini, R.; Masi, G.; Santorelli, F.M.; et al. Autism with Seizures and Intellectual Disability: Possible Causative Role of Gain-of-function of the Inwardly-Rectifying K+ Channel Kir4.1. *Neurobiol. Dis.* **2011**, *43*, 239–247. [CrossRef]

78. Laumonnier, F.; Eroger, S.; Guérin, P.; Molinari, F.; M'Rad, R.; Cahard, D.; Belhadj, A.; Halayem, M.; Persico, A.M.; Elia, M.; et al. Association of a Functional Deficit of the BKCa Channel, a Synaptic Regulator of Neuronal Excitability, With Autism and Mental Retardation. *Am. J. Psychiatry* **2006**, *163*, 1622. [CrossRef]

79. Deng, P.Y.; Rotman, Z.; Blundon, J.A.; Cho, Y.; Cui, J.; Cavalli, V.; Zakharenko, S.S.; Klyachko, V.A. FMRP Regulates Neurotransmitter Release and Synaptic Information Transmission by Modulating Action Potential Duration via BK Channels. *Neuron* **2013**, *77*, 696–711. [CrossRef]

80. Gonzalez–Gronow, M.; Cuchacovich, M.; Francos, R.; Cuchacovich, S.; Fernandez, M.D.P.; Blanco, A.; Bowers, E.V.; Kaczowka, S.; Pizzo, S.V. Antibodies against the voltage-dependent anion channel (VDAC) and its protective ligand hexokinase-I in children with autism. *J. Neuroimmunol.* **2010**, *227*, 153–161. [CrossRef]

81. Gvozdjáková, A.; Löw, H.; Sun, I.; Navas, P.; Crane, F.L. Plasma membrane coenzyme Q: Evidence for a role in autism. *Biol. Targets Ther.* **2014**, *8*, 199. [CrossRef]

82. Wong, C.C.Y.; Meaburn, E.L.; Ronald, A.; Price, T.S.; Jeffries, A.R.; Schalkwyk, L.C.; Plomin, R.; Mill, J. Methylomic analysis of monozygotic twins discordant for autism spectrum disorder and related behavioural traits. *Mol. Psychiatry* **2013**, *19*, 495–503. [CrossRef]

83. Nguyen, A.; Rauch, T.A.; Pfeifer, G.P.; Hu, V.W. Global methylation profiling of lymphoblastoid cell lines reveals epigenetic contributions to autism spectrum disorders and a novel autism candidate gene, RORA, whose protein product is reduced in autistic brain. *FASEB J.* **2010**, *24*, 3036–3051. [CrossRef]

84. Zhu, Y.; Mordaunt, C.E.; Yasui, D.H.; Marathe, R.; Coulson, R.L.; Dunaway, K.; Jianu, J.M.; Walker, C.K.; Ozonoff, S.; Hertz-Picciotto, I.; et al. Placental DNA methylation levels at CYP2E1 and IRS2 are associated with child outcome in a prospective autism study. *Hum. Mol. Genet.* **2019**, *28*, 2659–2674. [CrossRef]

85. Andrews, S.V.; Sheppard, B.; Windham, G.C.; Schieve, L.A.; Schendel, D.E.; Croen, L.E.; Chopra, P.; Alisch, R.S.; Newschaffer, C.J.; Warren, S.T.; et al. Case-control meta-analysis of blood DNA methylation and autism spectrum disorder. *Mol. Autism* **2018**, *9*, 40. [CrossRef]

86. Siu, M.T.; Butcher, D.T.; Turinsky, A.L.; Cytrynbaum, C.; Stavropoulos, D.J.; Walker, S.; Caluseriu, O.; Carter, M.; Lou, Y.; Nicolson, R.; et al. Functional DNA methylation signatures for autism spectrum disorder genomic risk loci: 16p11.2 deletions and CHD8 variants. *Clin. Epigenetics* **2019**, *11*, 1–19. [CrossRef]

87. Kimura, R.; Nakata, M.; Funabiki, Y.; Suzuki, S.; Awaya, T.; Murai, T.; Hagiwara, M. An epigenetic biomarker for adult high-functioning autism spectrum disorder. *Sci. Rep.* **2019**, *9*, 13662–13667. [CrossRef] [PubMed]

88. Saeliw, T.; Tangsuwansri, C.; Thongkorn, S.; Chonchaiya, W.; Suphapeetiporn, K.; Mutirangura, A.; Tencomnao, T.; Hu, V.W.; Sarachana, T. Integrated genome-wide Alu methylation and transcriptome profiling analyses reveal novel epigenetic regulatory networks associated with autism spectrum disorder. *Mol. Autism* **2018**, *9*, 27. [CrossRef]

89. Wong, C.C.Y.; Smith, R.G.; Hannon, E.; Ramaswami, G.; Parikshak, N.N.; Assary, E.; Troakes, C.; Poschmann, J.; Schalkwyk, L.C.; Sun, W.; et al. Genome-wide DNA methylation profiling identifies convergent molecular signatures associated with idiopathic and syndromic autism in post-mortem human brain tissue. *Hum. Mol. Genet.* **2019**, *28*, 2201–2211. [CrossRef]

90. Stathopoulos, S.; Gaujoux, R.; Lindeque, Z.; Mahony, C.; Van Der Colff, R.; Van Der Westhuizen, F.; O'Ryan, C. DNA Methylation Associated with Mitochondrial Dysfunction in a South African Autism Spectrum Disorder Cohort. *Autism Res.* **2020**, *13*, 1079–1093. [CrossRef]

91. Hu, Z.; Yang, Y.; Zhao, Y.; Yu, H.; Ying, X.; Zhou, D.; Zhong, J.; Zheng, Z.; Liu, J.; Pan, R.; et al. APOE hypermethylation is associated with autism spectrum disorder in a Chinese population. *Exp. Ther. Med.* **2018**, *15*, 4749–4754. [CrossRef]

92. Hranilović, D.; Blažević, S.; Stefulj, J.; Zill, P. DNA Methylation Analysis of HTR2A Regulatory Region in Leukocytes of Autistic Subjects. *Autism Res.* **2015**, *9*, 204–209. [CrossRef]

93. Hu, Z.; Ying, X.; Huang, L.; Zhao, Y.; Zhou, D.; Liu, J.; Zhong, J.; Huang, T.; Zhang, W.; Cheng, F.; et al. Association of human serotonin receptor 4 promoter methylation with autism spectrum disorder. *Medicine* **2020**, *99*, e18838. [CrossRef]

94. Lu, Z.; Liu, Z.; Mao, W.; Wang, X.; Zheng, X.; Chen, S.; Cao, B.; Huang, S.; Zhang, X.; Zhou, T.; et al. Locus-specific DNA methylation of Mecp2 promoter leads to autism-like phenotypes in mice. *Cell Death Dis.* **2020**, *11*, 85. [CrossRef]

95. Hicks, S.D.; Middleton, F.A. A Comparative Review of microRNA Expression Patterns in Autism Spectrum Disorder. *Front. Psychiatry* **2016**, *7*, 176. [CrossRef]

96. Hicks, S.D.; Carpenter, R.L.; Wagner, K.E.; Pauley, R.; Barros, M.; Tierney-Aves, C.; Barns, S.; Greene, C.D.; Middleton, F.A. Saliva MicroRNA Differentiates Children with Autism from Peers with Typical and Atypical Development. *J. Am. Acad. Child. Adolesc. Psychiatry* **2020**, *59*, 296–308. [CrossRef]

97. Sehovic, E.; Spahic, L.; Smajlovic-Skenderagic, L.; Pistoljevic, N.; Dzanko, E.; Hajdarpasic, A. Identification of developmental disorders including autism spectrum disorder using salivary miRNAs in children from Bosnia and Herzegovina. *PLoS ONE* **2020**, *15*, e0232351. [CrossRef]

98. Hagiwara, M.; Kimura, R.; Funabiki, Y.; Awaya, T.; Murai, T.; Hagiwara, M. MicroRNA profiling in adults with high-functioning autism spectrum disorder. *Mol. Brain* **2019**, *12*, 82–84. [CrossRef]

99. Ozkul, Y.; Taheri, S.; Bayram, K.K.; Sener, E.F.; Mehmetbeyoglu, E.; Öztop, D.B.; Aybuga, F.; Tufan, E.; Bayram, A.; Dolu, N.; et al. A heritable profile of six miRNAs in autistic patients and mouse models. *Sci. Rep.* **2020**, *10*, 1–14. [CrossRef]

100. Vasu, M.M.; Anitha, A.; Thanseem, I.; Suzuki, K.; Yamada, K.; Takahashi, T.; Wakuda, T.; Iwata, K.; Tsujii, M.; Sugiyama, T.; et al. Serum microRNA profiles in children with autism. *Mol. Autism* **2014**, *5*, 40. [CrossRef]

101. Vatsa, N.; Kumar, V.; Singh, B.K.; Kumar, S.S.; Sharma, A.; Jana, N.R. Down-Regulation of miRNA-708 Promotes Aberrant Calcium Signaling by Targeting Neuronatin in a Mouse Model of Angelman Syndrome. *Front. Mol. Neurosci.* **2019**, *12*, 35. [CrossRef]

102. Urdinguio, R.G.; Fernández, A.F.; López-Nieva, P.; Rossi, S.; Huertas, D.; Kulis, M.; Liu, C.-G.; Croce, C.M.; Calin, G.A.; Esteller, M. Disrupted microRNA expression caused by Mecp2 loss in a mouse model of Rett syndrome. *Epigenetics* **2010**, *5*, 656–663. [CrossRef]

103. Edbauer, D.; Neilson, J.R.; Foster, K.A.; Wang, C.-F.; Seeburg, D.P.; Batterton, M.N.; Tada, T.; Dolan, B.M.; Sharp, P.A.; Sheng, M. Regulation of Synaptic Structure and Function by FMRP-Associated MicroRNAs miR-125b and miR-132. *Neuron* **2010**, *65*, 373–384. [CrossRef]

104. Gaugler, T.; Klei, L.; Sanders, S.J.; Bodea, C.A.; Goldberg, A.P.; Lee, A.B.; Mahajan, M.C.; Manaa, D.; Pawitan, Y.; Reichert, J.G.; et al. Most genetic risk for autism resides with common variation. *Nat. Genet.* **2014**, *46*, 881–885. [CrossRef]

105. Deng, W.; Zou, X.; Deng, H.; Li, J.; Tang, C.; Wang, X.; Guo, X. The Relationship Among Genetic Heritability, Environmental Effects, and Autism Spectrum Disorders. *J. Child Neurol.* **2015**, *30*, 1794–1799. [CrossRef]

106. Edelson, L.R.; Saudino, K.J. Genetic and environmental influences on autistic-like behaviors in 2-year-old twins. *Behav. Genet.* **2009**, *39*, 255–264. [CrossRef]

107. Bölte, S.; Girdler, S.; Marschik, P.B. The contribution of environmental exposure to the etiology of autism spectrum disorder. *Cell. Mol. Life Sci.* **2019**, *76*, 1275–1297. [CrossRef]

108. Janecka, M.; Mill, J.; Basson, M.A.; Goriely, A.; Spiers, H.; Reichenberg, A.; Schalkwyk, L.; Fernandes, C. Advanced paternal age effects in neurodevelopmental disorders—Review of potential underlying mechanisms. *Transl. Psychiatry* **2017**, *7*, e1019. [CrossRef]

109. Wu, S.; Wu, F.; Ding, Y.; Hou, J.; Bi, J.; Zhang, Z. Advanced parental age and autism risk in children: A systematic review and meta-analysis. *Acta Psychiatr. Scand.* **2016**, *135*, 29–41. [CrossRef]

110. Atsem, S.; Reichenbach, J.; Potabattula, R.; Dittrich, M.; Nava, C.; Depienne, C.; Böhm, L.; Rost, S.; Hahn, T.; Schorsch, M.; et al. Paternal age effects on spermFOXK1andKCNA7methylation and transmission into the next generation. *Hum. Mol. Genet.* **2016**, *25*, 4996–5005. [CrossRef]

111. Kojima, M.; Yassin, W.; Owada, K.; Aoki, Y.; Kuwabara, H.; Natsubori, T.; Iwashiro, N.; Gonoi, W.; Takao, H.; Kasai, K.; et al. Neuroanatomical Correlates of Advanced Paternal and Maternal Age at Birth in Autism Spectrum Disorder. *Cereb. Cortex* **2018**, *29*, 2524–2532. [CrossRef]

112. Foldi, C.J.; Eyles, D.; McGrath, J.J.; Burne, T.H.J. Advanced paternal age is associated with alterations in discrete behavioural domains and cortical neuroanatomy of C57BL/6J mice. *Eur. J. Neurosci.* **2010**, *31*, 556–564. [CrossRef] [PubMed]

113. Sampino, S.; Juszczak, G.R.; Zacchini, F.; Swiergiel, A.H.; Modlinski, J.A.; Loi, P.; Ptak, G. Grand-paternal age and the development of autism-like symptoms in mice progeny. *Transl. Psychiatry* **2014**, *4*, e386. [CrossRef]

114. Gardener, H.; Spiegelman, D.; Buka, S.L. Prenatal risk factors for autism: Comprehensive meta-analysis. *Br. J. Psychiatry* **2009**, *195*, 7–14. [CrossRef]

115. Gardener, H.; Spiegelman, D.; Buka, S.L. Perinatal and Neonatal Risk Factors for Autism: A Comprehensive Meta-analysis. *Pediatrics* **2011**, *128*, 344–355. [CrossRef]

116. Wang, C.; Geng, H.; Liu, W.; Zhang, G. Prenatal, perinatal, and postnatal factors associated with autism. *Medicine* **2017**, *96*, e6696. [CrossRef]

117. Bejerot, S.; Eriksson, J.M.; Bonde, S.; Carlström, K.; Humble, M.B.; Eriksson, E. The extreme male brain revisited: Gender coherence in adults with autism spectrum disorder. *Br. J. Psychiatry* **2012**, *201*, 116–123. [CrossRef]

118. Baron-Cohen, S.; Auyeung, B.; Nørgaard-Pedersen, B.; Hougaard, D.M.; Abdallah, M.W.; Melgaard, L.; Cohen, A.S.; Chakrabarti, B.; Ruta, L.; Lombardo, M.V. Elevated fetal steroidogenic activity in autism. *Mol. Psychiatry* **2015**, *20*, 369–376. [CrossRef]

119. Baron-Cohen, S.; Tsompanidis, A.; Auyeung, B.; Nørgaard-Pedersen, B.; Hougaard, D.M.; Abdallah, M.; Cohen, A.; Pohl, A. Foetal oestrogens and autism. *Mol. Psychiatry* **2020**, *25*, 2970–2978. [CrossRef] [PubMed]

120. Crider, A.; Thakkar, R.; Ahmed, A.O.; Pillai, A. Dysregulation of estrogen receptor beta (ERβ), aromatase (CYP19A1), and ER co-activators in the middle frontal gyrus of autism spectrum disorder subjects. *Mol. Autism* **2014**, *5*, 46. [CrossRef]

121. Chakrabarti, B.; Dudbridge, F.; Kent, L.; Wheelwright, S.; Hill-Cawthorne, G.; Allison, C.; Banerjee-Basu, S.; Baron-Cohen, S. Genes related to sex steroids, neural growth, and social-emotional behavior are associated with autistic traits, empathy, and Asperger syndrome. *Autism Res.* **2009**, *2*, 157–177. [CrossRef]

122. Jackson, A.A.; Robinson, S.M. Dietary guidelines for pregnancy: A review of current evidence. *Public Health Nutr.* **2001**, *4*, 625–630. [CrossRef]

123. Van Eijsden, M.; Smits, L.J.M.; Van Der Wal, M.F.; Bonsel, G.J. Association between short interpregnancy intervals and term birth weight: The role of folate depletion. *Am. J. Clin. Nutr.* **2008**, *88*, 147–153. [CrossRef] [PubMed]

124. Magnusson, C.; Kosidou, K.; Dalman, C.; Lundberg, M.; Lee, B.K.; Rai, D.; Karlsson, H.; Gardner, R.; Arver, S. Maternal vitamin D deficiency and the risk of autism spectrum disorders: Population-based study. *BJPsych Open* **2016**, *2*, 170–172. [CrossRef]

125. Robea, M.; Luca, A.-C.; Ciobica, A. Relationship between Vitamin Deficiencies and Co-Occurring Symptoms in Autism Spectrum Disorder. *Medicine* **2020**, *56*, 245. [CrossRef]

126. Saghazadeh, A.; Ahangari, N.; Hendi, K.; Saleh, F.; Rezaei, N. Status of essential elements in autism spectrum disorder: Systematic review and meta-analysis. *Rev. Neurosci.* **2017**, *28*, 783–809. [CrossRef]

127. Schmidt, R.J.; Tancredi, D.J.; Krakowiak, P.; Hansen, R.L.; Ozonoff, S. Maternal Intake of Supplemental Iron and Risk of Autism Spectrum Disorder. *Am. J. Epidemiol.* **2014**, *180*, 890–900. [CrossRef]

128. Hagmeyer, S.; Mangus, K.; Boeckers, T.M.; Grabrucker, A.M. Effects of Trace Metal Profiles Characteristic for Autism on Synapses in Cultured Neurons. *Neural Plast.* **2015**, *2015*, 1–16. [CrossRef]

129. Goyal, D.K.; Neil, J.R.; Simmons, S.D.; Mansab, F.; Benjamin, S.; Pitfield, V.; Boulet, S.; Miyan, J.A. Zinc Deficiency in Autism: A Controlled Study. *Insights Biomed.* **2019**, *4*, 4. [CrossRef]

130. Yasuda, H.; Yoshida, K.; Yasuda, Y.; Tsutsui, T. Infantile zinc deficiency: Association with autism spectrum disorders. *Sci. Rep.* **2011**, *1*, 129. [CrossRef]

131. Li, S.-O.; Wang, J.-L.; Bjørklund, G.; Zhao, W.-N.; Yin, C.-H. Serum copper and zinc levels in individuals with autism spectrum disorders. *NeuroReport* **2014**, *25*, 1216–1220. [CrossRef]

132. Grabrucker, S.; Boeckers, T.M.; Grabrucker, A.M. Gender Dependent Evaluation of Autism like Behavior in Mice Exposed to Prenatal Zinc Deficiency. *Front. Behav. Neurosci.* **2016**, *10*, 37. [CrossRef]

133. Grabrucker, S.; Jannetti, L.; Eckert, M.; Gaub, S.; Chhabra, R.; Pfaender, S.; Mangus, K.; Reddy, P.P.; Rankovic, V.; Schmeisser, M.J.; et al. Zinc deficiency dysregulates the synaptic ProSAP/Shank scaffold and might contribute to autism spectrum disorders. *Brain* **2013**, *137*, 137–152. [CrossRef] [PubMed]

134. Grabrucker, A.M.; Knight, M.J.; Proepper, C.; Bockmann, J.; Joubert, M.; Rowan, M.; Nienhaus, G.U.; Garner, C.C.; Bowie, J.U.; Kreutz, M.R.; et al. Concerted action of zinc and ProSAP/Shank in synaptogenesis and synapse maturation. *EMBO J.* **2011**, *30*, 569–581. [CrossRef]

135. Frederickson, C.J.; Koh, J.-Y.; Bush, A.I. The neurobiology of zinc in health and disease. *Nat. Rev. Neurosci.* **2005**, *6*, 449–462. [CrossRef] [PubMed]

136. Vyas, Y.; Lee, K.; Jung, Y.; Montgomery, J.M. Influence of maternal zinc supplementation on the development of autism-associated behavioural and synaptic deficits in offspring Shank3-knockout mice. *Mol. Brain* **2020**, *13*, 1–18. [CrossRef]

137. Shih, P.-Y.; Hsieh, B.-Y.; Lin, M.-H.; Huang, T.-N.; Tsai, C.-Y.; Pong, W.-L.; Lee, S.-P.; Hsueh, Y.-P. CTTNBP2 Controls Synaptic Expression of Zinc-Related Autism-Associated Proteins and Regulates Synapse Formation and Autism-like Behaviors. *Cell Rep.* **2020**, *31*, 107700. [CrossRef]

138. Velie, E.M.; Block, G.; Shaw, G.M.; Samuels, S.J.; Schaffer, D.M.; Kulldorff, M. Maternal supplemental and dietary zinc intake and the occurrence of neural tube defects in California. *Am. J. Epidemiol.* **1999**, *150*, 605–616. [CrossRef]

139. Gardner, R.M.; Lee, B.K.; Magnusson, C.; Rai, D.; Frisell, T.; Karlsson, H.; Idring, S.; Dalman, C. Maternal body mass index during early pregnancy, gestational weight gain, and risk of autism spectrum disorders: Results from a Swedish total population and discordant sibling study. *Int. J. Epidemiol.* **2015**, *44*, 870–883. [CrossRef]

140. Wang, Y.; Tang, S.; Xu, S.; Weng, S.; Liu, Z. Maternal Body Mass Index and Risk of Autism Spectrum Disorders in Offspring: A Meta-analysis. *Sci. Rep.* **2016**, *6*, 34248. [CrossRef] [PubMed]

141. Getz, K.D.; Anderka, M.T.; Werler, M.M.; Jick, S.S. Maternal Pre-pregnancy Body Mass Index and Autism Spectrum Disorder among Offspring: A Population-Based Case-Control Study. *Paediatr. Périnat. Epidemiol.* **2016**, *30*, 479–487. [CrossRef]

142. Li, M.; Fallin, M.D.; Riley, A.; Landa, R.; Walker, S.O.; Silverstein, M.; Caruso, D.; Pearson, C.; Kiang, S.; Dahm, J.L.; et al. The Association of Maternal Obesity and Diabetes with Autism and Other Developmental Disabilities. *Pediatrics* **2016**, *137*, e20152206. [CrossRef]

143. Tang, S.; Wang, Y.; Gong, X.; Wang, G.-H. A Meta-Analysis of Maternal Smoking during Pregnancy and Autism Spectrum Disorder Risk in Offspring. *Int. J. Environ. Res. Public Health* **2015**, *12*, 10418–10431. [CrossRef]

144. Rosen, B.N.; Lee, B.K.; Lee, N.L.; Yang, Y.; Burstyn, I. Maternal Smoking and Autism Spectrum Disorder: A Meta-analysis. *J. Autism Dev. Disord.* **2014**, *45*, 1689–1698. [CrossRef]

145. Visser, J.C.; Rommelse, N.; Vink, L.; Schrieken, M.; Oosterling, I.J.; Van Der Gaag, R.J.; Buitelaar, J.K. Narrowly Versus Broadly Defined Autism Spectrum Disorders: Differences in Pre- and Perinatal Risk Factors. *J. Autism Dev. Disord.* **2012**, *43*, 1505–1516. [CrossRef]

146. Perrone-McGovern, K.; Simon-Dack, S.; Niccolai, L. Prenatal and Perinatal Factors Related to Autism, IQ, and Adaptive Functioning. *J. Genet. Psychol.* **2015**, *176*, 1–10. [CrossRef]

147. Eliasen, M.H.; Tolstrup, J.S.; Andersen, A.-M.N.; Gronbaek, M.; Olsen, J.; Strandberg-Larsen, K.; Grønbæk, M. Prenatal alcohol exposure and autistic spectrum disorders—A population-based prospective study of 80 552 children and their mothers. *Int. J. Epidemiol.* **2010**, *39*, 1074–1081. [CrossRef] [PubMed]

148. Gallagher, C.; McCarthy, F.P.; Ryan, R.M.; Khashan, A.S. Maternal Alcohol Consumption during Pregnancy and the Risk of Autism Spectrum Disorders in Offspring: A Retrospective Analysis of the Millennium Cohort Study. *J. Autism Dev. Disord.* **2018**, *48*, 3773–3782. [CrossRef]

149. Meador, K.J. Effects of in Utero Antiepileptic Drug Exposure. *Epilepsy Curr.* **2008**, *8*, 143–147. [CrossRef] [PubMed]

150. Veroniki, A.A.; Cogo, E.; Rios, P.; Straus, S.E.; Finkelstein, Y.; Kealey, R.; Reynen, E.; Soobiah, C.; Thavorn, K.; Hutton, B.; et al. Comparative safety of anti-epileptic drugs during pregnancy: A systematic review and network meta-analysis of congenital malformations and prenatal outcomes. *BMC Med.* **2017**, *15*, 1–20. [CrossRef]

151. Kobayashi, T.; Matsuyama, T.; Takeuchi, M.; Ito, S. Autism spectrum disorder and prenatal exposure to selective serotonin reuptake inhibitors: A systematic review and meta-analysis. *Reprod. Toxicol.* **2016**, *65*, 170–178. [CrossRef]

152. Wan, H.; Zhang, C.; Li, H.; Luan, S.; Liu, C. Association of maternal diabetes with autism spectrum disorders in offspring. *Medicine* **2018**, *97*, e9438. [CrossRef] [PubMed]

153. Xu, G.; Jing, J.; Bowers, K.; Liu, B.; Bao, W. Maternal diabetes and the risk of autism spectrum disorders in the offspring: A systematic review and meta-analysis. *J. Autism Dev. Disord.* **2014**, *44*, 766–775. [CrossRef]

154. Jiang, H.-Y.; Xu, L.-L.; Shao, L.; Xia, R.-M.; Yu, Z.-H.; Ling, Z.; Yang, F.; Deng, M.; Ruan, B. Maternal infection during pregnancy and risk of autism spectrum disorders: A systematic review and meta-analysis. *Brain Behav. Immun.* **2016**, *58*, 165–172. [CrossRef]

155. Zerbo, O.; Qian, Y.; Yoshida, C.; Grether, J.K.; Van De Water, J.; Croen, L.A. Maternal Infection during Pregnancy and Autism Spectrum Disorders. *J. Autism Dev. Disord.* **2015**, *45*, 4015–4025. [CrossRef]

156. Atladóttir, H.Ó.; Thorsen, P.; Østergaard, L.; Schendel, D.E.; Lemcke, S.; Abdallah, M.; Parner, E.T. Maternal Infection Requiring Hospitalization During Pregnancy and Autism Spectrum Disorders. *J. Autism Dev. Disord.* **2010**, *40*, 1423–1430. [CrossRef]

157. Chen, S.-W.; Zhong, X.-S.; Jiang, L.-N.; Zheng, X.-Y.; Xiong, Y.-Q.; Ma, S.-J.; Qiu, M.; Huo, S.-T.; Ge, J.; Chen, Q. Maternal autoimmune diseases and the risk of autism spectrum disorders in offspring: A systematic review and meta-analysis. *Behav. Brain Res.* **2016**, *296*, 61–69. [CrossRef]

158. Wu, S.; Ding, Y.; Wu, F.; Li, R.; Xie, G.; Hou, J.; Mao, P. Family history of autoimmune diseases is associated with an increased risk of autism in children: A systematic review and meta-analysis. *Neurosci. Biobehav. Rev.* **2015**, *55*, 322–332. [CrossRef]

159. Brown, A.S.; Sourander, A.; Hinkka-Yli-Salomäki, S.; McKeague, I.W.; Sundvall, J.; Surcel, H.-M. Elevated maternal C-reactive protein and autism in a national birth cohort. *Mol. Psychiatry* **2013**, *19*, 259–264. [CrossRef]

160. Brown, A.S.; Surcel, H.-M.; Hinkka-Yli-Salomäki, S.; Cheslack-Postava, K.; Bao, Y.; Sourander, A. Maternal thyroid autoantibody and elevated risk of autism in a national birth cohort. *Prog. Neuro-Psychopharmacol. Biol. Psychiatry* **2015**, *57*, 86–92. [CrossRef]

161. Meyer, U.; Feldon, J.; Fatemi, S.H. In-vivo rodent models for the experimental investigation of prenatal immune activation effects in neurodevelopmental brain disorders. *Neurosci. Biobehav. Rev.* **2009**, *33*, 1061–1079. [CrossRef]

162. Comi, A.M.; Zimmerman, A.W.; Frye, V.H.; Law, P.A.; Peeden, J.N. Familial Clustering of Autoimmune Disorders and Evaluation of Medical Risk Factors in Autism. *J. Child Neurol.* **1999**, *14*, 388–394. [CrossRef]

163. Atladóttir, H.O.; Pedersen, M.G.; Thorsen, P.; Mortensen, P.B.; Deleuran, B.; Eaton, W.W.; Parner, E.T.; Sutton, R.M.; Niles, D.; Nysaether, J.; et al. Association of Family History of Autoimmune Diseases and Autism Spectrum Disorders. *Pediatrics* **2009**, *124*, 687–694. [CrossRef]

164. Sanna, A.; Firinu, D.; Zavattari, P.; Valera, P. Zinc Status and Autoimmunity: A Systematic Review and Meta-Analysis. *Nutrients* **2018**, *10*, 68. [CrossRef] [PubMed]

165. Napoli, E.; Hung, C.; Wong, S.; Giulivi, C. Toxicity of the Flame-Retardant BDE-49 on Brain Mitochondria and Neuronal Progenitor Striatal Cells Enhanced by a PTEN-Deficient Background. *Toxicol. Sci.* **2013**, *132*, 196–210. [CrossRef]

166. Rossignol, D.A.; Frye, R.E. Mitochondrial dysfunction in autism spectrum disorders: A systematic review and meta-analysis. *Mol. Psychiatry* **2012**, *17*, 290–314. [CrossRef]

167. Yoshimasu, K.; Kiyohara, C.; Takemura, S.; Nakai, K. A meta-analysis of the evidence on the impact of prenatal and early infancy exposures to mercury on autism and attention deficit/hyperactivity disorder in the childhood. *NeuroToxicology* **2014**, *44*, 121–131. [CrossRef]

168. Shelton, J.F.; Geraghty, E.M.; Tancredi, D.; Delwiche, L.D.; Schmidt, R.J.; Ritz, B.; Hansen, R.L.; Hertz-Picciotto, I. Neurodevelopmental Disorders and Prenatal Residential Proximity to Agricultural Pesticides: The CHARGE Study. *Environ. Health Perspect.* **2014**, *122*, 1103–1109. [CrossRef]

169. Jeddi, M.Z.; Janani, L.; Memari, A.H.; Akhondzadeh, S.; Yunesian, M. The role of phthalate esters in autism development: A systematic review. *Environ. Res.* **2016**, *151*, 493–504. [CrossRef]

170. Dingemans, M.M.; Berg, M.V.D.; Westerink, R.H.S. Neurotoxicity of Brominated Flame Retardants: (In)direct Effects of Parent and Hydroxylated Polybrominated Diphenyl Ethers on the (Developing) Nervous System. *Environ. Health Perspect.* **2011**, *119*, 900–907. [CrossRef]

171. Wayman, G.A.; Bose, D.D.; Yang, N.; Lesiak, A.; Bruun, N.; Impey, S.; LeDoux, V.; Pessah, I.N.; Lein, P.J. PCB-95 Modulates the Calcium-Dependent Signaling Pathway Responsible for Activity-Dependent Dendritic Growth. *Environ. Health Perspect.* **2012**, *120*, 1003–1009. [CrossRef]

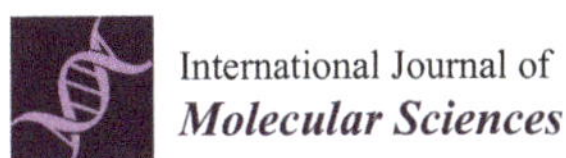 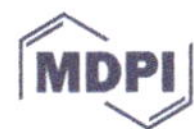

International Journal of
Molecular Sciences

Case Report

New Cav1.2 Channelopathy with High-Functioning Autism, Affective Disorder, Severe Dental Enamel Defects, a Short QT Interval, and a Novel *CACNA1C* Loss-of-Function Mutation

Dominique Endres [1,2,*,†], Niels Decher [3,†], Isabell Röhr [3], Kirsty Vowinkel [3], Katharina Domschke [2,4], Katalin Komlosi [5], Andreas Tzschach [5], Birgitta Gläser [5], Miriam A. Schiele [2], Kimon Runge [1,2], Patrick Süß [6], Florian Schuchardt [7], Kathrin Nickel [1,2], Birgit Stallmeyer [8], Susanne Rinné [3], Eric Schulze-Bahr [8,‡] and Ludger Tebartz van Elst [1,2,‡]

[1] Section for Experimental Neuropsychiatry, Department of Psychiatry and Psychotherapy, Medical Center-University of Freiburg, Faculty of Medicine, University of Freiburg, 79104 Freiburg, Germany; kimon.runge@uniklinik-freiburg.de (K.R.); kathrin.nickel@uniklinik-freiburg.de (K.N.); tebartzvanelst@uniklinik-freiburg.de (L.T.v.E.)

[2] Department of Psychiatry and Psychotherapy, Medical Center-University of Freiburg, Faculty of Medicine, University of Freiburg, 79104 Freiburg, Germany; katharina.domschke@uniklinik-freiburg.de (K.D.); miriam.schiele@uniklinik-freiburg.de (M.A.S.)

[3] Institute for Physiology and Pathophysiology, Vegetative Physiology and Marburg Center for Mind, Brain and Behavior-Philipps-University Marburg, 35037 Marburg, Germany; decher@staff.uni-marburg.de (N.D.); info@isabell-roehr.de (I.R.); kirsty.vowinkel@staff.uni-marburg.de (K.V.); rinne@staff.uni-marburg.de (S.R.)

[4] Center for Basics in Neuromodulation, Faculty of Medicine, University of Freiburg, 79106 Freiburg, Germany

[5] Institute of Human Genetics, Medical Center-University of Freiburg, Faculty of Medicine, University of Freiburg, 79106 Freiburg, Germany; katalin.komlosi@uniklinik-freiburg.de (K.K.); andreas.tzschach@uniklinik-freiburg.de (A.T.); birgitta.glaeser@uniklinik-freiburg.de (B.G.)

[6] Department of Molecular Neurology, University Hospital Erlangen, 91054 Erlangen, Germany; Patrick.Suess@uk-erlangen.de

[7] Department of Neurology, Medical Center-University of Freiburg, Faculty of Medicine, University of Freiburg, 79106 Freiburg, Germany; florian.schuchardt@uniklinik-freiburg.de

[8] Institute for Genetics of Heart Diseases, Department of Cardiovascular Medicine, University Hospital Münster, 48149 Münster, Germany; Birgit.Stallmeyer@ukmuenster.de (B.S.); eric.schulze-bahr@ukmuenster.de (E.S.-B.)

* Correspondence: dominique.endres@uniklinik-freiburg.de; Tel.: +49-761-270-66360
† These authors contributed equally to this work.
‡ These authors contributed equally to this work.

Received: 20 September 2020; Accepted: 7 November 2020; Published: 15 November 2020

Abstract: Complex neuropsychiatric-cardiac syndromes can be genetically determined. For the first time, the authors present a syndromal form of short QT syndrome in a 34-year-old German male patient with extracardiac features with predominant psychiatric manifestation, namely a severe form of secondary high-functioning autism spectrum disorder (ASD), along with affective and psychotic exacerbations, and severe dental enamel defects (with rapid wearing off his teeth) due to a heterozygous loss-of-function mutation in the *CACNA1C* gene (NM_000719.6: c.2399A > C; p.Lys800Thr). This mutation was found only once in control databases; the mutated lysine is located in the Cav1.2 calcium channel, is highly conserved during evolution, and is predicted to affect protein function by most pathogenicity prediction algorithms. L-type Cav1.2 calcium channels are widely expressed in the brain and heart. In the case presented, electrophysiological studies revealed a prominent reduction in the current amplitude without changes in the gating behavior of the Cav1.2 channel, most likely due to a trafficking defect. Due to the demonstrated loss of function, the p.Lys800Thr variant was finally classified as pathogenic (ACMG class 4 variant) and is likely to cause a newly described Cav1.2 channelopathy.

Keywords: CACNA1C; CaV1.2; autism; short QT syndrome; dental enamel defect

---

1. Introduction

Autism spectrum disorders (ASD) are frequent neurodevelopmental disorders characterized by social interaction difficulties, stereotypical procedures, routines and rituals, or special interests caused predominantly idiopathic or of unknown cause ("primary forms"); in a subset, a specific cause can be identified, and some of these secondary cases ("secondary forms") are part of genetically determined syndromes, e.g., fragile X syndrome [1]. Within these, Timothy syndrome is an extremely rare one characterized by long QT syndrome (LQTS) in the surface electrocardiography (ECG), skeletal abnormalities (e.g., cutaneous syndactyly), and neuropsychiatric features, such as autism [2–4], and is caused by gain-of-function mutations in the *CACNA1C* gene. Of note, some *CACNA1C* mutations may have an isolated cardiac, non-syndromal phenotype (only with QTc prolongation [5]). In contrast, patients with a short QT syndrome (SQTS) have not been described with extra-cardiac features so far.

2. Case Presentation

The authors present for the first time a syndromal form of SQTS in a 34-year-old German male patient that is characterized by extracardiac features, namely a severe form of secondary ASD together with affective and psychotic exacerbations, wearing of his teeth, and a short QT interval in the surface ECG due to a heterozygous loss-of-function mutation in the *CACNA1C* gene. The functional consequences of the genetic mutation were further analyzed using electrophysiological investigations of the mutant Cav1.2 calcium channel expressed in Xenopus oocytes [2]. The patient has given his signed written informed consent for this case report, including the presented images, the genetic information, and all other data, to be published.

2.1. Clinical Case Description

Since the first decade, the patient has suffered from the whole spectrum of autistic symptoms. The detailed diagnosis was performed according to the scheme established by the Freiburg Center for the Diagnosis and Treatment of Autism (http://www.uniklinik-freiburg.de/psych/live/patientenversorgung/schwerpunkte/schwerpunkt-asperger.html, accessed on 14 November 2020 [6–8]). His medical history showed alterations in (1) gaze control and holistic visual recognition (he had to learn to look into the eyes of others, uses analytical facial expression recognition, recognizes other people by certain characteristics); (2) problems with social communication (he lacks the tools to build relationships, is burdened by social contacts, small talk and telephoning cause him problems, plans social situations in detail in advance); (3) reduced social integration (has only a few close friends, needs his time alone); (4) interactional imagination abnormalities and sense of justice (he hated "doing things as if he were playing games", his sense of justice is 10/10, he is very honest); (5) linguistic pragmatics (as a child, he read dictionaries to understand proverbs, is often interpreting things literally); (6) routines and rituals (plans his everyday life in detail, is stressed by changes of plan, usually eats and drinks the same things); (7) motor clumsiness (he always had difficulties in sports, he had two "left hands" and two "left feet"); (8) sensory hypersensitivity (for loud noises and light, tormented in former times already by stroking by the mother); (9) strong perception of details (e.g., finds comma errors in texts, has difficulties with the "overall picture"); (10) special memory capacity (always knows exactly where what stood when he had read something); and (11) special interests for computer science [6]. The Autism Diagnostic Observation Schedule, Second Edition (ADOS-2; at the age of the patient of 34 years) confirmed clear autistic communication and interaction behavior confirming a syndrome diagnosis (14 points; cut off > 10 [9]). The testing of the recognition of emotions ("gnosis facialis") revealed indications of relative deficits in recognizing fear (http://www.gnosisfacialis.de/infoERT.html, accessed on 14 November 2020. In the Movie for the Assessment of Social Cognition (MASC), the patient scored borderline [10]. Difficulties in communication in social intuition were partially compensated by the patient in an analytical–cognitive way. In summary, two expert raters confirmed the presence of a high-functional ASD syndrome. His intelligence level was above average (he reached high school graduation "Abitur" in Germany with average grade 1.3; range: 1–6, optimal: 1, worst: 6) and later studied computer science.

At the age of 15 years, the patient developed his first depressive episode and, at the age of 17 years, his first hypomanic episode. Until publication of this case report, the patient suffered from recurrent depressive episodes, but hypomanic phases did not occur anymore after the age of 21 years. His first psychiatric presentation took place at the age of 18 years following mutistic states (i.e., he was unable to speak); there were no indications of schizophrenia or causation by illegal drugs. Video telemetry revealed no evidence of epileptic seizures. At the age of 18 years, monomorphic ventricular extrasystoles (VES) were noticed for the first time during a physical examination for military service suitability. At the age of 29 years, the teeth suddenly discolored and then receded (Figure 1A). During this time, the patient suffered from significant polydipsia (requiring around 10 L of drinks/day) and was treated with lithium, methylphenidate, pregabalin, and lorazepam. Polydipsia was mainly caused by lithium treatment with increased serum levels at that time (1.6–1.8 mmol/L; reference 0.4–1.2 mmol/L). Calcium serum levels were within the normal range, and, thereby, phosphate and parathyroid levels were not determined. In the further course, 13 teeth had to be extracted and were supplemented by dental prostheses; other teeth were crowned. At the age of 29 years, he also developed a paranoid hallucinatory episode with hearing voices and ideas of persecution under the treatment with methylphenidate, nortriptyline, quetiapine, pregabalin, and lorazepam. Recurrently, the patient received benzodiazepines, but, after this was stopped (by antagonization with flumazenil), a generalized tonic-clonic seizure occurred at the age of 29 years.

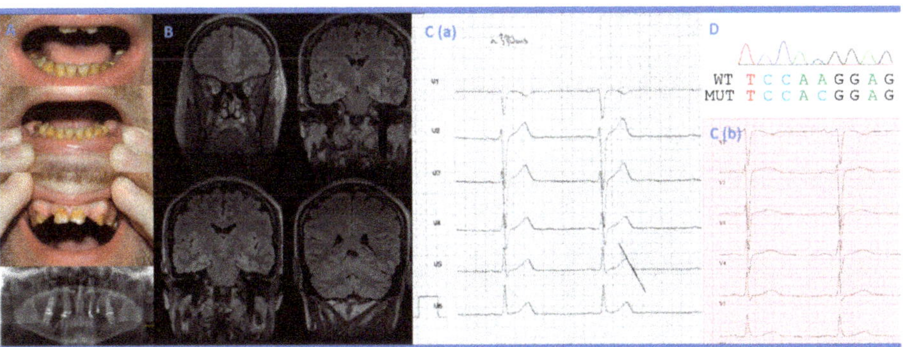

Figure 1. (**A**) The dental status at 29 years of age and the corresponding dental radiography showed a reduced density of several coronas and mild hypoplasia of the maxilla and mandible. (**B**) The cerebral magnetic resonance imaging of the patient revealed slight hippocampal damage on the left in the area of the corpus and the cauda, together with otherwise inconspicuous cerebral anatomic findings. (**C**) The baseline electrocardiography displayed a short QTc interval (heart rate 57/min, QT 330 ms, QTc: 324 ms; reference: > 350 ms; 3a) and normalization during treatment with quinidine (3 × 200 mg/d; QTc: 425 ms; reference: < 350 ms; 3b). (**D**) The DNA sequence electropherogram revealed a heterozygous state at position 2399 (c.2399A > C) in the *CACNA1C* gene predicted to result in p.Lys800Thr.

Electroencephalography at age 29, 33, and 34 years was inconspicuous. Analysis of the cerebrospinal fluid (CSF) revealed a borderline blood-brain barrier dysfunction (with CSF protein levels of 579 mg/L; reference: < 450 mg/L). The immunological screening showed an antinuclear antibody (ANA) titer of 1:100 (reference: < 1:50) and an IgA deficiency (0.26 g/L; reference: 0.7–4 g/L).

A highly symptomatic occurrence of the monomorphic VES was noted again during the subsequent in-patient hospital treatment at the age of 29 years. Further cardiologic evaluation showed ~12,000 VES/day during Holter ECG, and subsequently, due to the severe overall clinical course, the patient underwent ablation therapy in the area of the middle cardiac vein or coronary sinus twice, which reduced VES burden (remaining: 3600 VES/day). There was no evidence of a structural heart disease as assessed by transthoracic echocardiography. The family history was positive with his father suffering from depression, alcohol-dependency, tachycardia (treated with ß-blockers), and unclear dental damage (the patient had no contact with the father; therefore, further information is missing). The age of the mother at birth of the patient was 41 years, and the age of the father was 35 years.

Over the years, due to the severe course of the psychiatric symptoms, multiple psychopharmacological treatment trials have been carried out using varying and sometimes high doses (sertraline, fluoxetine, escitalopram, paroxetine, venlafaxine, vortioxetine, bupropion, nortriptyline, amitriptyline, clomipramine, lithium, methylphenidate, haloperidol, aripiprazole, perazine, promethazine, quetiapine, valproate, lamotrigine, carbamazepine, oxcarbazepine, pregabalin, levetiracetam, zonisamide, lacosamide, lorazepam, clonazepam, oxazepam, clobazam).

After complete discontinuation of psychotropic medication at the age of 31 years, a cardiac re-evaluation was performed, and a short QTc interval of 324 ms (Figure 1C; reference: > 350 ms) was noted for the first time. Overall, this resembled a (paradoxical) shortening of the QTc interval during a heart rate (HR) of 57 bpm; at a HR of 111 bpm, the QTc interval normalized (408 ms). There was no evidence of T-wave alternans. Due to suspected SQTS, quinidine treatment (3 × 200 mg/day) has been initialized to normalize repolarization, but also to reduce symptomatic VES burden and thereby indirectly to improve mental strength and personal stability. Of note, during treatment QTc intervals completely recovered (at 57/min: QRS 114 ms, QTc around 425 ms; T-wave: broad-based, biphasic; no early repolarization signs or Brugada sign; Figure 1C), and the burden of symptomatic VES was nearly absent (now: 16 VES/day).

2.2. Genetic Analyses

Genetic testing of genes related to SQTS (*KCNQ1*, *KCNH2*, *KCNJ2*, *CACNA1C*) revealed a heterozygous nucleotide variant in *CACNA1C* (NM_000719.6: c.2399A > C; p.Lys800Thr), which was very rare in control databases (MAF gnomAD: 0.00043%) and predicted to affect protein function by 16 of the 23 pathogenicity prediction algorithms (VarCards). The mutated lysine is located in the cytoplasmic loop between repeat II and repeat III of the Cav1.2 calcium channel and is highly conserved. To exclude pathogenic copy number variations (CNV) as a possible additional cause of ASD and the psychiatric symptoms, microarray-analysis was performed (CytoSureTM Constitutional v3 Array 180k, Oxford Gene Technology) in the patient. Molecular karyotyping did not show any pathogenic or relevant CNVs.

2.3. Electrophysiological Analyses

Heterologous expression studies of the mutant Cav1.2 calcium channel in *Xenopus* oocytes showed an isolated reduction in the current amplitude of the L-type calcium channels (Figure 2B,C) without a change in kinetic properties (Figure 2D–I) when compared with native (wild-type) channels. Here, the normalized bell-shaped current-voltage relationship and the voltage-dependence of activation were unaltered (Figure 2D–E). In addition, the voltage-dependence of inactivation (Figure 2F–G), the extent of inactivation (Figure 2H), and the kinetics of inactivation (Figure 2I) were similar as in wild-type channels. Thus, the genetic variant is responsible for an isolated reduction of the macroscopic current amplitudes of approximately 40% (Figure 2C). The lack of changes in the channel kinetics and maintained voltage-dependence of channel gating behavior suggest that this reduced current amplitude is most likely caused by an intracellular trafficking defect of the mutant Cav1.2 calcium channel.

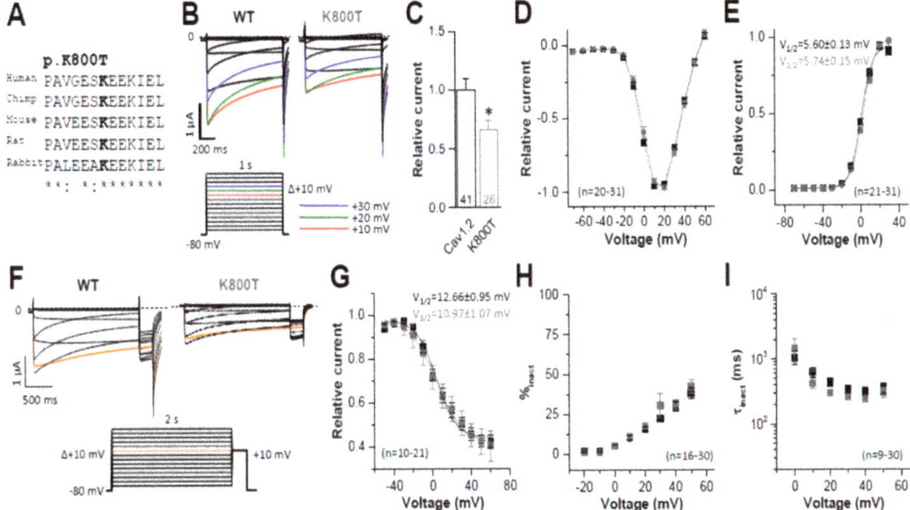

Figure 2. Own experimental analyses in the presented patient illustrated an isolated reduction in the current amplitude of L-type calcium channels without a change in kinetic properties. Two-electrode voltage-clamp measurements were performed in *Xenopus* oocytes, as previously described [2]. Ba^{2+} was used as a charge carrier, and for all experiments, Cav1.2 was co-expressed with the $\alpha 2\delta$ and $\beta 2b$ subunits [2]. In detail, the figure shows the following: (**A**) High evolutionary conservation of the K800 residue between different orthologues. (**B**) Representative current traces of wild-type (WT) Cav1.2 and mutant Cav1.2^{K800T} recorded with the indicated voltage protocol, in order to analyze the current amplitudes and the voltage-dependence of activation properties. (**C**) Reduced peak current amplitudes, analyzed at + 20 mV. (**D**) Normalized bell-shaped current voltage-relationship and (**E**) conductance-voltage (GV) relationship. The voltage of half-maximal activation (V1/2 act.) is indicated in the upper corner. (**F**) Representative current traces of wild-type Cav1.2 and Cav1.2^{K800T} recorded with the indicated voltage protocol, in order to analyze the inactivation properties. (**G**) Analyses of the voltage of half-maximal inactivation (V1/2 inact.). The V1/2 inact. values are provided in the upper corner. (**H**) Percentage of voltage-dependent inactivation of wild-type and Cav1.2^{K800T} analyzed at different voltage potentials. (**I**) Analyses of the time constant of voltage-dependent inactivation (τ inact.) of wild-type and Cav1.2^{K800T} analyzed at different voltage potentials. Numbers of experiments are indicted in the panels. Data are presented as mean $\pm$ s.e.m. * indicates $p < 0.05$.

With respect to these functional data, the p.Lys800Thr variant was classified as likely pathogenic (class 4 variant) according to the ACMG guidelines [11].

3. Discussion

The authors present a patient with a previously unpublished loss-of-function mutation of the *CACNA1C* gene with a novel, syndromal phenotype characterized by ASD, affective and psychotic exacerbations, dental enamel defect, and a short QT interval in the surface ECG.

The mutated *CACNA1C* gene (Chr. 12p13.3; 2,138 amino acids) encodes the α-subunit of the L-type calcium channel CaV1.2. These calcium channels are highly expressed in the brain and heart [3]. Genetic changes in *CACNA1C* are associated with Timothy syndrome or early repolarization disturbances/Brugada-like electrocardiography. However, patients with Timothy syndrome typically have gain-of-function mutations in the *CACNA1C* gene (e.g., p.Gly406Arg [2]), leading to maintained depolarizing L-type calcium current with long QT syndrome in the surface ECG and early sudden cardiac death (at an average age of 2.5 years; 3). Additionally, other cardiac features (AV conduction block with bradycardia, tachyarrhythmia, or congenital heart defects), neuropsychiatric involvement (developmental delays, seizures, ASD), hand/foot and facial findings (e.g., cutaneous syndactyly, low-set ears), hypoglycemia, and infections can be found in patients with Timothy syndrome [2]. Poor dental enamel was also reported earlier [3,12].

The presented case also suffered from high-functioning ASD, but he additionally presented with depressive and hypomanic episodes, as well as one paranoid hallucinatory episode. Such complex psychiatric syndromes are often found in patients with secondary, organic forms [1]. The genetic variant that has been classified finally as a likely pathogenic variant could explain the poor response to different psychotropic drugs in the patient's history. However, pharmacogenetic studies, e.g., on drug metabolism, have not been carried out. There were no signs of dysmorphia on the hands/feet or face in the presented patient. In addition, he suffered from poor dental enamel with severe caries, initially misinterpreted as "meth mouth" because of high-dose methylphenidate medication. Surprisingly, a short QT interval was first noted when the patient was off psychotropic drugs that typically prolong the QT interval and, in this particular case, led to a normalization. He also had a high burden of VES. Only just about 250 cases with short QT syndrome are currently known, however, these have either isolated cardiac phenotypes or acquired, concomitant conditions (e.g., electrolyte disturbances or carnitine deficiency), and to date only about 30 genetic variants in eight potential disease genes were identified (summarized in [13]). Most of these cases are due to gain-of-function mutations in the potassium channel genes (*KCNH2, KCNQ1, and KCNJ2*), whereas loss-of-function mutations in *CACNA1C* leading to SQTS are extremely rare, and, in these cases, the shortened QT interval is accompanied with a Brugada ECG phenotype (not seen in the present case). Due to controversial or absent functional data and contradictory in silico predictions, some of variants were re-classified as variants of uncertain significance following ACMG criteria (class 3 variant) in a recent publication [14]. Very recently, a *CACNA1C* loss-of-function variant has been linked with SQTS in combination with early repolarization patterns in the surface ECG [15].

The heterozygous c.2399 A > C variant in the presented patient is yet unreported, leading to a non-synonymous amino acid exchange in the α-subunit of the L-type calcium channel CaV1.2 (p.(Lys800Thr)). A causality of the mutation is possible because the gene mutation is located in a conserved gene region and is very rare in control databases. Most pathogenicity prediction programs that evaluate amino acid exchange in silico suggest a biochemical and thus pathogenic effect (VarCards: 16/23) as it has been shown by the in vitro data upon heterologous expression experiments. The variant finally could be classified as a class 4 variant ("likely pathogenic") according to the ACMG/AMP guideline [11]. Our functional studies revealed an isolated reduction of the current amplitudes (Figure 2C) without changes in the gating behavior of the channel. Therefore, a weak trafficking defect is the most likely mechanism of action for this atypical Cav1.2 channelopathy with brain, cardiac and dental enamel involvement.

4. Conclusions

In summary, this is a paradigmatic case of a secondary genetic variant of a complex, partially atypical mental disorder with heart and dental involvement. Many such secondary genetic variants probably occur, each of which is very rare, but, taken together, these rare variants might be causing a relevant subgroup of mental disorders. In the presented patient, a pathological variant can be assumed, which led to an atypical form of SQTS with a clinical spectrum that partially overlaps with that of Timothy syndrome. Associations between CaV1.2 channel (*CACNA1C*) polymorphisms and different psychiatric disorders, including autism, depression, bipolar disorder, and schizophrenia, were recently reported [16–19]. Further research will need to show whether similar cases exist and elucidate the therapeutic consequences that can be inferred from mutant Cav1.2 channel.

Author Contributions: D.E., P.S., F.S., E.S.-B., and L.T.v.E. treated the patient. D.E. performed the data research and wrote the paper. F.S. supported the literature search. N.D., I.R., K.V., and S.R. performed the experimental tests of calcium channels. E.S.-B. and B.S. performed *CACNA1C* testing and cardiac investigations and interpretation. E.S.-B. strongly revised the initial version of the paper. K.K. and A.T. examined the patient for signs of dysmorphia. B.G. performed and interpreted the microarray-analysis. N.D., M.A.S., K.R., K.N., and K.D. supported the overall interpretation and critically revised the manuscript. All authors were critically involved in the theoretical discussion and composition of the manuscript. All authors read and approved the final version of the manuscript.

Funding: The article processing charge was funded by the Baden-Wuerttemberg Ministry of Science, Research and Art and the University of Freiburg in the funding program Open Access Publishing.

Acknowledgments: Dominique Endres was funded by the Berta-Ottenstein-Programme for Advanced Clinician Scientists, Faculty of Medicine, University of Freiburg. Patrick Süß is a member of the research training group GRK2162 funded by the DFG (270949263/GRK2162) and is supported by the University Hospital Erlangen (ELAN project P059, IZKF clinician scientist program). Niels Decher was funded by the DFG (DE 1482/9-1). Florian Schuchardt received financial support from Forschungskommission, Medical Faculty, Albert-Ludwigs-University Freiburg.

Conflicts of Interest: Dominique Endres: None. Niels Decher: None. Isabell Röhr: None. Kirsty Vowinkel: None. Katharina Domschke: Steering Committee Neurosciences, Janssen. Katalin Komlosi: None. Andreas Tzschach: None. Birgitta Gläser: None. Miriam A. Schiele: None. Kimon Runge: None. Patrick Süß: None. Florian Schuchardt: None. Kathrin Nickel: None. Birgit Stallmeyer: None. Susanne Rinné: None. Eric Schulze-Bahr: None. Ludger Tebartz van Elst: Advisory boards, lectures, or travel grants within the last three years: Roche, Eli Lilly, Janssen-Cilag, Novartis, Shire, UCB, GSK, Servier, Janssen and Cyberonics.

References

1. Tebartz van Elst, L.; Pick, M.; Biscaldi, M.; Fangmeier, T.; Riedel, A. High-functioning autism spectrum disorder as a basic disorder in adult psychiatry and psychotherapy: Psychopathological presentation, clinical relevance and therapeutic concepts. *Eur. Arch. Psychiatry Clin. Neurosci.* **2013**, *263* (Suppl. S2), 189–196. [CrossRef] [PubMed]

2. Splawski, I.; Timothy, K.W.; Sharpe, L.M.; Decher, N.; Kumar, P.; Bloise, R.; Napolitano, C.; Schwartz, P.J.; Joseph, R.M.; Condouris, K.; et al. CaV1.2 Calcium Channel Dysfunction Causes a Multisystem Disorder Including Arrhythmia and Autism. *Cell* **2004**, *119*, 19–31. [CrossRef] [PubMed]

3. Napolitano, C.; Splawski, I.; Timothy, K.W.; Bloise, R.; Priori, S.G. Timothy Syndrome. In *GeneReviews®*; Adam, M.P., Ardinger, H.H., Pagon, R.A., Wallace, S.E., Bean, L.J.H., Stephens, K., Amemiya, A., Eds.; University of Washington: Seattle, WA, USA, 2006.

4. Walsh, M.A.; Turner, C.; Timothy, K.W.; Seller, N.; Hares, D.L.; James, A.F.; Hancox, J.C.; Uzun, O.; Boyce, D.; Stuart, A.G.; et al. A multicentre study of patients with Timothy syndrome. *Europace* **2018**, *20*, 377–385. [CrossRef] [PubMed]

5. Wemhöner, K.; Friedrich, C.; Stallmeyer, B.; Coffey, A.J.; Grace, A.; Zumhagen, S.; Seebohm, G.; Ortiz-Bonnin, B.; Rinné, S.; Sachse, F.B.; et al. Gain-of-function mutations in the calcium channel CACNA1C (Cav1.2) cause non-syndromic long-QT but not Timothy syndrome. *J. Mol. Cell. Cardiol.* **2015**, *80*, 186–195. [CrossRef] [PubMed]

6. Tebartz van Elst, L. *Das Asperger-Syndrom im Erwachsenenalter und Andere Hochfunktionale Autismus-Spektrum-Störungen*, 2nd ed.; Medizinisch Wissenschaftliche Verlagsgesellschaft: Berlin, Germany, 2015.

7. Tebartz van Elst, L.; Maier, S.E.; Fangmeier, T.; Endres, D.; Mueller, G.T.; Nickel, K.; Ebert, D.; Lange, T.; Hennig, J.; Biscaldi, M.; et al. Disturbed cingulate glutamate metabolism in adults with high-functioning autism spectrum disorder: Evidence in support of the excitatory/inhibitory imbalance hypothesis. *Mol. Psychiatry* **2014**, *19*, 1314–1325. [CrossRef] [PubMed]

8. Endres, D.; Tebartz van Elst, L.; Meyer, S.A.; Feige, B.; Nickel, K.; Bubl, A.; Riedel, A.; Ebert, D.; Lange, T.; Glauche, V.; et al. Glutathione metabolism in the prefrontal brain of adults with high-functioning autism spectrum disorder: An MRS study. *Mol. Autism* **2017**, *8*, 10. [CrossRef] [PubMed]

9. Lord, C.; Risi, S.; Lambrecht, E.H., Jr.; Leventhal, B.; DiLavore, P.C.; Pickles, A.; Rutter, M. The Autism Diagnostic Observation Schedule—Generic: A Standard Measure of Social and Communication Deficits Associated with the Spectrum of Autism. *J. Autism Dev. Disord.* **2000**, *30*, 205–223. [CrossRef] [PubMed]

Int. J. Mol. Sci. **2020**, *21*, 9029

Keywords: bioinformatics; human genetics; pharmacogenomics; autism

---

1. Introduction

Autism spectrum disorder (ASD) is a heterogeneous neurodevelopmental condition characterized by impairments in social interactions, delays in language development and patterns of restricted interests and/or repetitive behaviors [1]. ASD manifests along a wide distribution of core symptom severity and numerous health conditions present with ASD [2,3]. It is well-established that ASD has a predominantly genetic etiology, and genetic factors influence many of the medical conditions diagnosed with ASD [4,5]. Advancements in genomic technology are continually generating large amounts of data implicating various biological processes dysregulated in ASD. Notably, ASD is one of the most complex and prevalent neurodevelopmental conditions observed in humans, with a worldwide prevalence estimated at one in 160 children [6]. Furthermore, insufficient evidence exists substantiating efficacy of pharmaceutical treatment of specific symptoms and co-occurring conditions in ASD with many reported adverse events [7–9]. Informing more effective, personalized approaches for treatment of these heterogeneous conditions is a necessary area of research. An important next step is to better understand how current data can inform diagnosis and treatment of co-occurring conditions in ASD [10].

Fortunately, excellent tools are available to help circumvent challenges related to interpreting results from human genetic studies and offer immediate insight into mechanisms that are most likely to translate in the clinic setting [11–19]. While the definition of what constitutes 'clinically actionable' genetic information can vary and is dynamic [10], it is defined in this project as any functionally relevant, disease-implicated gene with evidence indicating a patient may have co-occurring condition that requires direct intervention, or that variation in the gene (or genetic mechanism) may influence how a patient will respond to a drug.

To initially identify all of the potential genetic factors that contribute to expression of a complex condition like ASD, it is necessary to compile results from many sources. These include statistical associations (e.g., genome-wide association study (GWAS) hits, rare variant burden test results, transmission disequilibrium test results) and functional evidence in humans and model organisms. Centralized repositories, like DisGeNET (https://www.disgenet.org/), integrate and uniformly annotate data and allow easy access to comprehensive knowledge of the genetic underpinnings of disease [17].

One way to facilitate interpretation of genetic results is to focus on implicated genes expressed in tissues relevant to the disease etiology [13,20–23]. As most evidence indicates that ASD relates to neurodevelopment [24], identifying ASD-associated genes that are expressed at appreciable levels in human brain tissue can rapidly prioritize genes that are more likely to be functionally relevant. Integrated databases, such as the Expression Atlas (https://www.ebi.ac.uk/gxa/home), offer results from large microarray and RNA-sequencing studies in humans (e.g., the Genotype Tissue Expression (GTEx) Project) and allow for efficient mining of data related to tissue-specific gene expression [13,22].

To further annotate those genes that are more likely to be functionally related to ASD etiology, it is useful to focus on genetic mechanisms evidenced to underlie ASD symptom expression. Notably, the biological functions of different genes implicated in ASD point to convergent mechanisms [25–27]. By identifying biological processes enriched for genes implicated in ASD and then focusing specifically on genes that influence these processes, genes of particular interest for functional follow-up and drug target repurposing or discovery can be readily classified [28–30]. Efforts to consistently describe gene products across databases, like the Gene Ontology (GO) Consortium [16], allow for identification of these larger, multi-gene processes. Furthermore, transgenic techniques in model organisms are incredibly useful for identifying genes with functional consequences relevant to human disease [31–33] and drug discovery [34]. On-going efforts by groups like the International Mouse Phenotyping Consortium (IMPC) offer web portals which allow for rapid mining of mouse phenotype data from knockout mutant strains for eventually every protein-coding gene in mice [35]. Determining the traits that are associated with knocking out specific genes may also offer insight into which genes are more likely to influence expression of co-occurring conditions in ASD.

The ultimate goal of precision medicine is to prevent disease; however, realization of this vision is likely many years away [36]. A key opportunity in precision medicine is to incorporate drug ontology and pharmacogenomics data to inform care and tailor treatment (i.e., maximize efficacy, minimize adverse events) [37,38]. An approach toward this goal is to determine if any of the proteins encoded by ASD candidate genes are targets for pharmaceutical compounds that are currently approved to treat symptoms and co-occurring conditions in ASD, or are potential novel targets based on evidence that they are chemically similar or function in the same mechanisms as approved drug targets [39,40]; integrated knowledge bases, like Pharos (https://pharos.nih.gov/), exist to identify these proteins [14]. It is also of interest to know whether a patient with a given variant will respond differently to medications. Resources such as the Pharmacogenomics Knowledge Base (PharmGKB; https://www.pharmgkb.org/) coalesce these data into a common portal [41].

To prioritize genes that may be clinically relevant, specifically with regard to co-occurring conditions, but have yet to be confirmed as having a causal relationship with human disease (i.e., pathogenic), it is advantageous to incorporate evidence related to genes with known pathogenic variants. Resources that define the clinical relevance of variants, like the American College of Medical Genetics (ACMG) [42] and ClinVar [18], can be used to identify these 'clinically actionable' genes. Furthermore, protein-protein interaction databases, like STRINGdb (https://string-db.org/), can be used to identify different genes with disparate variants that impact a common network [43]. By extension, protein interaction knowledge may identify candidate genes more likely to house pathogenic variants via revealing direct connections between their protein products and the products of genes with known pathogenic variants.

A major goal of our study is to develop an automated bioinformatics pipeline using the databases referenced above that can identify genes pulled from all published studies of ASD where variation may indicate a patient has a co-occurring condition that is important to treat, or are more likely to be useful for drug development and/or pharmacogenomics approaches to treatment of symptoms and comorbidities in patients with ASD. Each step of the pipeline is evaluated by comparing results for genes cited in connection with ASD to results for 1000 sets of *n* = 956 randomly selected human protein coding genes of equal number to the ASD gene set. Prioritized ASD genes are then queried against a gold standard, defined as expert curated evidence in ClinVar indicating that the gene has a pathogenic variant.

2. Results

At the time of these analyses, there were 956 unique protein coding genes with evidence for associations with ASD in the DisGeNET, which reflects expansive evidence from candidate gene studies, genome-wide genotyping, whole-exome/genome sequencing, and functional studies in human cell lines and model organisms (Supplementary Table S1). Notably, this initial list of ASD candidate genes included genes implicated via evidence from genetic studies of idiopathic ASD cases (e.g., *NLGN1*, *NLGN2*, *NLGN3*, *NLGN4X* and *NLGN4Y*), as well as genes pulled from studies evaluating syndromic cases of ASD (e.g., *FMR1*, *MECP2*, and *SHANK3*). All of the functional attributes used in our approach for prioritizing candidate genes had more ASD-related genes when compared to 1000 random sets, each with a random selection of 956 genes (Table 1). Ultimately, 18 ASD candidate genes were prioritized based on annotation in each step of the pipeline, which was more than the average number of genes from random gene sets ($X^2 = 11.30$, $p = 7.75 \times 10^{-4}$; Table 1).

Table 1. Comparisons of Functional Annotations for Autism Spectrum Disorder Candidate Genes to Random Genes.

Gene Attribute	ASD (*n*)	Random (mean ± sd)	X^2 (95%CI)	*p*-Value	*p*-Value$_{corrected}$
Brain Expressed	861	808.94 ± 11.01	21.36 (0.88, 0.92)	3.80×10^{-6}	5.07×10^{-6}
Associated Mouse Trait	88	68.89 ± 7.83	5.42 (0.07, 0.11)	1.99×10^{-2}	1.99×10^{-2}
Encodes Tclin	113	31.19 ± 5.45	219.18 (0.10, 0.14)	1.37×10^{-49}	6.98×10^{-49}
Encodes Tchem	148	80.76 ± 8.43	60.25 (0.13, 0.18)	8.35×10^{-15}	1.34×10^{-14}
Encodes Tbio	615	574.56 ± 14.99	6.96 (0.61, 0.67)	8.34×10^{-3}	9.53×10^{-3}
Encodes Tdark	51	253.28 ± 13.02	218.69 (0.04, 0.07)	1.74×10^{-49}	6.98×10^{-49}
Pharmacogenomic	124	52.15 ± 50.23	103.25 (0.11, 0.15)	2.96×10^{-24}	5.92×10^{-24}
ACMG Network	475	313.53 ± 13.25	122.98 (0.46, 0.53)	1.41×10^{-28}	3.76×10^{-28}
All Attributes	18	8.02 ± 2.56	11.30 (0.01, 0.03)	7.75×10^{-4}	-

Shown are the number of genes cited in connection with ASD in DisGeNET with pipeline attributes compared to the average number of genes across 1000 random sets. Included for each attribute are results of chi-square tests comparing the proportion of genes annotated in the ASD list (*n* = 956) to the average proportion of genes across all random lists. Uncorrected and Benjamini-Hochberg corrected *p*-values are included. Tclin = FDA-approved compound targets, Tchem = molecules with known properties similar to approved drug targets, Tbio = proteins with known biological or molecular functions but no known drug target properties, Tdark = proteins with relatively unknown function, sd = standard deviation, CI = confidence interval.

2.1. ASD Candidate Gene Expression in Human Brain

There were 861 (90.1%) ASD genes which were expressed at TPM $\geq$ 0.5 in at least one of the brain regions evaluated using available RNA-sequencing data from typical human tissue. This was increased when compared to random gene sets (84.6%, X^2 = 21.36, $p_{corrected}$ = 5.07×10^{-6}; Table 1). Notably, ASD-related genes were expressed at different levels in human brain tissue available in GTEx when compared to expression patterns of the random gene sets ($F_{(13,\ 13117)}$ = 2.19, Pillai = 0.002, p = 7.83×10^{-3}). These differences related almost entirely to increased levels of ASD gene expression in the pituitary gland ($F_{(1,\ 15317)}$ = 14.10, $p_{corrected}$ = 2.24×10^{-3}; Figure 1). No other evaluated brain regions showed evidence of differential expression of ASD genes compared to genes in the random sets (Supplementary Table S2).

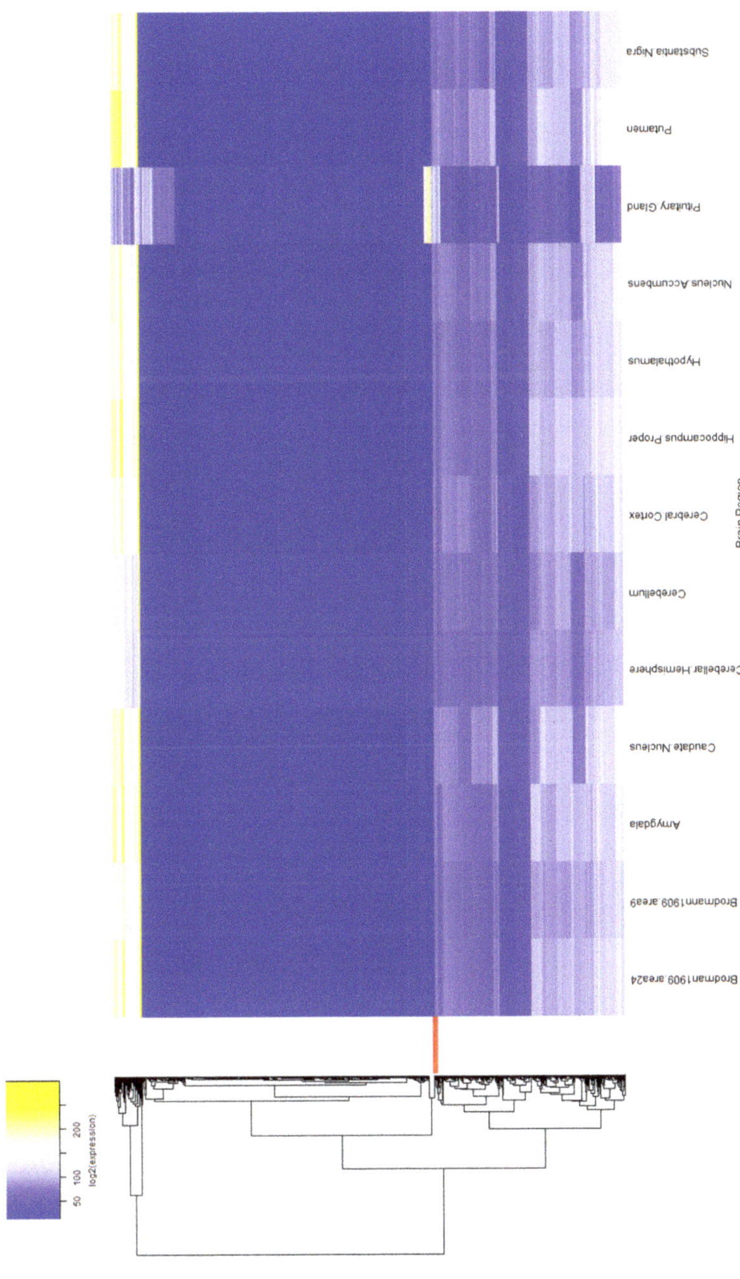

Figure 1. Brain Expression Profiles of ASD Candidate Gene Set and Random Gene Sets. Shown are average expression levels for ASD and random gene sets, based on transcripts per million, for each brain region obtained from typical human tissue in GTEx. Average expression of each gene set in the respective brain region are clustered based on Euclidean measures. The ASD risk gene cluster has been amplified for easier visualization and is highlighted in red on the *y*-axis.

2.2. ASD Candidate Genes Associated with Mammalian Phenotypes

There were 225 biological processes defined in humans and overrepresented in ASD candidate genes. There were also 258 processes defined in mice that were overrepresented among ASD gene mouse orthologs; 200 of these overlapped with biological processes overrepresented for ASD genes in humans (Supplementary Table S3). Products from 931 genes (96.5% of all ASD genes) were involved in these processes. Seven terms reflecting Mammalian Phenotypes (MP) defined in the IMPC were mapped to a GO-defined biological process overrepresented among the ASD genes. Phenotypes included 'abnormal postnatal growth/weight/body size' (MP:0002089), 'decreased body size' (MP:0001265), 'increased body size' (MP:0001264), 'abnormal nervous system morphology' (MP:0003632), 'abnormal brain development' (MP:0000913), and 'abnormal embryo development' (MP:0001672). These traits were represented by three top level terms (i.e., 'growth/size/body region phenotype' [MP:0005378], 'nervous system phenotype' [MP:0003631], 'embryo phenotype' [MP:0005380]). More ASD genes (9.2%) were associated with at least one trait under these top-level terms in mouse knockouts when compared to genes in the random sets (Table 1, $X^2 = 5.42$, $p_{corrected} = 1.99 \times 10^{-2}$). Specifically, more ASD genes were associated with abnormal postnatal growth/size/body region phenotypes when knocked out in mouse models (Table 2, $X^2 = 8.60$, $p_{corrected} = 1.01 \times 10^{-2}$). The most prevalent of these types of traits was 'decreased lean body mass' (MP:0002089), followed by 'decreased body length' (MP:0002089; Figure 2).

Table 2. Proportions of Autism Spectrum Disorder Genes Associated with Specific Top Level Mammalian Phenotypes.

Associated Mouse Trait	ASD (*n*)	Random (mean ± sd)	X^2 (95%CI)	*p*-Value	*p*-Value$_{corrected}$
Growth phenotype	63	43.59 ± 6.32	8.60 (0.05, 0.08)	3.37×10^{-3}	1.01×10^{-2}
Nervous system phenotype	18	12.16 ± 3.36	2.37 (0.01, 0.03)	1.23×10^{-1}	1.85×10^{-1}
Embryo phenotype	17	18.46 ± 4.18	0.05 (0.01, 0.03)	8.21×10^{-1}	8.21×10^{-1}

Shown are results comparing the number of ASD candidate genes that were associated with a mammalian phenotype reflecting overrepresented Gene Ontology Biological Processes defined in humans, compared to the average number of genes across 1000 random sets. Chi-square test results are based on the proportion of genes in the ASD list ($n = 956$) compared to the average proportion of genes across all random lists. Uncorrected and Benjamini-Hochberg corrected *p*-values are included. sd = standard deviation.

2.3. ASD Candidate Genes Influencing Drug Response

Compared to random genes, ASD candidate genes encoded more potential drug targets or contain variants that may inform pharmaceutical treatment (Table 1). Specifically, an increased proportion of genes cited in connection with ASD (11.8%) encode FDA-approved drug targets ($X^2 = 219.18$, $p_{corrected} = 6.98 \times 10^{-49}$), or had molecular properties similar to approved targets (15.5%, $X^2 = 60.25$, $p_{corrected} = 1.34 \times 10^{-14}$). Furthermore, more ASD genes (13.0%) contained variants with evidence for significant pharmacogenetic effects ($X^2 = 103.25$, $p_{corrected} = 5.92 \times 10^{-24}$).

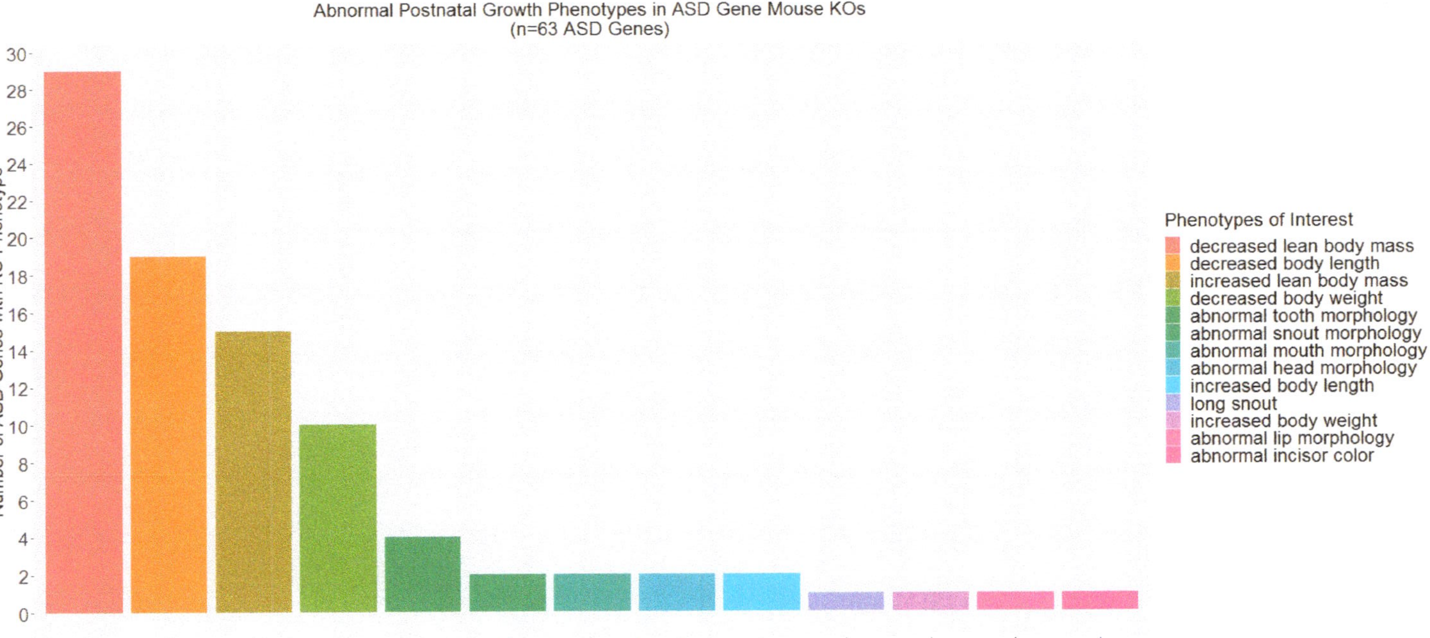

Figure 2. Frequency of Autism Spectrum Disorder-related Genes Associated with Abnormal Postnatal Growth Phenotypes. Shown are the specific traits that were associated more often with knocking out the 63 ASD candidate genes associated with growth phenotypes in mice (see Supplementary Table S1 for mouse trait associated genes) when compared to genes from random sets. Traits are presented in descending order based on the number of associated ASD genes.

2.4. ASD-ACMG Protein Interactions

There were nine ASD risk genes with evidenced pathogenic variants for which the ACMG recommends clinical testing (Supplementary Table S1). In addition, an increased proportion of proteins encoded by candidate genes (49.7%) had predicted direct interactions with proteins encoded by ACMG-recommended genes compared to proteins encoded by genes in the 1000 random sets (Table 1, $X^2 = 122.98$, $p_{corrected} = 3.76 \times 10^{-28}$). On average, ASD-related proteins formed six connections ($x = 6.32$, sd $= 14.20$) with ACMG proteins; however, there was no evidence that candidate proteins formed more connections when compared to proteins encoded by genes in any of the random sets ($X^2 = 824.34$, $p = 9.99 \times 10^{-1}$).

2.5. Evaluation of Pathogenic Variants in Prioritized ASD Candidate Genes

Of the 27,622 total genes harboring variants as curated in the September 2020 update of ClinVar (https://www.ncbi.nlm.nih.gov/clinvar/), 900 were genes cited in connection with ASD and 487 of these had a variant reported to be pathogenic or likely pathogenic. This represents approximately half (50.9%) of the full list of 956 ASD-related genes included in the DisGeNET. Of the 18 ASD-related genes that were prioritized via our pipeline (Figure 3), 78% ($n = 14$) had a variant reported to be pathogenic or likely pathogenic (Table 3, Supplementary Table S1).

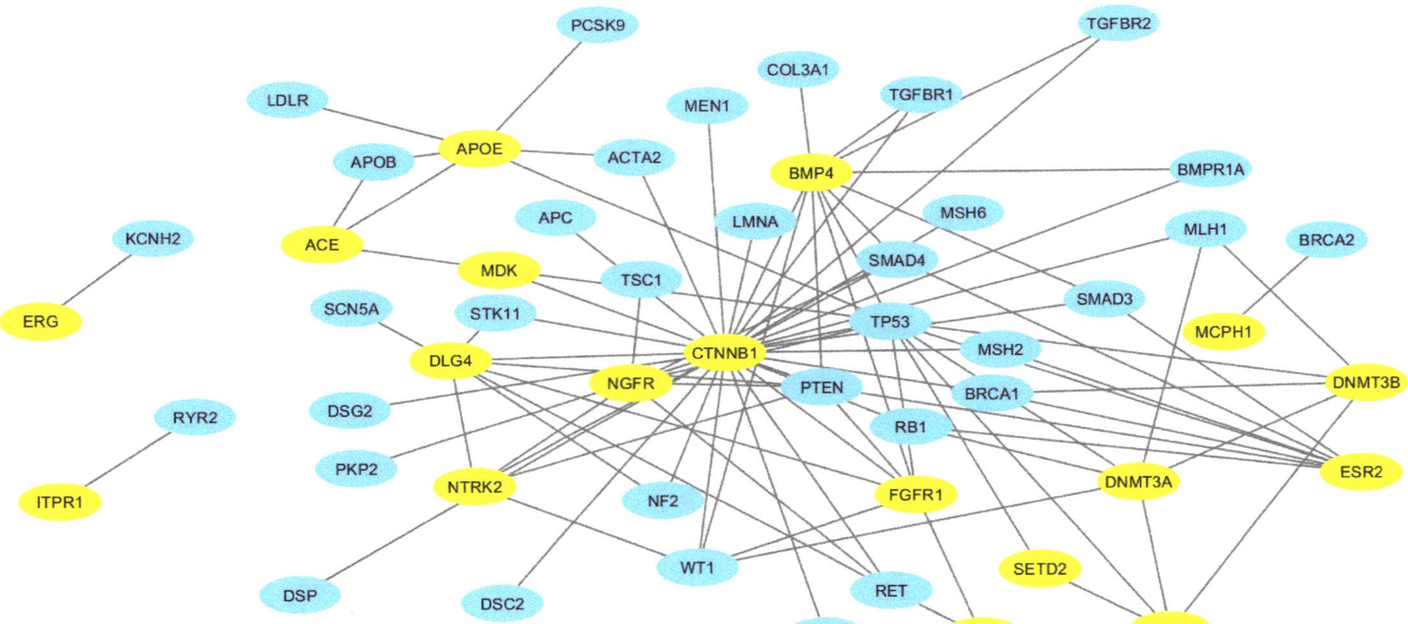

Figure 3. Prioritized ASD Proteins and ACMG Proteins Interaction Network. Shown are direct interactions predicted between proteins encoded by ASD candidate genes annotated in all pipeline categories and proteins encoded by American College of Medical Genetics (ACMG) recommended actionable genes. Top ASD-related proteins are highlighted in yellow, ACMG-recommended proteins in blue. Notably, none of the prioritized ASD genes were represented among the 59 genes compiled by the ACMG.

Table 3. Prioritized Genes with Pathogenic/Likely Pathogenic Variants.

ASD Gene	Brain Region (TPM)	Associated Mouse Trait (s)	Mapped GO BP	Drug Development	PharmGKB
APOE	Substantia Nigra (1141)	postnatal growth	growth	NA	PA55
DLG4	Cerebellar Hemisphere (232)	postnatal growth	growth	Tchem	NA
CTNNB1	Cerebellar Hemisphere (188)	postnatal growth	growth	Tchem	PA27013
FGFR1	Cerebellum (92)	embryo development	organism development	Tclin	NA
NTRK2	Brodman1909 area24 (91)	postnatal growth, nervous system morphology	growth, CNS development	Tchem	PA31818
ITPR1	Cerebellum (73)	embryo development	organism development	Tchem	NA
SETD2	Cerebellar Hemisphere (41)	postnatal growth, nervous system morphology	growth, CNS development	Tchem	NA
DNMT3A	Cerebellum (21)	postnatal growth, embryo development	growth, organism development	Tclin	PA27445
EHMT1	Cerebellum (14)	postnatal growth	growth	Tchem	NA
BMP4	Cerebellar Hemisphere (8)	nervous system morphology	CNS development	Tchem	NA
ACE	Pituitary (7)	embryo development	organism development	Tclin	PA139
DNMT3B	Cerebellar Hemisphere (6)	embryo development	organism development	Tchem	NA
MCPH1	Cerebellar Hemisphere (6)	postnatal growth	growth	NA	PA30701
ESR2	Pituitary (0.8)	postnatal growth	growth	Tclin	PA27886

Details are shown for the 14 Autism Spectrum Disorder (ASD) genes annotated in all functional categories included in the pipeline that had pathogenic variants defined in ClinVar. Included are human gene symbols, the brain region of highest expression in Genotype Tissue Expression (GTEx), traits associated in mouse knockouts, the corresponding Gene Ontology (GO) Biological Process (BP) defined in humans, the drug development level, and the PharmGKB ID for pharmacogenetic variant guidelines. TPM = transcripts per million, Tclin = FDA-approved compound targets, Tchem = molecules with known properties similar to approved targets, CNS = central nervous system, NA = not available.

3. Discussion

The central goal of this study was to build a bioinformatics pipeline to rapidly detect specific candidate genes that are more likely to be clinically relevant based on functional evidence and drug target properties. Compared to random gene sets, more ASD-related genes were expressed in control post-mortem brain tissue. In addition, more ASD genes were associated with postnatal growth phenotypes when knocked out in mice. Furthermore, ASD genes encoded more targets for FDA-approved drugs or bioactive molecules with drug-like properties, and more had a pharmacogenetic variant. Proteins encoded by ASD genes also showed more evidence for direct interactions with proteins encoded by the ACMG recommended clinically actionable genes. These results suggest that all of the functional categories incorporated in our pipeline were useful in identifying the candidate genes most likely to be functionally and clinically relevant. While there are numerous challenges limiting the clinical utility of information from genetic studies of complex conditions, the pipeline we developed addresses a key issue related to knowledge gaps among physicians regarding the benefits of genetic testing [44]. As incorporating genomic technology into patient care is largely dependent on clinicians' perspectives of its utility, it is important to identify ways to better inform clinicians about relevant genetic findings beneficial to optimizing treatment. Developing tools that summarize the extensive amounts of data available and present them in a manner that offers more immediate insights into the benefits for patient care is a necessary step toward more efficient integration of this knowledge into the clinic. Ultimately, we expect evidence from our pipeline will be useful in supporting clinical decisions regarding the benefits of genetic testing for optimizing treatment. Results from our work may also inform future research focused on drug repurposing, characterizing pleiotropic genetic effects connecting clinically distinct conditions or prioritizing genes for in vitro or in vivo studies aimed at elucidating molecular mechanisms underlying expression of symptoms in ASD.

3.1. ASD-Related Gene Expression in the Pituitary Is Increased Compared to Random Sets

Although more ASD genes overall were expressed in the brain, evidence of differential expression was limited to the pituitary. Genes cited in connection with ASD were expressed at higher levels here compared to genes included in the random sets. During embryogenesis, non-dysfunctional genetic regulation of pituitary gland development results in typical production of numerous hormones and the appropriate release of neuropeptides, like oxytocin and arginine vasopressin [45]. Many of the hormones and neuropeptides produced and regulated by the pituitary have been suspected to be disrupted in individuals with ASD, as well as other neuropsychiatric disorders [46]. Notably, brain region specific gene expression data were obtained from individuals without evidence of disease [13]. It is possible that in individuals with ASD, dysregulation of these pituitary-expressed genes results in the development of a dysfunctional pituitary and subsequent issues with neurotransmission of molecules important to expression of social and repetitive behaviors, which are core symptoms of ASD [47]. It is unclear why other brain regions did not show evidence of differential expression of ASD candidate genes when compared to random sets of genes. While we chose to use the GTEx resource, as these data are more readily accessible—and likely more generalizable to other conditions—compared to resources containing data generated from ASD brain tissue, this may limit the ability to understand genetic differences that may be unique to the brains of individuals with ASD. Specifically, it is hypothesized that brain regions involved in social behavior drive ASD symptomatology; these include the amygdala, orbitofrontal cortex, temporoparietal cortex and insula [48]. With the exception of the amygdala, gene expression in the precise brain regions that are proposed biomarkers for ASD are not quantified in the GTEx resource potentially explaining why our results were limited to the pituitary. As opposed to prioritizing genes solely based on brain expression, focusing future work on prioritizing genes that are differentially expressed in the brains of patients with ASD may be more useful to pinpointing clinically relevant genetic data for ASD specifically.

3.2. ASD-Related Genes Associated with Abnormal Postnatal Growth in Mouse Knockouts

ASD candidates were also more likely to be associated with growth/size/body region phenotypes when knocked out in mouse models included in the Knockout Mouse Phenotyping (KOMP) project. This result supports a risk model for neurodevelopmental disorders that reflects deviations from typical body size during development [49]. However, it should be noted that while the ambitious goal of the KOMP project is to eventually test for associations between the extensive phenotypes included in the pipeline and every protein coding gene in the mouse, a number of genes have yet to be evaluated. For example, the *Phosphatase and Tensin Homolog (PTEN)* gene was excluded during this annotation step. *PTEN* is well-known to contain pathogenic clinically-actionable variants and has not yet been tested via the KOMP pipeline (https://www.mousephenotype.org/data/genes/MGI:109583). This is likely due to the fact that this gene is an essential gene and is homozygous lethal as a null resulting in a limited embryo phenotype [50]. Notably, *PTEN* has been well studied in disease-specific mouse KO projects and these data are available via the Mouse Genome Informatics (MGI) resource (http://www.informatics.jax.org/marker/key/31908). Unfortunately, MGI data are not readily accessible via an application program interface (API), like the IMPC data, making it more difficult to incorporate into an automated pipeline. Furthermore, there may be bias introduced when incorporating evidence obtained from data generated in disease-specific studies as many of these focus on confirming reports in humans and may only test for specific traits reflecting the implicated human disease [51,52]. It is expected that as the IMPC database expands to include more genes, the automated gene prioritization pipeline we developed will also improve. Future work may focus on determining the level of contribution mouse model data adds to the prioritization accuracy of our pipeline. In addition, we may specifically incorporate information regarding embryonic lethal phenotypes as part of the gene annotations.

3.3. More ASD Genes Are Implicated in Drug Response

Also notable is more ASD genes encode molecules that are useful to drug development, supporting the ability to maximize drug efficacy while minimizing adverse events. As mentioned above, numerous treatment regimens using pharmaceutical compounds have been developed to address specific symptoms and co-occurring conditions in ASD; however, there is insufficient evidence supporting efficacy for many compounds with many reported adverse events [7–9]. Functional characterization of implicated genes that encode targets for drugs not currently used to treat symptoms in ASD may offer opportunity for repurposing [53]. Additionally, identifying genes that encode similar molecules to current targets may help pinpoint genes and pathways that should be fast-tracked for functional study as novel targets. Furthermore, as many individuals carry pharmacogenetic variants that influence drug response [54], identifying these variants in ASD genes that encode targets for drugs used to treat ASD symptoms is an important avenue of research that may provide results helpful toward more effective personalized treatment of symptoms in ASD.

3.4. More ASD-Related Proteins Interact with ACMG Gene Encoded Proteins

Genes that are recommended for testing by the ACMG are almost entirely those containing variants having a strong relationship with increased cancer risk [42,55]. Given the mounting evidence that much of the genetic architecture underlying expression of cancer is shared with ASD [56], it is interesting that more ASD proteins were predicted to directly interact with ACMG proteins. It is possible that these results support a connection between ASD and cancer etiology. Regardless, identifying specific ASD-related proteins that interact with cancer susceptibility proteins may be important for recognizing genes with disease-causing variants that should be evaluated at the bench and in the clinic.

3.5. Prioritized ASD Candidate Genes More Likely to Have Pathogenic Variants

Ultimately, the pipeline we developed identified a subset of ASD-related genes with a higher proportion of pathogenic or likely pathogenic variants compared to the initial list of genes cited in connection with ASD. This suggests the approach is useful to deciphering clinically relevant genetic results from all of the currently available evidence. Notably, the pipeline is also useful in a broader sense for functional annotation of gene lists to select genes that are worthy of further study. By automating this process as much as possible, clinically useful results for hundreds of genes implicated in ASD can be delivered rapidly.

3.6. Limitations and Future Directions

Limitations for each step in the pipeline and future work aimed at overcoming these limitations have been noted throughout. Additional limitations of the approach include the inability to automate the pipeline in its entirety. This is due to the availability of many of the resources utilized. As detailed in the Material and Methods, resources that were considered important for ensuring accuracy of the pipeline (e.g., DRSC Integrative Ortholog Prediction Tool, Ontology Mapping repository) did not have an API thereby requiring direct downloads of these data. A future goal to circumvent automation issue is to establish a database with cached data to allow for complete automation. In addition, the genetic landscape is dynamic, meaning results obtained at one specific time point represent only a snapshot of the available information, and this may be potentially misleading. Future work will focus on regularly incorporating updates into pipeline automation to ensure the most current evidence is incorporated.

4. Materials and Methods

A schematic of the entire functional annotation pipeline developed is provided in Figure 4. More specifically, an initial list of ASD candidate genes was identified by querying data available in the DisGeNET 6.0 database of human gene-disease associations [17], v1.1.0 update May 2019 (http://www.disgenet.org). The benefits of this database include gene-disease associations identified via text-mining of multiple sources and includes evidence from studies of idiopathic ASD cases (including cases from multiplex families and sporadic cases from simplex families), as well as studies conducted in individuals with underlying familial and non-familial syndromes. All Unified Medical Language System Concept Unique Identifiers (CUI) that relate to ASD were selected from the disease mappings file provided by DisGeNET and a data frame of genes with evidence for a relationship with CUIs relating to ASD was created. CUIs queried in DisGeNET were as follows: Autism Spectrum Disorders [C1510586], Autistic behavior [C0856975], and Autistic Disorder [C0004352], Autistic features [C1846135], Autistic spectrum disorder with isolated skills [C1298684].

Next, the list of 'ASD-related' genes were annotated to identify those expressed in the human brain. We used RNA-sequencing data from non-diseased brain tissue made available via the Genotype-Tissue Expression (GTEx) project, an ongoing collaborative effort to build a comprehensive public resource to study tissue-specific gene expression and regulation [13,57]. Genes expressed at a default cut-off of $\geq$ 0.5 transcripts per million (TPM) across all available brain regions in GTEx were downloaded from the Expression Atlas (https://www.ebi.ac.uk/gxa/home) and queried for ASD-related genes. Available brain regions included the amygdala ($n = 129$ individuals), anterior cingulate cortex ($n = 147$), caudate ($n = 194$), cerebellar hemisphere ($n = 175$), cerebellum ($n = 209$), frontal cortex ($n = 175$), hippocampus ($n = 165$), hypothalamus ($n = 170$), nucleus accumbens ($n = 202$), putamen ($n = 170$) and substantia nigra ($n = 114$).

To further identify genes encoding proteins that function in biological processes relevant to ASD etiology, conditional gene set overrepresentation analyses were conducted comparing candidate genes to all human protein coding genes included in Ensembl release 99 [58]. We used the parent-child algorithm from the TopGO R package version 2.38.1 (The R Foundation for Statistical Computing, Vienna, Austria) for overrepresentation analyses which incorporates knowledge about hierarchical relationships between GO terms into the calculation of statistical significance [59,60]. Significance was determined using Fisher's exact test and set at a Bonferroni-adjusted level of $\alpha = 0.05/n$ where n is the number of nodes tested. As a goal was to find genes with a phenotypic consequence when knocked out in mice, we then mapped human genes to the most likely mouse orthologs using the best match from all prediction tools available via the DRSC Integrative Ortholog Prediction Tool (Version 8.0 August 2019; https://www.flyrnai.org/diopt). Only orthologs that had a high rank, indicating that the number of tools that support the orthologous gene-pair relationship was ≥ 2, and that this ortholog had the best score in both forward and reverse mapping, were included in subsequent analyses [61]. Overrepresentation analyses were then conducted comparing mouse orthologs for ASD genes to all mouse protein coding genes as described above for human genes. Biological processes overrepresented for human ASD genes and mouse ASD gene orthologs were cross-referenced to identify overlap. We then mapped significantly overrepresented GO terms defined in both humans and mice to mammalian phenotype terms (MP) using direct mapping (i.e., distance = 1) from the

Ontology Mapping repository, OxO (https://www.ebi.ac.uk/spot/oxo, updated 11 September 2020), which is hosted by the Ontology Lookup Service [62]. The genotype-phenotype representational state transfer API from the IMPC (http://www.mousephenotype.org/) [63] was subsequently queried using the jsonlite R package v1.6.1 (The R Foundation for Statistical Computing, Vienna, Austria) [64] to prioritize genes that have a phenotypic consequence—associated with $p \leq 0.05$ in KOs of either sex—representing top level MP terms that reflect the ASD gene overrepresented GO-defined processes.

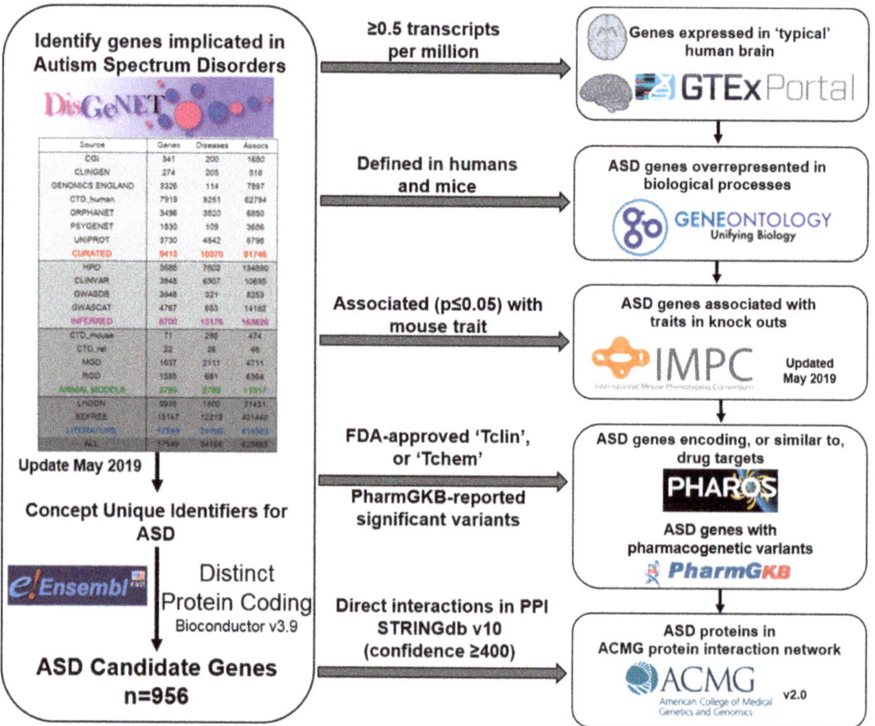

Figure 4. Candidate Gene Identification and Annotation Pipeline. All human protein coding genes defined in Ensembl, with evidence for influencing risk for concept unique identifiers reflecting Autism Spectrum Disorder (ASD) were identified from the DisGeNET resource which compiles evidence from all sources included in the corresponding table on the left side of the schematic. The initial list of 956 ASD candidate genes was then annotated using the publicly available resources included on the right side of the schematic, based on the criteria indicated above each arrow for each annotation step. TPM = transcripts per million, Tclin = FDA-approved compound targets, Tchem = molecules with properties similar to approved targets.

To identify genes encoding currently approved drug targets or those that may be novel drug targets, we used jsonlite to query the Pharos database (https://pharos.nih.gov/idg/api). Available drug development levels included: FDA-approved compound targets (Tclin), molecules with known properties similar to approved drug targets (Tchem), proteins with known biological or molecular functions but no known drug target properties (Tbio), and proteins with relatively unknown function (Tdark). To identify genes with pharmacogenetic variants evidenced to influence individual responses to drugs, we directly downloaded variant and clinical annotations data from PharmGKB (https://www.pharmgkb.org/downloads), update 20 March 2020. Only those associations that were reported in the literature as significant were used in annotations.

To decipher genes that are potentially actionable, protein-protein interactions between ASD candidate proteins and proteins currently recommend as clinically actionable by the ACMG were predicted using STRINGdb R package v10 (The R Foundation for Statistical Computing, Vienna, Austria) [65]. The ACMG 2016 update SF v2.0 [42] was used for network prediction (https://www. ncbi.nlm.nih.gov/clinvar/docs/acmg/). We focused on ASD-related proteins with evidence for direct interactions with proteins encoded by ACMG-recommended genes. We also calculated the quantity of direct interactions between proteins in this network. ACMG-ASD protein interaction networks were visualized using Cytoscape v3.5.1 (The Cytoscape Consortium, San Diego, CA, USA) [66].

To help show that the pipeline was useful for prioritizing clinically relevant candidate genes, we selected 1000 random sets of protein coding genes in humans (Ensembl release 99), while allowing for replacement, of equal number to the ASD gene list from biomaRt R package v 2.42.1 (The R Foundation for Statistical Computing, Vienna, Austria) [67] and annotated as described above. The one proportion test was used to determine if the proportion of genes in the ASD set that were annotated was increased compared to the average proportions of genes across all random sets (i.e., the expected proportion). Significance was based on a Benjamin-Hochberg false discovery rate corrected at $p \leq 0.05$. To determine if specific brain regions were enriched for ASD candidate gene expression compared to random genes, we used the limma package in R v 3.38.3 (The R Foundation for Statistical Computing, Vienna, Austria) [68]. The average expression of each gene set in the respective brain regions was clustered based on Euclidean measures. Tests for differences in the average gene expression of ASD genes and the average expression across genes in the random sets among brain regions were done using multivariate analysis of variance. Significance was based on a Benjamini-Hochberg false discovery rate corrected at $p < 0.05$. Kruskal-Wallis test was used to determine if the number of direct connections between ACMG-recommended gene encoded proteins were different across the ASD and random sets. Evidence included in ClinVar expanding upon current ACMG recommendations was also used as a gold standard reference to determine how often ASD genes with confirmed pathogenic or likely pathogenic variants were prioritized.

Supplementary Materials: Supplementary Materials can be found at http://www.mdpi.com/1422-0067/21/23/9029/s1.

Author Contributions: Conceptualization, O.J.V., M.G.B., S.H.E., B.A.M., J.S.S., J.H.M.; methodology, validation, investigation, formal analysis, data curation, and writing—original draft preparation, O.J.V.; writing—review and editing, M.G.B., S.H.E., B.A.M., J.S.S., J.H.M.; supervision, J.H.M.; funding acquisition, O.J.V. and J.H.M. All authors have read and agreed to the published version of the manuscript.

Funding: This research was funded by the National Library of Medicine, K01LM012870 (OJV) and R01LM010098 (JHM). The funders had no role in the design of the study; in the collection, analyses or interpretation of data; in the writing of the manuscript, or in the decision to publish the results.

Conflicts of Interest: The authors declare no conflict of interest.

Abbreviations

ACMG	American College of Medical Genetics
API	Application program interface
ASD	Autism spectrum disorder
CUI	Concept Unique Identifiers
FDA	Food and Drug Administration
GO	Gene ontology
GTEx	Genotype tissue expression
GWAS	Genome-wide association study
IMPC	International Mouse Phenotyping Consortium
KOMP	Knockout Mouse Phenotyping project
MGI	Mouse Genome Informatics
MP	Mammalian phenotype
PharmGKB	Pharmacogenomics Knowledge Base

References

1. American Psychiatric Association. *Diagnostic and Statistical Manual of Mental Disorders*, 5th ed.; American Psychiatric Association: Arlington, VA, USA, 2013.
2. Hyman, S.L.; Levy, S.E.; Myers, S.M.; Council on children with disabilities, section on developmental and behavioral pediatrics. Identification, Evaluation, and Management of Children with Autism Spectrum Disorder. *Pediatrics* **2020**, *145*. [CrossRef] [PubMed]
3. Bishop-Fitzpatrick, L.; Movaghar, A.; Greenberg, J.S.; Page, D.; DaWalt, L.S.; Brilliant, M.H.; Mailick, M.R. Using machine learning to identify patterns of lifetime health problems in decedents with autism spectrum disorder. *Autism Res. Off. J. Int. Soc. Autism Res.* **2018**, *11*, 1120–1128. [CrossRef] [PubMed]
4. Robert, C.; Pasquier, L.; Cohen, D.; Fradin, M.; Canitano, R.; Damaj, L.; Odent, S.; Tordjman, S. Role of Genetics in the Etiology of Autistic Spectrum Disorder: Towards a Hierarchical Diagnostic Strategy. *Int. J. Mol. Sci.* **2017**, *18*, 618. [CrossRef] [PubMed]
5. Hodges, H.; Fealko, C.; Soares, N. Autism spectrum disorder: Definition, epidemiology, causes, and clinical evaluation. *Transl. Pediatr.* **2020**, *9*, S55–S65. [CrossRef] [PubMed]
6. Elsabbagh, M.; Divan, G.; Koh, Y.-J.; Kim, Y.S.; Kauchali, S.; Marcín, C.; Montiel-Nava, C.; Patel, V.; Paula, C.S.; Wang, C.; et al. Global prevalence of autism and other pervasive developmental disorders. *Autism Res. Off. J. Int. Soc. Autism Res.* **2012**, *5*, 160–179. [CrossRef]
7. Scott, L.J.; Dhillon, S. Spotlight on risperidone in irritability associated with autistic disorder in children and adolescents. *CNS Drugs* **2008**, *22*, 259–262. [CrossRef]
8. Kolevzon, A.; Mathewson, K.A.; Hollander, E. Selective serotonin reuptake inhibitors in autism: A review of efficacy and tolerability. *J. Clin. Psychiatry* **2006**, *67*, 407–414. [CrossRef]
9. McPheeters, M.L.; Warren, Z.; Sathe, N.; Bruzek, J.L.; Krishnaswami, S.; Jerome, R.N.; Veenstra-Vanderweele, J. A systematic review of medical treatments for children with autism spectrum disorders. *Pediatrics* **2011**, *127*, e1312–e1321. [CrossRef]
10. Carter, T.C.; He, M.M. Challenges of Identifying Clinically Actionable Genetic Variants for Precision Medicine. *J. Healthc. Eng.* **2016**, *2016*. [CrossRef]
11. Cooper, D.N.; Stenson, P.D.; Chuzhanova, N.A. The Human Gene Mutation Database (HGMD) and Its Exploitation in the Study of Mutational Mechanisms. *Curr. Protoc. Bioinform.* **2005**, *12*, 1–13. [CrossRef]
12. Rouillard, A.D.; Gundersen, G.W.; Fernandez, N.F.; Wang, Z.; Monteiro, C.D.; McDermott, M.G.; Ma'ayan, A. The harmonizome: A collection of processed datasets gathered to serve and mine knowledge about genes and proteins. *Database J. Biol. Databases Curation* **2016**, *2016*. [CrossRef] [PubMed]
13. GTEx Consortium. The Genotype-Tissue Expression (GTEx) project. *Nat. Genet.* **2013**, *45*, 580–585. [CrossRef] [PubMed]
14. Nguyen, D.-T.; Mathias, S.; Bologa, C.; Brunak, S.; Fernandez, N.; Gaulton, A.; Hersey, A.; Holmes, J.; Jensen, L.J.; Karlsson, A.; et al. Pharos: Collating protein information to shed light on the druggable genome. *Nucleic Acids Res.* **2017**, *45*, D995–D1002. [CrossRef] [PubMed]
15. Eppig, J.T.; Smith, C.L.; Blake, J.A.; Ringwald, M.; Kadin, J.A.; Richardson, J.E.; Bult, C.J. Mouse Genome Informatics (MGI): Resources for Mining Mouse Genetic, Genomic, and Biological Data in Support of Primary and Translational Research. In *Systems Genetics*; Schughart, K., Williams, R.W., Eds.; Methods in Molecular Biology; Springer: New York, NY, USA, 2017; Volume 1488, pp. 47–73. ISBN 978-1-4939-6425-3.
16. Gene Ontology Consortium. Gene Ontology Consortium: Going forward. *Nucleic Acids Res.* **2015**, *43*, D1049–D1056. [CrossRef]
17. Piñero, J.; Bravo, À.; Queralt-Rosinach, N.; Gutiérrez-Sacristán, A.; Deu-Pons, J.; Centeno, E.; García-García, J.; Sanz, F.; Furlong, L.I. DisGeNET: A comprehensive platform integrating information on human disease-associated genes and variants. *Nucleic Acids Res.* **2017**, *45*, D833–D839. [CrossRef] [PubMed]
18. Landrum, M.J.; Lee, J.M.; Riley, G.R.; Jang, W.; Rubinstein, W.S.; Church, D.M.; Maglott, D.R. ClinVar: Public archive of relationships among sequence variation and human phenotype. *Nucleic Acids Res.* **2014**, *42*, D980–D985. [CrossRef] [PubMed]
19. Mooney, S.D.; Krishnan, V.G.; Evani, U.S. Bioinformatic tools for identifying disease gene and SNP candidates. *Methods Mol. Biol. Clifton NJ* **2010**, *628*, 307–319. [CrossRef]

20. Ferreira, M.A.R.; Jansen, R.; Willemsen, G.; Penninx, B.; Bain, L.M.; Vicente, C.T.; Revez, J.A.; Matheson, M.C.; Hui, J.; Tung, J.Y.; et al. Gene-based analysis of regulatory variants identifies 4 putative novel asthma risk genes related to nucleotide synthesis and signaling. *J. Allergy Clin. Immunol.* **2017**, *139*, 1148–1157. [CrossRef] [PubMed]

21. Pers, T.H.; Timshel, P.; Ripke, S.; Lent, S.; Sullivan, P.F.; O'Donovan, M.C.; Franke, L.; Hirschhorn, J.N.; Schizophrenia Working Group of the Psychiatric Genomics Consortium. Comprehensive analysis of schizophrenia-associated loci highlights ion channel pathways and biologically plausible candidate causal genes. *Hum. Mol. Genet.* **2016**, *25*, 1247–1254. [CrossRef]

22. Petryszak, R.; Keays, M.; Tang, Y.A.; Fonseca, N.A.; Barrera, E.; Burdett, T.; Füllgrabe, A.; Fuentes, A.M.-P.; Jupp, S.; Koskinen, S.; et al. Expression Atlas update—An integrated database of gene and protein expression in humans, animals and plants. *Nucleic Acids Res.* **2016**, *44*, D746–D752. [CrossRef]

23. Hardison, R.C. A guide to translation of research results from model organisms to human. *Genome Biol.* **2016**, *17*, 161. [CrossRef]

24. Ecker, C.; Bookheimer, S.Y.; Murphy, D.G.M. Neuroimaging in autism spectrum disorder: Brain structure and function across the lifespan. *Lancet Neurol.* **2015**, *14*, 1121–1134. [CrossRef]

25. Sanders, S.J.; He, X.; Willsey, A.J.; Ercan-Sencicek, A.G.; Samocha, K.E.; Cicek, A.E.; Murtha, M.T.; Bal, V.H.; Bishop, S.L.; Dong, S.; et al. Insights into Autism Spectrum Disorder Genomic Architecture and Biology from 71 Risk Loci. *Neuron* **2015**, *87*, 1215–1233. [CrossRef] [PubMed]

26. Voineagu, I.; Wang, X.; Johnston, P.; Lowe, J.K.; Tian, Y.; Horvath, S.; Mill, J.; Cantor, R.M.; Blencowe, B.J.; Geschwind, D.H. Transcriptomic analysis of autistic brain reveals convergent molecular pathology. *Nature* **2011**, *474*, 380–384. [CrossRef] [PubMed]

27. Johnson, M.R.; Shkura, K.; Langley, S.R.; Delahaye-Duriez, A.; Srivastava, P.; Hill, W.D.; Rackham, O.J.L.; Davies, G.; Harris, S.E.; Moreno-Moral, A.; et al. Systems genetics identifies a convergent gene network for cognition and neurodevelopmental disease. *Nat. Neurosci.* **2016**, *19*, 223–232. [CrossRef] [PubMed]

28. Mi, H.; Muruganujan, A.; Casagrande, J.T.; Thomas, P.D. Large-scale gene function analysis with the PANTHER classification system. *Nat. Protoc.* **2013**, *8*, 1551–1566. [CrossRef] [PubMed]

29. Rutherford, K.D.; Mazandu, G.K.; Mulder, N.J. A systems-level analysis of drug-target-disease associations for drug repositioning. *Brief. Funct. Genom.* **2018**, *17*, 34–41. [CrossRef]

30. Mohs, R.C.; Greig, N.H. Drug discovery and development: Role of basic biological research. *Alzheimers Dement.* **2017**, *3*, 651–657. [CrossRef]

31. Shulman, J.M.; Shulman, L.M.; Weiner, W.J.; Feany, M.B. From fruit fly to bedside: Translating lessons from Drosophila models of neurodegenerative disease. *Curr. Opin. Neurol.* **2003**, *16*, 443–449. [CrossRef]

32. Wang, J.; Al-Ouran, R.; Hu, Y.; Kim, S.-Y.; Wan, Y.-W.; Wangler, M.F.; Yamamoto, S.; Chao, H.-T.; Comjean, A.; Mohr, S.E.; et al. MARRVEL: Integration of Human and Model Organism Genetic Resources to Facilitate Functional Annotation of the Human Genome. *Am. J. Hum. Genet.* **2017**, *100*, 843–853. [CrossRef]

33. Ji, X.; Kember, R.L.; Brown, C.D.; Bućan, M. Increased burden of deleterious variants in essential genes in autism spectrum disorder. *Proc. Natl. Acad. Sci. USA* **2016**, *113*, 15054–15059. [CrossRef] [PubMed]

34. Sacca, R.; Engle, S.J.; Qin, W.; Stock, J.L.; McNeish, J.D. Genetically Engineered Mouse Models in Drug Discovery Research. In *Mouse Models for Drug Discovery*; Proetzel, G., Wiles, M.V., Eds.; Methods in Molecular Biology; Humana Press: Totowa, NJ, USA, 2010; Volume 602, pp. 37–54. ISBN 978-1-60761-057-1.

35. Koscielny, G.; Yaikhom, G.; Iyer, V.; Meehan, T.F.; Morgan, H.; Atienza-Herrero, J.; Blake, A.; Chen, C.-K.; Easty, R.; Di Fenza, A.; et al. The International Mouse Phenotyping Consortium Web Portal, a unified point of access for knockout mice and related phenotyping data. *Nucleic Acids Res.* **2014**, *42*, D802–D809. [CrossRef] [PubMed]

36. Collins, F.S.; Varmus, H. A new initiative on precision medicine. *N. Engl. J. Med.* **2015**, *372*, 793–795. [CrossRef] [PubMed]

37. Evans, W.E.; Relling, M.V. Pharmacogenomics: Translating functional genomics into rational therapeutics. *Science* **1999**, *286*, 487–491. [CrossRef] [PubMed]

38. Butler, M.G. Pharmacogenetics and Psychiatric Care: A Review and Commentary. *J. Ment. Health Clin. Psychol.* **2018**, *2*, 17–24. [CrossRef] [PubMed]

39. Hopkins, A.L.; Groom, C.R. The druggable genome. *Nat. Rev. Drug Discov.* **2002**, *1*, 727–730. [CrossRef]

40. Yang, H.; Qin, C.; Li, Y.H.; Tao, L.; Zhou, J.; Yu, C.Y.; Xu, F.; Chen, Z.; Zhu, F.; Chen, Y.Z. Therapeutic target database update 2016: Enriched resource for bench to clinical drug target and targeted pathway information. *Nucleic Acids Res.* **2016**, *44*, D1069–D1074. [CrossRef]

41. Thorn, C.F.; Klein, T.E.; Altman, R.B. Pharmacogenomics and bioinformatics: PharmGKB. *Pharmacogenomics* **2010**, *11*, 501–505. [CrossRef]

42. Kalia, S.S.; Adelman, K.; Bale, S.J.; Chung, W.K.; Eng, C.; Evans, J.P.; Herman, G.E.; Hufnagel, S.B.; Klein, T.E.; Korf, B.R.; et al. Recommendations for reporting of secondary findings in clinical exome and genome sequencing, 2016 update (ACMG SF v2.0): A policy statement of the American College of Medical Genetics and Genomics. *Genet. Med. Off. J. Am. Coll. Med. Genet.* **2017**, *19*, 249–255. [CrossRef]

43. Chen, J.Y.; Youn, E.; Mooney, S.D. Connecting protein interaction data, mutations, and disease using bioinformatics. *Methods Mol. Biol. Clifton NJ* **2009**, *541*, 449–461. [CrossRef]

44. Raghavan, S.; Vassy, J.L. Do physicians think genomic medicine will be useful for patient care? *Pers. Med.* **2014**, *11*, 424–433. [CrossRef] [PubMed]

45. McCabe, M.J.; Dattani, M.T. Genetic aspects of hypothalamic and pituitary gland development. *Handb. Clin. Neurol.* **2014**, *124*, 3–15. [CrossRef] [PubMed]

46. Iovino, M.; Messana, T.; De Pergola, G.; Iovino, E.; Dicuonzo, F.; Guastamacchia, E.; Giagulli, V.A.; Triggiani, V. The Role of Neurohypophyseal Hormones Vasopressin and Oxytocin in Neuropsychiatric Disorders. *Endocr. Metab. Immune Disord. Drug Targets* **2018**, *18*, 341–347. [CrossRef] [PubMed]

47. Harony, H.; Wagner, S. The contribution of oxytocin and vasopressin to mammalian social behavior: Potential role in autism spectrum disorder. *Neurosignals* **2010**, *18*, 82–97. [CrossRef]

48. Weston, C.S.E. Four Social Brain Regions, Their Dysfunctions, and Sequelae, Extensively Explain Autism Spectrum Disorder Symptomatology. *Brain Sci.* **2019**, *9*, 130. [CrossRef]

49. Raznahan, A. Sizing up the search for autism spectrum disorder (ASD) risk markers during prenatal and early postnatal life. *J. Am. Acad. Child Adolesc. Psychiatry* **2014**, *53*, 1045–1047. [CrossRef]

50. Di Cristofano, A.; Pesce, B.; Cordon-Cardo, C.; Pandolfi, P.P. Pten is essential for embryonic development and tumour suppression. *Nat. Genet.* **1998**, *19*, 348–355. [CrossRef]

51. Meehan, T.F.; Conte, N.; West, D.B.; Jacobsen, J.O.; Mason, J.; Warren, J.; Chen, C.-K.; Tudose, I.; Relac, M.; Matthews, P.; et al. Disease model discovery from 3,328 gene knockouts by The International Mouse Phenotyping Consortium. *Nat. Genet.* **2017**, *49*, 1231–1238. [CrossRef]

52. Brommage, R.; Powell, D.R.; Vogel, P. Predicting human disease mutations and identifying drug targets from mouse gene knockout phenotyping campaigns. *Dis. Model. Mech.* **2019**, *12*. [CrossRef]

53. Pushpakom, S.; Iorio, F.; Eyers, P.A.; Escott, K.J.; Hopper, S.; Wells, A.; Doig, A.; Guilliams, T.; Latimer, J.; McNamee, C.; et al. Drug repurposing: Progress, challenges and recommendations. *Nat. Rev. Drug Discov.* **2019**, *18*, 41–58. [CrossRef]

54. Van Driest, S.L.; Shi, Y.; Bowton, E.A.; Schildcrout, J.S.; Peterson, J.F.; Pulley, J.; Denny, J.C.; Roden, D.M. Clinically actionable genotypes among 10,000 patients with preemptive pharmacogenomic testing. *Clin. Pharmacol. Ther.* **2014**, *95*, 423–431. [CrossRef] [PubMed]

55. Green, R.C.; Berg, J.S.; Grody, W.W.; Kalia, S.S.; Korf, B.R.; Martin, C.L.; McGuire, A.L.; Nussbaum, R.L.; O'Daniel, J.M.; Ormond, K.E.; et al. ACMG recommendations for reporting of incidental findings in clinical exome and genome sequencing. *Genet. Med. Off. J. Am. Coll. Med. Genet.* **2013**, *15*, 565–574. [CrossRef] [PubMed]

56. Gabrielli, A.P.; Manzardo, A.M.; Butler, M.G. GeneAnalytics Pathways and Profiling of Shared Autism and Cancer Genes. *Int. J. Mol. Sci.* **2019**, *20*, 1166. [CrossRef] [PubMed]

57. GTEx Consortium. The GTEx Consortium atlas of genetic regulatory effects across human tissues. *Science* **2020**, *369*, 1318–1330. [CrossRef]

58. Aken, B.L.; Ayling, S.; Barrell, D.; Clarke, L.; Curwen, V.; Fairley, S.; Fernandez Banet, J.; Billis, K.; García Girón, C.; Hourlier, T.; et al. The Ensembl gene annotation system. *Database J. Biol. Databases Curation* **2016**, *2016*. [CrossRef]

59. Grossmann, S.; Bauer, S.; Robinson, P.N.; Vingron, M. Improved detection of overrepresentation of Gene-Ontology annotations with parent child analysis. *Bioinformatics* **2007**, *23*, 3024–3031. [CrossRef]

60. Alexa, A.; Rahnenführer, J.; Lengauer, T. Improved scoring of functional groups from gene expression data by decorrelating GO graph structure. *Bioinformatics* **2006**, *22*, 1600–1607. [CrossRef]

61. Hu, Y.; Flockhart, I.; Vinayagam, A.; Bergwitz, C.; Berger, B.; Perrimon, N.; Mohr, S.E. An integrative approach to ortholog prediction for disease-focused and other functional studies. *BMC Bioinform.* **2011**, *12*, 357. [CrossRef]

62. Perez-Riverol, Y.; Ternent, T.; Koch, M.; Barsnes, H.; Vrousgou, O.; Jupp, S.; Vizcaíno, J.A. OLS Client and OLS Dialog: Open Source Tools to Annotate Public Omics Datasets. *Proteomics* **2017**, *17*. [CrossRef]

63. Dickinson, M.E.; Flenniken, A.M.; Ji, X.; Teboul, L.; Wong, M.D.; White, J.K.; Meehan, T.F.; Weninger, W.J.; Westerberg, H.; Adissu, H.; et al. High-throughput discovery of novel developmental phenotypes. *Nature* **2016**, *537*, 508–514. [CrossRef]

64. Ooms, J. The jsonlite Package: A Practical and Consistent Mapping Between JSON Data and R Objects. *arXiv* **2014**, arXiv:1403.2805.

65. Szklarczyk, D.; Franceschini, A.; Wyder, S.; Forslund, K.; Heller, D.; Huerta-Cepas, J.; Simonovic, M.; Roth, A.; Santos, A.; Tsafou, K.P.; et al. STRING v10: Protein-protein interaction networks, integrated over the tree of life. *Nucleic Acids Res.* **2015**, *43*, D447–D452. [CrossRef] [PubMed]

66. Shannon, P.; Markiel, A.; Ozier, O.; Baliga, N.S.; Wang, J.T.; Ramage, D.; Amin, N.; Schwikowski, B.; Ideker, T. Cytoscape: A software environment for integrated models of biomolecular interaction networks. *Genome Res.* **2003**, *13*, 2498–2504. [CrossRef] [PubMed]

67. Smedley, D.; Haider, S.; Ballester, B.; Holland, R.; London, D.; Thorisson, G.; Kasprzyk, A. BioMart—Biological queries made easy. *BMC Genom.* **2009**, *10*, 22. [CrossRef]

68. Ritchie, M.E.; Phipson, B.; Wu, D.; Hu, Y.; Law, C.W.; Shi, W.; Smyth, G.K. Limma powers differential expression analyses for RNA-sequencing and microarray studies. *Nucleic Acids Res.* **2015**, *43*, e47. [CrossRef]

Publisher's Note: MDPI stays neutral with regard to jurisdictional claims in published maps and institutional affiliations.

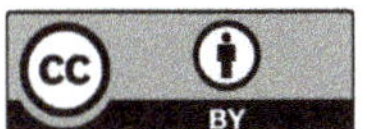

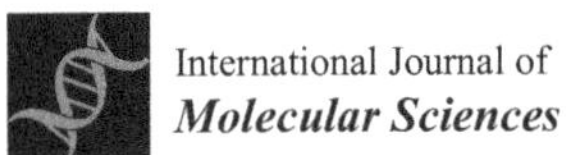

International Journal of
Molecular Sciences

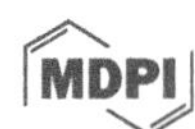

Article

Genomic, Clinical, and Behavioral Characterization of 15q11.2 BP1-BP2 Deletion (Burnside-Butler) Syndrome in Five Families

Isaac Baldwin [1,2,†], Robin L. Shafer [3,†], Waheeda A. Hossain [1,2], Sumedha Gunewardena [4], Olivia J. Veatch [1,4], Matthew W. Mosconi [3,5] and Merlin G. Butler [1,2,*]

[1] Department of Psychiatry & Behavioral Sciences, University of Kansas Medical Center, 3901 Rainbow Blvd. MS 4015, Kansas City, KS 66160, USA; ibaldwin2@kumc.edu (I.B.); whossain@kumc.edu (W.A.H.); oveatch@kumc.edu (O.J.V.)

[2] Department of Pediatrics, University of Kansas Medical Center, 3901 Rainbow Blvd. MS 4015, Kansas City, KS 66160, USA

[3] Schiefelbusch Institute for Life Span Studies and Kansas Center for Autism Research and Training, University of Kansas, Lawrence, KS 66045, USA; rshafer3@ku.edu (R.L.S.); mosconi@ku.edu (M.W.M.)

[4] Department of Molecular and Integrative Physiology, University of Kansas Medical Center, Kansas City, KS 66160, USA; sgunewardena@kumc.edu

[5] Clinical Child Psychology Program, University of Kansas, Lawrence, KS 66045, USA

* Correspondence: mbutler4@kumc.edu

† Represents co-first authorship.

Citation: Baldwin, I.; Shafer, R.L.; Hossain, W.A.; Gunewardena, S.; Veatch, O.J.; Mosconi, M.W.; Butler, M.G. Genomic, Clinical, and Behavioral Characterization of 15q11.2 BP1-BP2 Deletion (Burnside-Butler) Syndrome in Five Families. *Int. J. Mol. Sci.* **2021**, *22*, 1660. https://doi.org/10.3390/ijms22041660

Academic Editor: Paola Bonsi

Received: 15 January 2021
Accepted: 2 February 2021
Published: 7 February 2021

Publisher's Note: MDPI stays neutral with regard to jurisdictional claims in published maps and institutional affiliations.

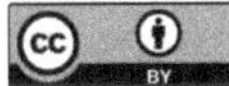

Abstract: The 15q11.2 BP1-BP2 deletion (Burnside-Butler) syndrome is emerging as the most common cytogenetic finding in patients with neurodevelopmental or autism spectrum disorders (ASD) presenting for microarray genetic testing. Clinical findings in Burnside-Butler syndrome include developmental and motor delays, congenital abnormalities, learning and behavioral problems, and abnormal brain findings. To better define symptom presentation, we performed comprehensive cognitive and behavioral testing, collected medical and family histories, and conducted clinical genetic evaluations. The 15q11.2 BP1-BP2 region includes the *TUBGCP5*, *CYFIP1*, *NIPA1*, and *NIPA2* genes. To determine if additional genomic variation outside of the 15q11.2 region influences expression of symptoms in Burnside-Butler syndrome, whole-exome sequencing was performed on the parents and affected children for the first time in five families with at least one parent and child with the 15q11.2 BP1-BP2 deletion. In total, there were 453 genes with possibly damaging variants identified across all of the affected children. Of these, 99 genes had exclusively de novo variants and 107 had variants inherited exclusively from the parent without the deletion. There were three genes (*APBB1*, *GOLGA2*, and *MEOX1*) with de novo variants that encode proteins evidenced to interact with CYFIP1. In addition, one other gene of interest (*FAT3*) had variants inherited from the parent without the deletion and encoded a protein interacting with CYFIP1. The affected individuals commonly displayed a neurodevelopmental phenotype including ASD, speech delay, abnormal reflexes, and coordination issues along with craniofacial findings and orthopedic-related connective tissue problems. Of the 453 genes with variants, 35 were associated with ASD. On average, each affected child had variants in 6 distinct ASD-associated genes ($\bar{x}$ = 6.33, sd = 3.01). In addition, 32 genes with variants were included on clinical testing panels from Clinical Laboratory Improvement Amendments (CLIA) approved and accredited commercial laboratories reflecting other observed phenotypes. Notably, the dataset analyzed in this study was small and reported results will require validation in larger samples as well as functional follow-up. Regardless, we anticipate that results from our study will inform future research into the genetic factors influencing diverse symptoms in patients with Burnside-Butler syndrome, an emerging disorder with a neurodevelopmental behavioral phenotype.

Keywords: 15q11.2 BP1-BP2 deletion; Burnside-Butler syndrome; clinical findings; cognition; neuropsychiatric behavior development; genomic characterization; exome sequencing; protein–protein interaction

147

1. Introduction

Chromosome 15 abnormalities have been reported for a number of years in the medical literature, specifically for Prader-Willi (PWS) and Angelman (AS) syndromes, the first examples of genomic imprinting in humans [1–4]. These disorders are generally due to a chromosome 15q11-q13 deletion depending on the parent-of-origin (i.e., PWS—paternal, AS—maternal). The typical 15q11-q13 deletions are classified as either Type I with deletions involving the proximal 15q breakpoint (BP1) and a distal 15q breakpoint (BP3), or Type II relating to a smaller 15q11-q13 deletion involving a second proximal breakpoint (BP2) and distal BP3. The larger Type I deletion is approximately 6 Mb and includes the *TUBGCP5*, *CYFIP1*, *NIPA1*, and *NIPA2* genes, while the smaller Type II deletion is approximately 5.5 Mb with all four genes intact [5].

Clinical and behavior differences have been reported for the past 15 years involving specific deletion classes in both PWS and AS. For example, individuals with PWS or AS having the Type I deletion, generally have more learning and behavioral problems compared to those with the Type II deletion [6,7]. Specifically, patients with PWS and larger deletions have more compulsions and maladaptive behaviors, as well as lower cognition, reading and math skills when compared to PWS patients with smaller deletions [3,5,6,8]. In AS, more impaired speech and seizure activity are noted in individuals with the larger deletion [4].

The emerging 15q11.2 BP1-BP2 microdeletion (Burnside-Butler) syndrome (BBS) encompasses the region between the PWS/AS chromosome 15q deletion breakpoints and includes the *TUBGCP5*, *CYFIP1*, *NIPA1*, and *NIPA2* genes. This microdeletion was consistently reported in early studies of patients presenting with unexplained behavioral, cognitive, and/or psychiatric problems [9–11]. Ho et al. [12] later summarized the results of ultra-high microarray single nucleotide polymorphism (SNP) analysis and found this microdeletion to be the most common cytogenetic finding observed in over 10,000 consecutive patients studied and presenting for genetic services with features of ASD or other neurodevelopmental disorders. Furthermore, a systematic literature review by Cox and Butler [10] found over 200 individuals reported with this microdeletion and grouped the clinical findings into five categories: (1) developmental, speech, and motor delays (73%, 67%, and 42% of cases, respectively); (2) dysmorphic ears and palatal anomalies (46%); (3) writing and reading impairment, memory problems, and verbal IQ scores $\leq$ 75 (50–60%); (4) general behavior problems, unspecified (55%); and (5) abnormal brain imaging, including a smaller brain surface with a thicker cortex (43%).

Notably, the four genes encoded in the 15q11.2 BP1-BP2 region are syntenic, bi-allelically conserved, and functionally predicted to interact with each other along with seven other genes (i.e., *IGFBP2*, *CFHR1*, *CFHR3*, *MNS1*, *SPG20*, *BMPR2*, and *SPAST*) recently reported and analyzed via in silico studies and STRING functional interactions network [13]. Rafi and Butler [13] also found that the encompassed four protein-coding genes showed 11 nodes and 34 edges. Network nodes represent proteins with splice isoforms or post-translational modifications collapsed into each node for all proteins produced by a single protein-coding gene. Edges represent protein–protein associations that jointly contribute to a shared function. These genes are at the center of our focus on genomics and clinical findings in individuals with the 15q11.2 BP1-BP2 deletion.

A major focus of our report is to identify variants if present in the non-deleted alleles of the four genes from the affected children in five unrelated families with the 15q11.2 BP1-BP2 microdeletion and characterize potential influences of genome-wide variation on symptom expression using whole-exome sequencing in trios. We assessed clinical, behavioral, and cognitive phenotypes as well as physical and motor development in relationship to genetic findings in each subject in separate families, the first study of its kind in this emerging syndrome.

2. Results

Five families were studied. Each family included one parent and at least one child with the 15q11.2 BP1-BP2 deletion, as confirmed by Methylation Specific-Multiplex Ligation Probe Amplification (MS-MLPA) assays. Each family was initially ascertained via the child having neurodevelopmental problems and/or ASD; chromosomal studies confirmed the 15q11.2 BP1-BP2 microdeletion. The parents were then cytogenetically analyzed to identify the deletion and five families with six affected children (three males and three females) were recruited for study.

2.1. Cognitive and Behavioral Features

Results of cognitive and behavioral testing obtained from members of five families with the 15q11.2 BP1-BP2 deletion are shown in Tables 1 and 2. In terms of general cognitive functioning, 9/11 individuals with 15q11.2 BP1-BP2 microdeletions performed in the average to superior range; whereas, one affected child (Subject 3) scored just below the normal range for full-scale IQ, and one affected child (Subject 11) was unable to complete cognitive testing due to limited receptive and expressive language understanding and severe developmental delay. Academic abilities (spelling, reading comprehension, and math) were broadly commensurate with individuals' cognitive abilities, though three individuals showed spelling abilities at least 1 standard deviation (SD) below their verbal abilities (Subjects 2, 3, and 9); one showed suppressed reading relative to verbal abilities (Subject 3), and one showed suppressed math relative to their nonverbal abilities (Subject 7). Verbal memory abilities appeared to be relatively intact among individuals. The majority of participants performed within 1 SD of the mean across subscales of the California Verbal Learning Test [14] (CVLT). Two participants (Subjects 1 and 3) scored below average on most subscales, however, and Subject 10 performed 1.5 SD below the mean on long delay recall and 3 SD below the mean on the recognition subscale. All individuals tested performed within the normal range or above on the Peabody Picture Vocabulary Test, Fourth Edition [15] (PPVT-4), indicating intact receptive language ability. Results from the Trail Making tests [16] indicated performance in the average to superior range across participants on Part A, demonstrating that psychomotor speed and planning was intact. In contrast, 4/10 participants showed performance on Part B that was greater than one 1 SD below their performance on Part A, suggesting the ability to rapidly and flexibly shift between response sets was selectively disrupted.

Results from Autism Diagnostic Observation Schedule, Second Edition [17,18] (ADOS-2) testing suggested 3/6 affected children met testing criteria for a classification of ASD (Subjects 2, 9, and 11; Subject 3 was 1 point below threshold). The Vineland Adaptive Behavior Scale, Third Edition [19] (VABS-III) indicated that all of the children in our cohort experienced deficits in a broad range of adaptive skills, with four of the six participants scoring two standard deviations below the population average on at least one subscale. For 6/7 affected children, rates and severity of repetitive behavior were comparable to children with ASD of similar ages [20]. The Broad Autism Phenotype Questionnaire [21] (BAP-Q) indicated autism-associated traits in 2/5 affected parents (Subjects 1 and 6) based on score thresholds defined by Sasson et al. [22]. Three of the five parents displayed repetitive behavior severity that was comparable to individuals with ASD of similar ages [20].

Table 1. Cognitive testing and results for families with 15q11.2 BP1-BP2 deletion.

Tests	Family A			Family B		Family C		Family D		Family E	
	52 yr Mother (Subject1)	15 yr Male (Subject2)	6 yr Male (Subject3)	54 yr Mother (Subject4)	16 yr Female (Subject5)	33 yr Mother (Subject6)	10 yr Male (Subject7)	37 yr Mother (Subject8)	9 yr Female (Subject9)	33 yr Father (Subject10)	6 yr Female (Subject11)
WASI-II IQ											
Perceptual	104	105	79	142	116	112	89	97	83	92	NT
Verbal	96	93	94	111	125	94	99	101	102	109	NT
Full Scale	100	99	84	128	124	103	93	99	92	101	NT
WRAT-IV											
Reading	92	103	75	98	115	95	99	99	112	128	NT
Math	96	82	88	124	116	97	72	90	100	105	NT
Spelling	96	75	79	125	134	109	85	106	87	102	NT
CVLT-II/CVLT-C											
Short Delay Free Recall	−1.5	0.5	−1.0	1.0	−0.5	0.5	0.0	1.0	−0.5	−0.5	NT
Short Delay Cued Recall	−1.5	0.5	−1.5	1.0	0.5	1.0	−1.0	0.5	−1.5	−0.5	NT
Long Delay Free Recall	−1.5	0.0	−2.5	1.0	0.5	1.0	−1.0	0.0	−0.5	−1.5	NT
Long Delay Cued Recall	−1.5	0.5	−2.5	1.0	0.5	0.5	−0.5	0.0	−1.0	−0.5	NT
Recognition	−2.5	0.5	0.5	0.0	−0.5	0.0	1.5	0.0	1.0	−3	NT
PPVT-4											
Total Score	99	119	120	107	130	106	107	97	104	104	NT
Trail Making Test											
Part A	130	129	92	126	99	110	88	111	107	119	NT
Part B	126	117	104	75	82	106	71	103	95	104	NT

Age in years (yr) and subject number for family members with the 15q11.2 BP1-BP2 deletion are indicated. NT: Not tested due to non-compliance. Scores for the CVLT are reported as z-scores (mean = 0, std = ±1), scores for all other measures are normed scores with mean = 100, std = ±15.

Table 2. Behavioral testing and results for families with 15q11.2 BP1-BP2 deletion syndrome.

Behavioral Tests	Family A			Family B		Family C		Family D		Family E	
	52 yr Mother (Subject1)	15 yr Male (Subject2)	6 yr Male (Subject3)	54 yr Mother (Subject4)	16 yr Female (Subject5)	33 yr Mother (Subject6)	10 yr Male (Subject7)	37 yr Mother (Subject8)	9 yr Female (Subject9)	33 yr Father (Subject10)	6 yr Female (Subject11)
ADOS-2											
RRB	NT	1	3	NT	0	NT	0	NT	4	NT	3 *
Social Affect	NT	11	3	NT	3	NT	4	NT	5	NT	19 *
Total (ASD Cutoff = 7)	NT	12	6	NT	3	NT	4	NT	9	NT	22 *
Classification	NT	Autism	Non-Autism	NT	Non-Autism	NT	Non-Autism	NT	Autism	NT	Autism
BAP-Q Total Score (cut-offs: M = 3.55, F = 3.17)	5.33	NT	NT	1.11	NT	3.67	NT	0.89	NT	3.28	NT
VABS-III (Standard Scores)											
Communication	NT	54	77	NT	97	NT	70	NT	69	NT	36
Daily Living	NT	60	82	NT	98	NT	92	NT	105	NT	46
Socialization	NT	40	82	NT	82	NT	80	NT	80	NT	51
Adaptive Behavior Composite	NT	55	78	NT	90	NT	59	NT	82	NT	48
RBS-R Overall Score	10	39	9	2	18	9	21	3	15	8	31

Age in years (yr) and subject number for family members with the 15q11.2 BP1-BP2 deletion are indicated. RRB: Restricted and repetitive behaviors, NT: not tested—measure was only administered to either parent or child cohort. * These results are from ADOS-2 Module 1 rather than Module 3.

151

2.2. Sensorimotor Ability

Group means, standard deviations, and effect sizes for postural control are reported in Table 3. Six children with the 15q11.2 BP1-BP2 deletion, six age- and sex-matched control children, five affected parents, and four age- and sex-matched control adults completed sensorimotor testing. Children with the 15q11.2 BP1-BP2 showed medium to large elevations in center of pressure (COP) length (d = −0.64) and variability in medial-lateral (ML) sway relative to control children (d = −0.70), and small increases in variability of anterior-posterior (AP) sway (d = −0.38). Affected parents showed large increases in COP length relative to control adults (d = −0.94), and these differences were medium for variability of AP sway (d = −0.61).

Table 3. Group comparisons of postural ability in children and adults with 15q11.2 BP1-BP2 deletion syndrome and matched controls.

Postural Control Variables	Children			Adults		
	BBS (*n* = 6)	Control (*n* = 6)		BBS (*n* = 5)	Control (*n* = 4)	
	Mean (SD)	Mean (SD)	Cohen's d	Mean (SD)	Mean (SD)	Cohen's d
COP Length (cm)	35.74 (21.37)	23.81 (15.36)	−0.641	19.45 (11.15)	11.95 (1.36)	−0.944
ML SD (log)	−0.49 (0.34)	−0.75 (0.40)	−0.702	−1.02 (0.31)	−1.06 (0.13)	−0.166
AP SD (log)	−0.32 (0.31)	−0.42 (0.15)	−0.383	−0.41 (0.32)	−0.57 (0.19)	−0.606

Group means and standard deviations (SD) for children and parents with the 15q11.2 BP1-BP2 deletion (BBS) and their matched controls as well as effect sizes (Cohen's *d*) for group comparisons. Negative effect sizes indicate greater variability for BBS children or adults relative to controls. COP: center of pressure, ML SD: medial-lateral standard deviation, AP SD: anterior-posterior standard deviation.

2.3. Whole-Exome Sequencing

The per sequence Phred quality scale was above 35 for all the samples and 99.5% of sequenced reads mapped to the genome, resulting in ~37.1 million mapped reads per sample. There were 67,994 variants identified across the dataset. Of these, 526 were identified as high confidence, potentially damaging variants (PDVs) located in 453 distinct genes in affected children (see Figure 1). Each affected child had an average of 100 PDVs ($\bar{x}$ = 100.33, sd = 15.97) affecting 88 different genes ($\bar{x}$ = 88.00, sd = 12.88). The most prevalent type of PDV were missense variants (36.009%), followed by frameshifts (15.83%), inframe insertions and deletions (InDels; 15.67%), splice site variants (9.17%), losses or gains of stop codons (10.84%), protein altering variants (0.67%), and losses of start codons (0.33%; Figure 2). Almost all types of variants had a proportion that were inherited, de novo, or of unknown inheritance (Figure 2). In total, 132 of PDVs identified in affected children were predicted de novo. Some variants that were de novo in one child were observed inherited in others. Notably, there were 99 distinct genes with PDVs that were exclusively de novo. In addition, there were 125 PDVs in 107 genes that were inherited exclusively from the parent without the deletion.

There were three genes with PDVs that were exclusively de novo evidenced to encode proteins that interact with the protein encoded by *CYFIP1* which is located in the region deleted in patients with BBS (Figure 3). These included an inframe deletion in *APBB1* in Subject 3, a missense mutation in *GOLGA2* in Subject 2, and a missense mutation in *MEOX1* in Subject 7. In particular, *APBB1* is associated with ASD (Supplemental Table S1). As noted above, Subject 3 was near the threshold for an ASD diagnosis based on the ADOS-2, and had a history of global developmental delay (Table 4). Notably, the location of the deletion identified in *APBB1* affects a region of the protein that contains simple sequence repeats (e.g., low-complexity region). As such, it is unclear whether or not this type of variation would influence phenotype expression.

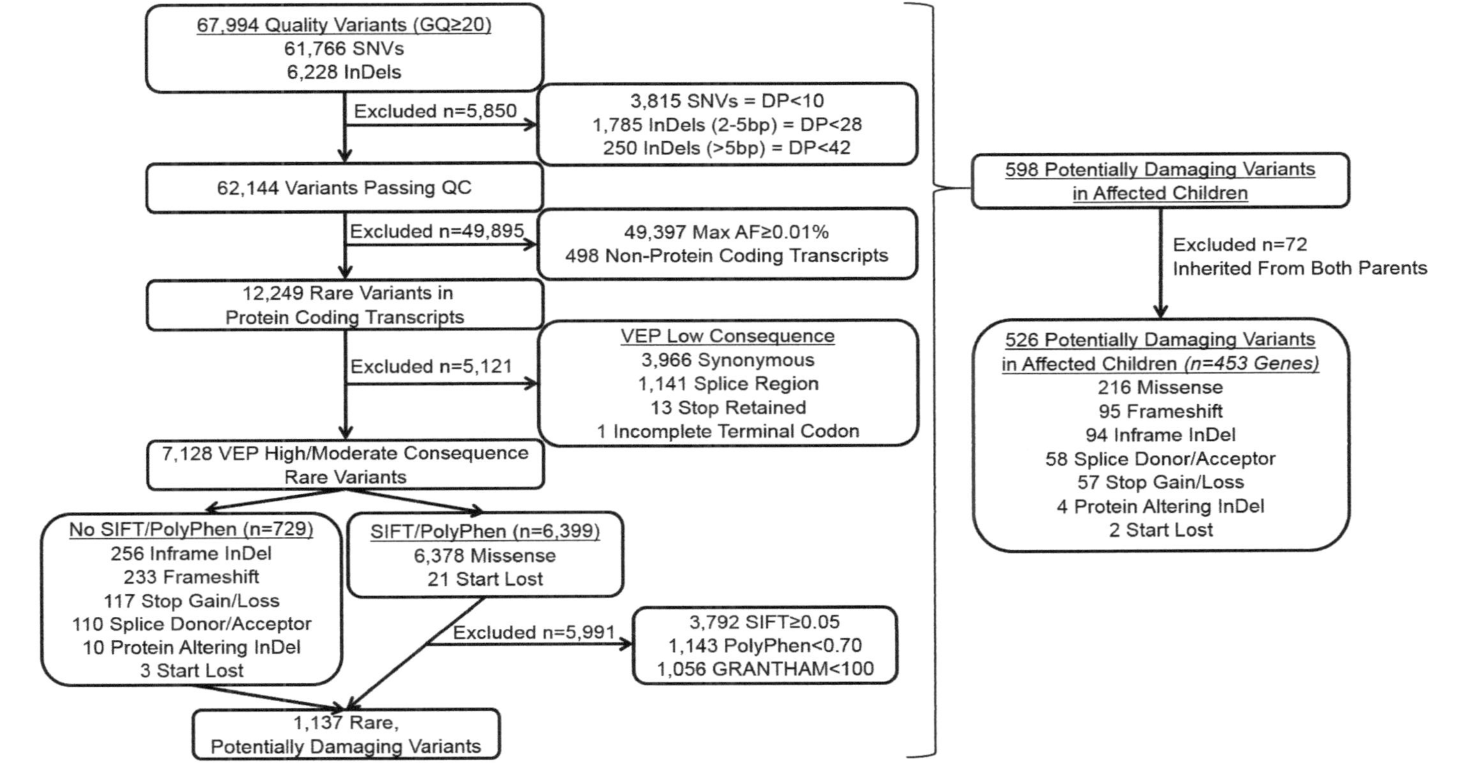

Figure 1. Quality control and variant selection. Overview of the criteria used to select high confidence, potentially damaging variants from whole-exome sequence data. Maximum allele frequencies (Max AF) were based on the maximum observed frequency across all reference populations available in the 1000 Genomes Project, the European Standard Population, and the Genome Aggregation Database. Abbreviations: GQ = genotype quality, SNVs=single nucleotide variant, InDels = insertion/deletion variant, DP = depth, VEP = Variant Effect Predictor.

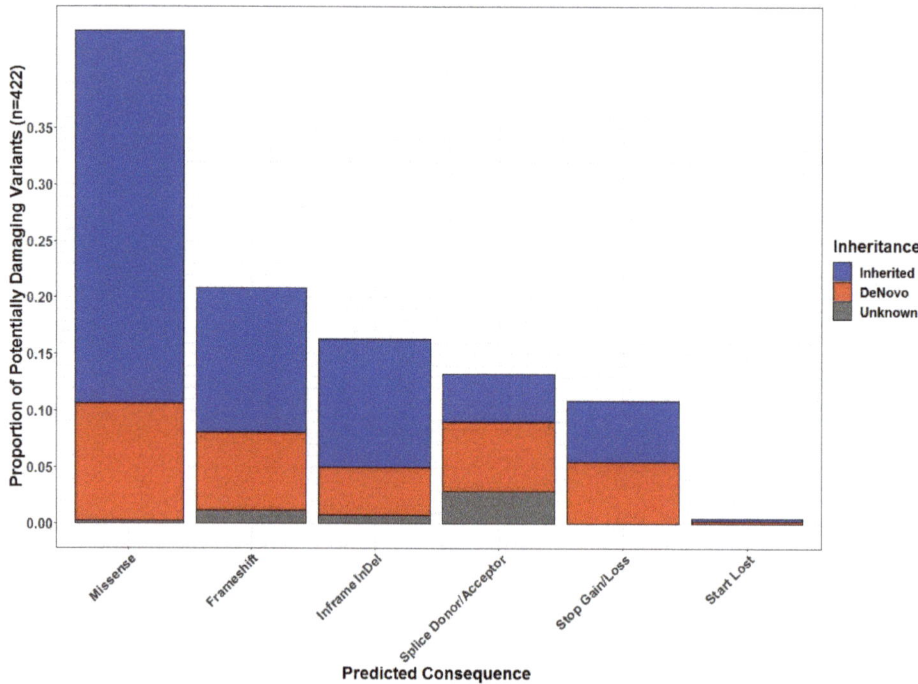

Figure 2. Predicted protein consequences of potentially damaging variants in affected children (Families A–D). Shown are the frequencies of Variant Effect Predictor consequences for variants identified in five affected children that were highly or moderately likely to damage the protein product. Data were not included for the affected child from Family E as the parents' data were unavailable. Colors indicate variant consequences that were inherited (blue), de novo (crimson), or unknown (grey = uncharacterized Mendelian violations, or improbable homozygous de novo).

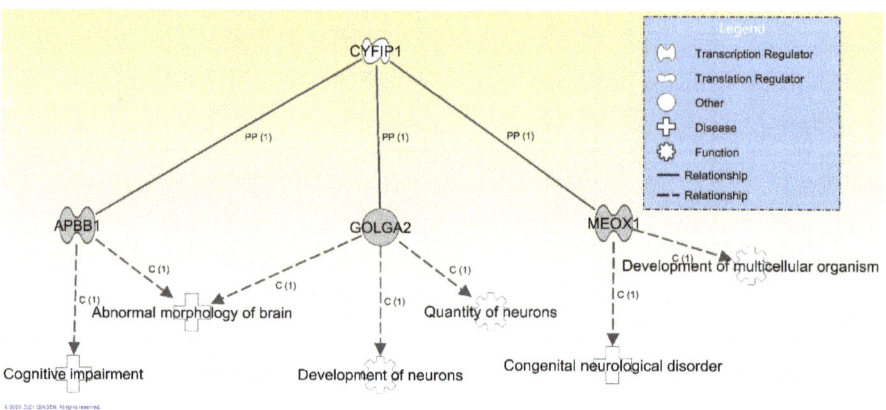

Figure 3. Genes with de novo variants with evidence for downstream relationships with *CYFIP1*. Shown are three genes prioritized following Ingenuity Pathway Analysis of all genes with de novo variants in affected children that were evidenced to be involved in the etiology of diseases relevant to symptoms observed in affected children. Included are protein–protein interactions (PP) and diseases and functions where variation in the gene is causal (C).

Table 4. Medical history of families with 15q11.2 BP1-BP2 deletion.

Medical History	Family A			Family B		Family C		Family D		Family E	
	52 yr Mother (Subject1)	15 yr Male (Subject2)	6 yr Male (Subject3)	54 yr Mother (Subject4)	16 yr Female (Subject5)	33 yr Mother (Subject6)	10 yr Male (Subject7)	37 yr Mother (Subject8)	9 yr Female (Subject9)	33 yr Father (Subject10)	6 yr Female (Subject11)
Prenatal	Mother age 46 yr			Pre-eclampsia		Gestational diabetes					
Birth		C-section	C-section		C-section		C-section				
Birth weight		3.4 kg (30th%)	3.6 kg (50th%)				3.7 kg (55th%)				3.8 kg (75th%)
Neuro-develop-mental	Learning difficulties	Autism spectrum disorder	Global develop-mental delay				Dyslexia, regression		Learning difficulties		Regression at 12mo
Neuro-psychiatric	Depression	ADHD, OCD, anxiety			ADHD, GAD, OCD, social phobia, selective mutism		ADHD, OCD, ODD				Sleep disturbance
Neurological			Non-essential tremor			Right calf paresthesia	Epilepsy		Hypotonia, fine and gross motor delay		Epilepsy (Lennox-Gastaut syndrome)
Eye				Astigmatism					Left strabismus		No retinal folds
Musculo-skeletal			Leg braces, ankle instability	Herniated disc lumbar 5	Kyphosis, hyper-flexible	Scoliosis		Scoliosis			
Motor		Weak postural control, walked at 16 mo	Fine and gross motor delay, walked at 25 mo				Walked at 12 months		Crawled at 20 months, walked at 26 months		Sat at 13mo, crawled at 18mo, poor balance and coordination
Cardio-vascular	Hyper-tension Hyper-lipidemia				Patent foramen ovale, Postural hypotension					Hyper-tension	
Respiratory					Asthma						
Gastro-intestinal			Consti-pation						Consti-pation		
Skin			Easy bruising, delayed healing		Eczema, delayed healing						
Endocrine	Diabetes mellitus			Post-partum thyroiditis	Delayed bone age, delayed growth	Gestational diabetes					
Reproductive	PCOS										
Immunologic				Thymic hyper-trophy	Anaphy-laxis						

Age in years (yr) and subject number for family members with the 15q11.2 BP1-BP2 deletion are indicated. PCOS—polycystic ovarian syndrome, ADHD—attention deficit hyperactivity disorder, OCD—obsessive compulsive disorder, ODD—oppositional defiant disorder, GAD—generalized anxiety disorder.

There were also genes with PDVs inherited exclusively from the parent without the 15q11.2 BP1-BP2 deletion that encoded proteins interacting with the products of two genes encoded in the deleted region, *CYFIP1* and *TUBGCP5* (Figure 4). Specifically, missense mutations were identified in two genes. These included *FAT3* where a PDV was observed in Subject 2; Subject 3 had the same variant in this gene and a variant in *GOLGA2*. Neither of these genes are associated with ASD or included on any of the evaluated clinical testing panels.

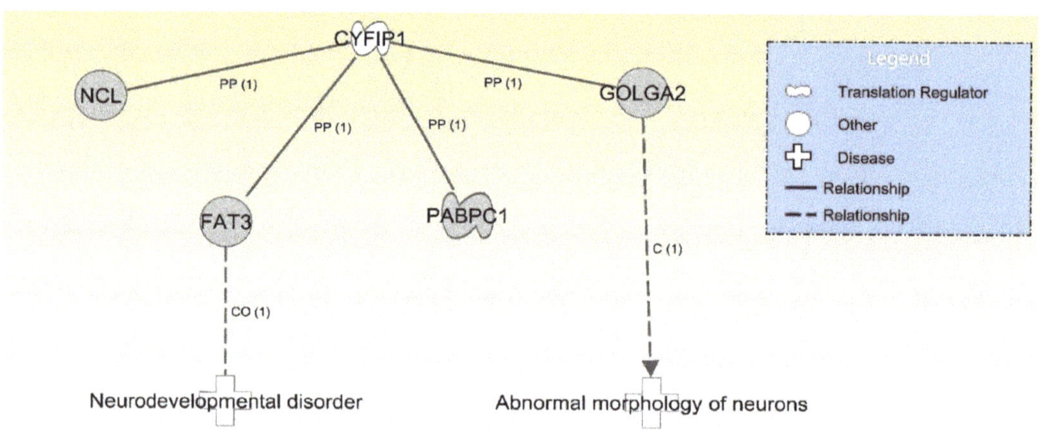

Figure 4. Genes with variants transmitted from non-deleted parents to affected children with evidence for downstream relationships with *CYFIP1*. Shown are genes prioritized following Ingenuity Pathway Analysis of all genes with variants in affected children that were inherited from parents without the 15q11.2 BP1-BP2 microdeletion that were also evidenced to be involved in the etiology of diseases relevant to symptoms observed in affected children. Included are protein–protein interactions (PP) and diseases and functions where variation in the gene is causal (C) or correlated (CO).

Other genes of interest with PDVs were identified based on associations with clinical and physical findings in affected subjects as described in Tables 1, 2, 4 and 5. Notably, an average of 17 genes ($\bar{x}$ = 17.3, sd = 5.3) with PDVs in each patient were associated with ASD. As seen in Figure 5, Subject 2 had the most ASD-associated genes with PDVs (n = 25). Compared to other affected children, Subject 2 also had the most severe repetitive behaviors measured via the Repetitive Behavior Scale – Revised [23] (RBS-R) and the most severe ADOS-2 score (Table 2). In addition, all affected children had PDVs in multiple genes that were included on clinical testing panels for intellectual disability ($\bar{x}$ = 8.7, sd = 4.7), ataxia ($\bar{x}$ = 6.8, sd = 2.9), epilepsy ($\bar{x}$ = 6.2, sd = 2.8), comprehensive cardiovascular defects ($\bar{x}$ = 2.8, sd = 1.1), and neuronal migration disorders ($\bar{x}$ = 2.0, sd = 1.1). There were four subjects with PDVs in genes included on the cerebral cortical malformations panel, almost all of whom had some evidence of neurological issues (Tables 4 and 5). Additionally, of note, both Subjects 7 and 11 had PDVs in genes included on the testing panel for cleft palate—*GLI2* and *FOXE1*, respectively— and had craniofacial malformations involving the mouth (Table 5). In addition, Subject 5 inherited a stop-loss variant in a connective tissue disorder gene, *FLCN*, from the parent with the deletion (Subject 4) both of whom had a history of musculoskeletal findings (Table 4). More details for all genes with PDVs meeting our inclusion criteria are provided in the Supplemental Table S1.

157

Table 5. Specific clinical evaluation and physical exam findings of families with 15q11.2 BP1-BP2 deletion.

Physical Exam	Family A			Family B		Family C		Family D		Family E	
	52 yr Mother (Subject1)	15 yr Male (Subject2)	6 yr Male (Subject3)	54 yr Mother (Subject4)	16 yr Female (Subject5)	33 yr Mother (Subject6)	10 yr Male (Subject7)	37 yr Mother (Subject8)	9 yr Female (Subject9)	33 yr Father (Subject10)	6 yr Female (Subject11)
Head circumference	57.3 cm (75th%)	56.6 cm (75th%)	51.5 cm (50th%)	56.8 cm (90th%)	53.3 cm (25th%)	56.2 cm (50th%)	54.2 cm (85th%)	55.5 cm (50th%)	55.7 cm (>97th%)	57.8 cm (75th%)	49.5 cm (25th%)
Inner canthal distance	3.3 cm (75th%)	2.9 cm (50th%)	2.7 cm (50th%)	3.2 cm (75th%)	3.2 cm (75th%)	2.5 cm (3rd%)	3.2 cm (75th%)			3.1 cm (50th%)	3.0 cm (50th%)
Outer canthal distance	8.3 cm (25th%)	8.6 cm (50th%)	7.3 cm (3rd%)	8.4 cm (25th%)	8.3 cm (25th%)	8.0 cm (3rd%)	8.4 cm (50th%)			9.2 cm (75th%)	8.7 cm (75th%)
Right hand length	19.2 cm (97th%)	20.2 cm (97th%)	15.6 cm (97th%)	16.3 cm (3rd%)	17.0 cm (25th%)	18.2 cm (75th%)	15.6 cm (25th%)	16.6 cm (25th%)	15.8 cm (75th%)	19.0 cm (75th%)	13.3 cm (50th%)
Right middle finger length	8.3 cm (75th%)	8.8 cm (97th%)	6.7 cm (97th%)	7.2 cm (3rd%)	7.6 cm (25th%)	7.6 cm (25th%)	6.9 cm (50th%)	7.2 cm (3rd%)	6.8 cm (75th%)	8.1 cm (75th%)	5.2 cm (25th%)
Right ear length	7.4 cm (75th%)	6.7 cm (75th%)	6.2 cm (75th%)	6.8 cm (75th%)	6.1 cm (50th%)	6.8 cm (75th%)	6.4 cm (75th%)	6.2 cm (50th%)	5.7 cm (25th%)	NA	5.7 cm (50th%)
Weight	110 kg (>95th%)	67.1 kg (80th%)	26.3 kg (90th%)	67.1 kg (75th%)	45.8 kg (10th%)	89.1 kg (>95th%)	32.5 kg (50th%)	79.3 kg (90th%)	35.5 kg (80th%)	123.2 kg (>95th%)	27.6 kg (>95th%)
Height	176 cm (>95th%)	182 cm (95th%)	137 cm (>95th%)	158 cm (20th%)	158 cm (20th%)	158.5 cm (20th%)	139 cm (50th%)	159 cm (25th%)	142 cm (90th%)	178 cm (50th%)	NA
BMI	35.5 (>95th%)	24.9 (90th%)	14.0 (5th%)	26.9 (85th%)	18.3 (20th%)	35.5 (>95th%)	16.8 (50th%)	31.4 (95th%)	17.6 (70th%)	38.9 (>95th%)	NA
Head/Facial features		Soft ears, fold easily	Broad, soft ears	Small upper incisor (#10)	Small upper incisor (#10)		Flat occiput, fleshy ears, thin upper lip, and flat philtrum		Right ear overfolded	Broad, round face	Broad, round face, broad nose, full lips, prominent jaw, forehead, and ears, depressed nasal bridge
Eyes		Pigment changes, Sensitive to light	Pigment changes, Sensitive to light		Left pupil larger than right	Mild left ptosis	Mild bilateral ptosis (L > R)			Myopia, right sided ptosis	
Back	No scoliosis	No scoliosis	Right shoulder higher than left, no scoliosis	Mild scoliosis	Kyphosis, right shoulder droop		Mild scoliosis				
Upper extremities			Hyper-extensibility: Beighton score 6/9		Hyper-extensibility: Beighton score 7/9, cubitus valgus					Broad hands	Soft fleshy, broad hands

Table 5. *Cont.*

Physical Exam	Family A			Family B		Family C		Family D		Family E	
	52 yr Mother (Subject1)	15 yr Male (Subject2)	6 yr Male (Subject3)	54 yr Mother (Subject4)	16 yr Female (Subject5)	33 yr Mother (Subject6)	10 yr Male (Subject7)	37 yr Mother (Subject8)	9 yr Female (Subject9)	33 yr Father (Subject10)	6 yr Female (Subject11)
Lower extremities			Second toes overlap third, plantar creases, flat feet, ankle instability on pronation	Left leg longer than right, knee-buttock asymmetry	Knee-buttock asymmetry, flat feet		Left leg longer than right	Flat feet	Flat feet		
Other musculo-skeletal							Pectus carinatum				Large body size
Skin	Birth mark on thigh	Soft, fleshy	Loose, soft, velvety	Eczema	Soft with freckles		Soft				Birth marks on thigh and forehead
Neurological					Increased deep tendon reflexes	Decreased sensation right lateral calf		Decreased deep tendon reflexes	Decreased muscle tone and reflexes in all extremities		Toe walking, poor coordination and balance

Age in years (yr) and subject number for family members with the 15q11.2 BP1-BP2 deletion are indicated.

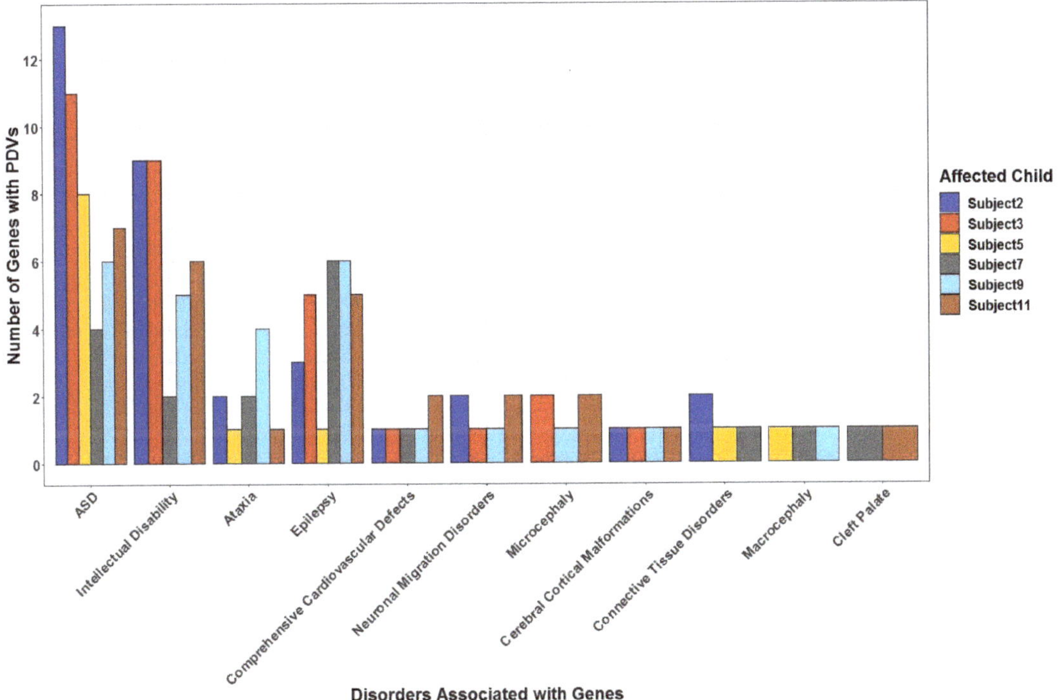

Figure 5. Number of genes with possibly damaging variants (PDVs) in each affected child associated with disorders of interest. Shown are the total number of genes with PDVs on the y-axis, that are also evidenced to be involved in the conditions on the x-axis. For autism spectrum disorder (ASD), evidence was based on the Simons Foundation for Autism Research Institute gene list. For other conditions, evidence was based on inclusion on clinical testing panels from Clinical Laboratory Improvement Amendments (CLIA) approved and accredited commercial laboratories.

3. Discussion

This study is the first of its kind to characterize phenotypic, behavioral, and cognitive measures combined with exome sequencing in families with the 15q11.2 BP1-BP2 deletion. An initial goal was to determine if the sequences of one or more of the four genes in the 15q11.2 BP1-BP2 region showed a variant inherited from the parent with the intact (non-deleted) chromosome. When disturbed, the four genes in the 15q11.2 region are associated with cognitive impairment, speech and/or motor delay, dyslexia, and psychiatric/behavioral problems (e.g., attention deficit hyperactivity disorder (ADHD), autism, schizophrenia, or psychosis). The cardinal disease associations for the four contiguous genes in the 15q11.2 BP1-BP2 region are: *NIPA1*—Spastic Paraplegia 6; *NIPA2*—Angelman syndrome and Prader-Willi syndrome; *CYFIP1*—fragile X syndrome and autism; and *TUBGCP5*—Prader-Willi syndrome. The four genes are individually associated with PWS, ASD, schizophrenia, epilepsy, and Down syndrome. Collectively, all four genes have been associated with up to 75% of patients with ten distinctive neurodevelopmental disorders [13].

The addition of newly reported findings including ataxia, poor coordination, seizures, and congenital anomalies including palatal, heart, and ear defects along with structural brain disturbances [11] which are also associated with the four genes in the 15q11.2 BP1-BP2 region raises the question of whether these genes interact with other genes, their biological processes or molecular functions. These related genes may play a role in the clinical presentation causing core features of Prader-Willi and Angelman syndromes as additional clinical structural differences are seen in those with the four genes deleted in the typical 15q11-q13 Type I deletion seen in these syndromes. For example, dysfunctional variation in the *NIPA1* and *NIPA2* genes could impair the function of magnesium transport as both genes encode magnesium transporters [24,25]. Their biological processes and molecular functions could regulate axonogenesis and axon extension via relationships with bone morphogenetic protein (BMP) and signaling pathways, regulations of cellular and developmental growth, and interaction with the *FMR1* gene causing fragile X syndrome [13]; all pertinent and relevant to the reported variable clinical phenotypes seen in this microdeletion syndrome. We used whole-exome sequence data to identify other genes outside of the deleted region with possibly damaging variants to help detect genetic effects underlying expression of symptoms in the affected child bringing the family to medical attention. Detailed physical examinations and family pedigrees were performed, for the first time, by an experienced clinical geneticist trained as a dysmorphologist to characterize the phenotype and review of systems on each subject. In addition, cognitive and behavior testing, including motor assessments for ataxia or balance disturbances of each family member, were performed using various validated techniques and tests by experts in the field. These studies were the major outcome measures for comparison with the genomic data and analysis for similarities among our families with the 15q11.2 BP1-BP2 deletion.

3.1. Clinical and Neuropsychiatric Behavior Developmental Findings

We did not identify consistent patterns of cognitive impairments across individuals with 15q11.2 BP1-BP2 microdeletion syndrome. General cognitive, academic, and receptive vocabulary abilities were relatively intact with only one participant, Subject 11, not able to complete standardized IQ testing, showing indications of intellectual/developmental delay. Similarly, verbal memory abilities appeared to be unaffected across the majority of participants, though 3/10 participants showed mild deficits in suggesting that more selective issues in verbal memory and learning may impact a subset of individuals with the 15q11.2 BP1-BP2 microdeletion. Similarly, multiple participants (4/10) showed executive deficits characterized by a reduced ability to flexibly shift response sets. These participants were largely nonoverlapping with those showing verbal memory issues indicating that these cognitive effects may be relatively distinct across individuals with 15q11.2 BP1-BP2 deletion syndrome. Several children had a history of learning problems reported by parents, school records, or neuropsychological evaluations.

Our results suggest that individuals with 15q11.2 BP1-BP2 deletions have increased risk for ASD. The prevalence of ASD in the general population is estimated to be 1 in 54 (1.8%) [26]; however, in our sample, we found that 3/6 (50%) of affected children met testing standards for a diagnosis of ASD and 2/5 (40%) of affected parents demonstrated elevated autistic traits (one additional child, Subject 3, and one additional parent, Subject 10, scored just below the cutoff for the ADOS-2 and BAP-Q, respectively). Consistent with high rates of ASD and ASD-related traits in our sample, we observed high rates of repetitive behavior in a majority of our participants with 5/6 affected children and 3/5 adults demonstrating severity of repetitive behavior that is comparable to similarly aged persons with ASD [20]. Of note, our sample of 15q11.2 BP1-BP2 deletion carriers (parents) may actually underrepresent the prevalence of ASD in the population of these carriers since persons who are parents and those who volunteer to participate in research and travel significant distances are likely to represent a cohort with relatively mild symptoms. Notably, all of the affected children were observed to have variants in multiple genes that were associated with ASD or found on the intellectual disability testing panel.

One limitation to classification of ASD in this sample is the use of only one observational diagnostic tool (the ADOS-2), rather than using a combination of clinical observation, parent interviews and strict DSM-V criteria to confirm diagnosis; however, scores on the ADOS-2 combined with scores on the Vineland and RBS-R strongly indicate elevated rates of ASD and ASD-related traits in our sample. Similar to findings from studies of individuals with idiopathic ASD, the majority of our participants (9/11) showed adaptive functioning abilities below the mean for their age. These findings suggest that the 15q11.2 BP1-BP2 deletion confers increased risk for ASD and functional impairments independent of selective impacts on cognitive abilities.

Most of the individuals in this sample presented with at least one dysmorphic feature, some of which were present across multiple families. Five had abnormal ear findings such as broad, soft, fleshy, or overfolded ears. The child of Family C also had a smooth upper lip and philtrum. In the case of Family E, both the father and child had a broad, round face as well as broad hands. Flat feet were present in three individuals. Both the mother and child of Family B had small upper incisors. Six of the participants had eye findings demonstrating ptosis including both affected individuals from Family C and the father of Family E. The connective tissue finding of mild scoliosis was observed in two unrelated individuals whereas kyphosis was found in one other participant. Hyperextensibility or instability of various joints was a common feature, with unrelated individuals demonstrating a positive Beighton hyperflexibility score of at least six out of nine showing hypermobile joints. The 6-year-old child of Family A had a history of ankle instability and wore leg braces. Leg asymmetry was also found in two unrelated individuals. Pectus carinatum was seen in one individual while four participants had loose, soft skin, and two unrelated individuals had birth marks. Two unrelated affected children had a reported history of delayed wound healing.

Neurological problems were also present in several children. Two were diagnosed with epilepsy, one had non-essential tremor, and the child of Family D had gross hypotonia. The mother and child of Family D were both found to have decreased deep tendon reflexes, whereas the child of Family B had increased deep tendon reflexes. Ataxia was seen in the child of Family E. Motor delay was also relatively common, with four affected children showing delayed motor milestones. Motor deficits in affected individuals were also evident in our tests of postural control. While this test does not have normed scores or clinical cutoffs, group averages and effect sizes indicate that both children and adults with the 15q11.2 BP1-BP2 microdeletion show increased variability of postural sway relative to non-affected controls. This is consistent with findings of increased variability of motor behavior in neurodevelopmental disorders including Prader-Willi syndrome [27], ASD [28,29], and fragile-X associated disorders [30], and involvement of ataxia-related genes in 15q11.2 BP1-BP2. Of note, all affected children had PDVs in genes evidenced to cause ataxia, epilepsy, comprehensive cardiovascular defects, and neuronal migration disorders. In addition, many children had PDVs in genes involved in connective tissue disorders, cerebral cortical malformations, micro/macrocephaly, and congenital malformations with craniofacial defects that are included on the clinical cleft palate DNA testing panel.

3.2. Protein–Protein Interactions and Functions Related to NIPA1, NIPA2, CYFIP1 and TUBGCP5 Genes in the 15q11.2 BP1-BP2 Region

Of particular interest are the genes that had either a de novo variant, or a variant inherited from the parent without the deletion that encode proteins that interact with products of the four genes in the 15q11.2 BP1-BP2 region. As reported by Rafi and Butler [13] when examining the protein–protein interactions of the four genes in the 15q11.2 BP1-BP2 region, the predicted biological processes can be summarized as follows: regulation of cell growth, magnesium ion transmembrane transport, regulation of axonogenesis, regulation of plasma membrane bounded cell projection organization, positive regulation of axon extension, regulation of cellular response to growth factor stimulus, regulation of developmental growth, positive regulation of cell projection organization, mitotic spindle organization, regulation of BMP signaling pathway, and positive regulation of plasma membrane bounded cell projection assembly.

Notably, NIPA1 protein was observed in our previous study to interact with 11 other proteins. Five (45%) of the 11 proteins were members of the BMP superfamily, three (27%) were BMP receptors and TGFB1 (9%) protein, indicating that three-fourths of the NIPA1 interacting proteins are important for developmental bone morphogenesis or multifunctional proteins that control proliferation, differentiation, and other functions in many cell types. The NIPA2 protein interacted with 19 other proteins with three (16%) involved with the BMP protein superfamily, three (16%) proteins interact with BMP receptors, ACVR1, TGFBR1, and six members of the SMAD superfamily of proteins (42%); all playing a role as intracellular signal transducers and transcriptional modulators activated by TGFB, thereby impacting bone morphogenesis and its related functions. Specifically, the Spastin protein, encoded by *SPAST,* was observed to interact with both NIPA1 and NIPA2. A variant in *SPAST* was found in Subject 9. This child had hypotonia and history of fine and gross motor delay as well as autism. Spastin severs polyglutamylated microtubules and likely has a role in axon growth and branching [31,32]. Mutations in both *SPAST* and *NIPA1* have been identified as causes of hereditary spastic paraplegia, a condition which causes progressive weakness and spasticity of the legs [33,34]. De novo variants in *SPAST* are evidenced to be associated with ASD with comorbid spastic paraplegia [35].

The CYFIP1 protein is also reported to interact with other proteins having a wide range of activity with functions related to cytoskeleton organization and actin filament binding with cell-matrix adhesion, MAP kinase signal transduction of cell growth, survival and differentiation, stimulation of glucose uptake, intracellular protein breakdown and tissue remodeling with mediation of translational repression [36]. We observed that five additional genes with either a de novo or non-deleted parent inherited variant in the affected child encode proteins that interact with CYFIP1. *GOLGA2* encodes a protein that acts as a membrane skeleton that maintains the structure of the Golgi apparatus. Mouse models of this gene indicate its involvement in brain morphology and the development and quantity of neurons [37,38]. Loss of this gene also resulted in ataxia in mice [37]. Subject 2 had a PDV in this gene as well as a disturbed motor phenotype, ASD, and neuropsychiatric behavior developmental phenotypes. *MEOX1* encodes a mesodermal transcription factor that plays a key role in somitogenesis, specifically sclerotome development. *MEOX1* is involved in overall organism development in humans [39] and mutations in mice result in evidence of congenital neurological disorders [40]. Subject 7 had a de novo PDV in *MEOX1* along with connective tissue defects, congenital malformations, epilepsy, and neuropsychiatric behavior developmental phenotypes. Finally, *FAT3* encodes an atypical cadherin protein and may play a role in the interactions between neurites derived from specific subsets of neurons during development. While *FAT3* was not included in any of the disease association categories we directly evaluated, missense mutations in this gene are associated with the neurodevelopmental disorder, Hirschsprung disease (https://www.ncbi.nlm.nih.gov/clinvar/RCV000201304.1/) (accessed on 6 February 2021). Both Subjects 2 and 3 had a PDV in this gene and evidence of a neurodevelopmental phenotype and should be monitored for gastrointestinal issues.

3.3. Identified Gene Variants with Potential Clinical Significance

As the first effort to identify variants in the four 15q11.2 BP1- BP2 genes in this microdeletion syndrome, we analyzed the non-deleted alleles in affected patients and assessed family members as well, using whole-exome sequencing in order to compare the genomic data of related genes with clinical, cognitive, and behavioral data. Some of these variants are identified by the gene panels as potentially contributing to multiple phenotypes in our subjects, as in the case of *MLC1,* which was a candidate for macrocephaly and motor delay in Subject 9 and for contribution to epilepsy in Subject 7. All variants passing inclusion criteria for possibly damaging the gene in which it is located, and the corresponding evidence for clinical significance of having a variant in the gene, can be found in Supplemental Table S1.

Other particular genes of interest with PDVs include numerous genes of the collagen or COL group which code for proteins that make up various subtypes of collagen. Disturbances in these genes are known to cause several connective tissue disorders [41]. For example, in addition to the stop-loss variant in the connective tissue disorder gene *FLCN,*

Subject 5—who had significant joint hyperextensibility—inherited a frameshift in *COL5A3* from the parent with the deletion. Additional missense variants in collagen-encoding genes, *COL21A1* and *COL6A2*, were inherited from the non-deleted parent in Subject 7, who had joint hyperflexibility. Specifically, variation in *COL6A2* is associated with Ullrich congenital muscular dystrophy 1 (https://omim.org/entry/254090) (accessed on 6 February 2021). Subject 9 had an inframe deletion in *COL4A3* and a missense variant in *COL6A6* that was inherited from the deleted parent. While no joint hyperflexibility was noted, this patient had flat feet which may reflect collapse of connective tissues of the midfoot. Dysfunction in collagen proteins may also manifest as other symptoms. *COL4A3*, for instance, is implicated in disorders resulting in renal failure (https://omim.org/entry/120070) (accessed on 6 February 2021) and Subject 9 was also noted to have a history of constipation. Furthermore, variation in *COL6A6* has been implicated in skin disorders [42]. Subject 11, also without joint hyperflexibility, had the same missense variant identified in *COL6A6* and had birthmarks noted on the thigh and forehead.

Finally, *CDK19* gene is another candidate explaining clinical findings in Subject 11 who had a de novo missense variant in this gene. A disturbance in this gene has been associated with bilateral congenital retinal folds, microcephaly, and intellectual disability [43]. Of these findings, intellectual disability was present in Subject 11.

4. Materials and Methods

4.1. Families with 15q11.2 BP1-BP2 Deletion or Burnside-Butler Syndrome (BBS)

A total of five families with an affected child diagnosed with the 15q11.2 BP1-BP2 microdeletion were recruited and extensively evaluated using a series of cognitive, behavioral and motor assessments, family and medical histories, physical examination, and exome sequencing analyses. All participants or their legal guardians signed informed consent forms approved by the Institutional Review Board at the University of Kansas Medical Center (KUMC) before entry into the study. The five families included six affected children (3 males and 3 females) with one family having two affected children (Family A, Subjects 2 and 3) with BBS. Four mothers and one father had a confirmed 15q 11.2 BP1-BP2 deletion. Methylation-specific multiplex ligation-dependent probe amplification (MS-MLPA) was performed on two families for confirmation of the parents' cytogenetic diagnoses using existing methodology [36].

4.2. Cognitive and Behavioral Measures

Cognitive and behavioral assessments were administered to all members of our study cohort (except where otherwise noted). All interviews and observational measures were conducted by trained members of our study team. The following cognitive and behavioral measures were administered:

The Wechsler Abbreviated Scales of Intelligence [44] (WASI-II) was used to assess general cognitive abilities including verbal, perceptual (nonverbal), and full-scale IQ.

The Wide Range Achievement Test-4 [45] (WRAT-4) was used to assess basic academic skills implicated previously in BBS, including sentence comprehension, word reading, spelling, and math computation.

The California Verbal Learning Test [14] (CVLT) is a comprehensive assessment of verbal learning and memory that specifically measures short delay free recall, short delay cued recall, long delay free recall, long delay cued recall, and long delay recognition. The CVLT-II was used in adolescents and adults (aged 16 to 89 years; N = 6), while the California Verbal Learning Test for Children (CVLT-C) was administered to children (aged 5 to 16 years; N = 4).

The Peabody Picture Vocabulary Test, Fourth Edition [15] (PPVT-4) was used to assess receptive vocabulary. During the PPVT-4, participants are instructed to identify the picture that best matches a target word. The number of correctly identified pictures was examined.

The Trail Making Test [16] is a commonly used assessment of visual search, processing speed, and cognitive flexibility consisting of two parts: Part A primarily measures visual search and processing speed as participants draw lines connecting numbers in sequential order as fast as possible. Part B assesses cognitive flexibility as participants must alternate between connecting letters and numbers as fast as possible (A-1-B-2-C-3, etc.). Reaction time and the number of errors made were examined for Parts A and B.

The Autism Diagnostic Observation Schedule, Second Edition [17,18] (ADOS-2) is a semi-structured play- and conversation-based assessment of the core social, communication, and repetitive behaviors in ASD. Module 3 (for children/adolescents with fluent speech) was used for all children in our study cohort except one non-verbal child, who as noted in Table 2, was administered Module 1 (for children 31 months or older who are preverbal or only use single words). The social-affective and total algorithm scores were examined. Higher scores reflect more severe symptoms of ASD.

Broad Autism Phenotype Questionnaire [21] (BAP-Q) measures traits relating to the broad autism phenotype—the presence of core diagnostic symptoms of ASD (e.g., social/communication impairments and restricted, repetitive behaviors) that occur below the threshold for a clinical diagnosis. This questionnaire consists of three subscales: social abnormalities, pragmatic language difficulties, and rigid personality and a desire for sameness. The BAP-Q was administered only to the parents in our study cohort. We used cutoff scores defined by Sasson et al. [22] (Males $\geq$ 3.55, Females $\geq$ 3.17), where higher scores indicate greater presence of ASD traits.

Vineland Adaptive Behavior Scales-Third Edition [19] (VABS-III) is a series of semi-structured caretaker interviews assessing current adaptive and daily living skills across four domains: communication, daily living skills, socialization, and motor skills.

The Repetitive Behavior Scale—Revised [23] (RBS-R) is a rating scale that assesses five categories of repetitive behavior (motor stereotypy, repetitive self-injury, compulsions, routines/sameness, restricted interests) commonly observed in individuals with developmental disabilities. Adult participants provided self-reported responses to the RBS-R, and a parent or caregiver provided responses on behalf of the child participants. Higher scores indicate greater severity of repetitive behavior. This measure does not have defined clinical thresholds, so we compared scores to age-dependent averages from a large cohort study of individuals with ASD [20].

4.3. Clinical Evaluation and Physical Examinations

A complete physical examination was performed by a clinical geneticist (MGB) with anthropometric measures (e.g., head circumference, ear length, inner and outer canthal distances, hand and mid-finger lengths) and data recorded including a three-generation family pedigree. Past medical histories and review of systems were included for cognition, behavior, seizures, pulmonary, cardiac, gastrointestinal, genitourinary, renal, musculoskeletal, cutaneous, immune, and hematology. Clinical photographs were obtained following written consent.

4.4. Postural Control Testing

Participants completed a postural control task to assess gross sensorimotor ability. Data for children and adult participants with the 15q11.2 BP1-BP2 deletion were compared to age- and sex-matched control participants who were unrelated to the families affected by the BBS deletion. Control participants completed postural control testing as part of larger studies taking place at two separate research sites. Where noted, some of the task parameters differed between these two sites.

Postural control was assessed using an AMTI (American Mechanical Technology, Inc., Watertown, MA, USA) AccuGait strain gauge force platform. Participants were tested bare footed in a well-lit room. They were instructed to stand as still as possible on the platform with their feet shoulder width apart and their arms resting at their sides. Participants completed three trials each lasting 30–45 s.

To standardize the duration of data analyzed, the first five seconds of each trial were removed and only the subsequent 20 s were included for analysis. Trials during which the participant lost balance or did not remain still for the duration of the trial (e.g., took a step, sneezed, spoke, walked away, etc.) were excluded from analysis. Participants who had fewer than two useable trials were excluded from analyses.

The center of pressure (COP) time series were derived from the force and moment data during standing posture. The time series of each trial was down-sampled to 100 Hz (for five control participants, data were down-sampled to 200 Hz) and low-pass filtered using a fourth-order double pass Butterworth filter with a cutoff frequency of 6 Hz.

The variability of each participant's postural sway was quantified using the standard deviation (SD) of the COP in both the medial-lateral (ML) and anterior-posterior (AP) directions, as has been done in previous studies [30]. SD values were log transformed to correct for skewed distributions.

Data analyses were conducted separately for adults and children. Due to the small sample size of this study, we limited our analyses to the calculation of group means, standard deviations, and effect sizes (Cohen's d) and interpreted as small (d = 0.2), medium (d = 0.5), or large (d = 0.8) according to Cohen's standards [46]. One child with the 15q11.2 BP1-BP2 deletion (Subject 11) did not complete any postural control testing, so data from this participant and the matched control were not included in the analyses.

4.5. DNA Extraction

Saliva and buccal cells were collected using a Saliva DNA Collection and Preservation Device (Norgen Biotek Corporation, Thorold, Ontario, CA, USA). Genomic DNA was isolated and purified using a Saliva DNA Isolation Kit (Norgen Biotek Corporation) according to manufacturer's protocol.

4.6. Methylation Specific-Multiplex Ligation Probe Amplification (MS-MLPA)

The MS-MLPA assay is a standard laboratory assay to examine for chromosome 15 deletions and was used to identify the presence or absence of the 15q11.2 BP1-BP2 deletion prior to enrolling individuals in this study. MS-MLPA was performed using reagents and kits obtained from MRC-Holland (Amsterdam, The Netherlands) including ME028-C1 kits containing sequence specific probes along the length of the 15q11.2-q13 region. The C1 kit contains 47 MLPA probes for copy number detection using fragment analysis following manufacturer's instructions and reported elsewhere [36].

4.7. Whole-Exome Sequencing

Genomic DNA (5 µg) samples from four families (5 affected children and 4 sets of parents) were exome sequenced at the KUMC Genomics Core facility, and one family was sequenced in a commercial laboratory (GeneDx, Gaithersburg, MD, USA). Exome sequencing was performed using the TruSeq Exome Library Prep Kit (Illumina FC-150-1001, San Diego, CA, USA). High molecular weight (HMW) genomic DNA (gDNA) was fragmented using the Covaris S2 Ultra-Sonication system. Following fragmentation, DNA was end-repaired and 3' adenylated prior to adaptor ligation using TruSeq DNA indexed adapters. The DNA libraries were equalized to 233 or 250 ng and pooled for two rounds of enrichment using the TruSeq Exome capture probes. TruSeq Exome capture probes target 45 Mb of coding sequence from >98% of RefSeq, Consensus CDS (CCDS), and Ensembl coding content. Following the final exome capture, the enriched libraries were amplified using polymerase chain reaction (PCR) to generate sufficient yield for sequencing. Enriched amplified libraries were validated using the Agilent Bioanalyzer 2100 system and quantitated using the Roche LightCycler96 RealTime PCR system. Final library concentration results were used to dilute the library pool to 2 nM and pooled for multiplexed sequencing on a NovaSeq 6000 sequencing machine (Illumina, San Diego, CA, USA). The onboard clonal clustering procedure was automated during the NovaSeq 6000 sequencing run. The 100-cycle paired end sequencing was performed using the NovaSeq 6000 S2 Reagent Kit—200 cycle (Illumina 20012861). Following sequencing, the raw base call files (.bcl) were converted to fastq files and de-multiplexed into individual libraries using Illumina's bcl2fastq2 software.

4.8. Variant Calling and Quality Control Procedures

The initial read quality was assessed using the FastQC software1 [47]. The sequenced reads were then aligned to the human genome (hg38) using the Burrows–Wheeler aligner (BWA) [48]. The initial read quality was assessed using the FastQC software1 [47]. The sequenced reads were then aligned to the human genome (hg38) using the BWA [48]. Variant analyses of these data were performed in accordance with the Genome Analysis Toolkit (GATK) variant calling best practices pipeline [49]. Variant calling was as follows: The "MergeBamAlignment" tool was used to incorporate metadata to the aligned BAM files. The "MarkDuplicates" tool was used to locate and tag duplicate reads in the BAM files. The "BaseRecalibrator" tool was used to generate a recalibration table for base quality score recalibration (BQSR). Known polymorphic sites obtained from the GATK resource bundle were provided to this tool (Mills and 1000 G gold standard insertions or deletions (InDels) hg38 vcf, Homo sapiens assembly38 dbsnp138 vcf). The "ApplyBQSR" tool was run next in the two-stage process of base quality score recalibration. SNPs and InDels were called using the "HaplotypeCaller" tool. The resulting gVCF files were combined using the "CombineGVCFs" tool to form a multi-sample gVCF file. This file was passed for Joint genotyping using the "GenotypeGVCFs" tool. A recalibration model to score variant quality was built separately for InDels and SNPs using the "VariantRecalibrator" tool. The tool "ApplyVQSR" was then used with these models in the second stage of the variant quality score recalibration (VQSR) process to filter the input variants based on the recalibration table. The resulting data were further processed using the Genotype Refinement Workflow with the goal of improving the accuracy of genotype calls and discarding unreliable genotype calls. The first step of this process was to calculate the genotype posterior probabilities given family and known population genotypes using the "CalculateGenotypePosteriors" tool. The pedigree information of the families and a high confidence SNP file was provided to this tool. Variant calls were hard filtered to exclude genotype quality scores less than 20 (GQ < 20.0).

Figure 1 shows additional quality control and variant selection details from the whole-exome sequencing analysis. Specifically, single nucleotide variants (SNVs) were required to have read depth $\geq$10, InDels were required to have depth $\geq$28X when 2–5 base pairs (bp) long and $\geq$42X when 5–200 bps. To identify SNVs and InDels passing all quality control that were potentially damaging, the functional effects of variants on encoded proteins were predicted using the "SnpEff [50]" and Ensembl Variant Effect Predictor (VEP) tools [51]. Rare variants—with a maximum allele frequency (AF) <0.01% based on reference populations available in the 1000 Genomes Project, the European Standard Population and the Genome Aggregation Database—located in protein coding gene transcripts were selected. Rare variants predicted by VEP to have consequences that were moderately (i.e., inframe InDels, missense, or protein altering) or highly likely (i.e., splice site alterations, gains or losses of stop codons, loss of start codons, or frameshifts) to damage the protein products were then prioritized. Missense and start loss SNVs were further evaluated for potential deleterious effects using Sorting Intolerant From Tolerant (SIFT) [52], PolyPhen [53], and Grantham substitution scores [54] with inclusion criteria as follows: SIFT score < 0.05, PolyPhen score $\geq$ 0.70, and Grantham score $\geq$ 100 [54]. We then prioritized variants in affected children that were predicted de novo, or inherited from only one parent as additional evidence for potential clinical relevance.

4.9. Functional and Clinical Characterization of Genes with Variants

The implicated diseases and biological functions of the genes with variants of interest were then identified using the Ingenuity Systems Pathway Analysis (IPA) tool [55]. Variant effects analyses were run considering molecules and/or direct relationships that were experimentally observed in mammals (i.e., humans, mice, rats) from all data sources. Two separate analyses were run on genes with de novo variants and genes with inherited variants. As it was expected that de novo variants were more likely to represent clinically relevant findings [56], variant effects analysis of genes with de novo PDVs were conducted using evidence from all possible mutation consequences, including unclassified and silent mutations. For genes with PDVs that were transmitted to affected children from the parent without the 15q11.2 BP1-BP2 microdeletion, only evidence from likely damaging mutation consequences (i.e., null, frameshift, loss of function, missense, gain-of-function, knockout, in-frame, or nonsense mutations) were considered. In addition, as the specific symptoms of affected children were diagnosed (see below for details on measures and clinical evaluations), genes overrepresented at a Benjamini–Hochberg corrected $p \leq 0.05$ in diseases and disorders reflecting these symptoms were selected for follow-up. These genes were then evaluated in Path Designer to determine if any direct or indirect relationships were observed or predicted downstream of the four genes encoded in the 15q11.2 BP1-BP2 deletion region.

To further evaluate genes with PDVs that may relate to symptoms observed in affected children, these genes were annotated based on evidence of associations with ASD using the 2020 Q2 release of the Simons Foundation for Autism Research Initiative (SFARI) gene list (https://gene.sfari.org/about-gene-scoring/) (accessed on 6 February 2021). In addition, genes were evaluated for inclusion on panels from Fulgent Genetics (https://www.fulgentgenetics.com/) (accessed on 6 February 2021) and Prevention Genetics (https://www.preventiongenetics.com/) (accessed on 6 February 2021), both Clinical Laboratory Improvement Amendments (CLIA) approved and accredited commercial laboratories. Interrogated panels from Fulgent Genetics included: epilepsy, intellectual disability, comprehensive cardiovascular defects, ataxia, microcephaly, macrocephaly, cerebral cortical malformations, neuronal migration disorders and malformations including cleft palate. Genes for connective tissue disorders reflected a combination of both the Fulgent Genetics and Prevention Genetics panels as the latter panel was more comprehensive.

5. Conclusions

Our study of the 15q11.2 BP1-BP2 deletion (Burnside-Butler) syndrome, an emerging disorder, found variants in genes beyond the four genes in the chromosome 15q11.2 BP1-BP2 region using exome sequencing with our inclusion criteria and correlations with reported gene and protein interactions with associated diseases or findings. Although we cannot claim that the gene variants found are causal for the clinical, behavioral, or cognitive findings observed (e.g., 9/11 subjects had adaptive functioning abilities below mean for age; 8/11 subjects demonstrated repetitive behavioral scores comparable to ASD subjects; 4 affected children tested had delayed motor milestones; joint instability or hyperextensibility was commonly observed) our data suggests that variants in genes encoded outside of the 15q11.2 BP1-BP2 region may be of interest to future research. Notably, four of the five probands in the five unrelated families inherited the 15q11.2 BP1-BP2 deletion from the mother while only one father (Family E) had the deletion. The affected child in Family E was also the most severely affected (ataxia, wheel-chair user, non-verbal, impaired cognition). This may indicate parent of origin effects, similar to those reported in Davis et al. [57], which included lower motor function and coordination when of paternal origin and more cognitive and behavioral disturbances and seizures when of maternal origin. It is also important to note that several families included in our study traveled long distances. The travel and testing required for participation may have selected for affected children and parents that are relatively less severe than others with this deletion. It is possible that many less severe symptoms reported in this analysis dataset relate primarily to dysfunction in the four core genes encoded in the 15q11.2 BP1-BP2 deleted region. Future studies focused on ascertaining individuals with more severe expression of the symptoms we report may identify more concrete evidence for damaging variants in other genes in addition to the four core genes. Importantly, replication and functional studies are needed to confirm these hypotheses. As noted in our study, a neurodevelopmental phenotype (autism, speech delay, abnormal reflexes, and coordination) was most commonly found along with craniofacial findings (ear anomalies), and orthopedic or connective tissue problems (flat feet, scoliosis, hypermobile joints). These clinical, cognitive, behavioral, and genomic characterizations with reported protein interactions of the four genes of interest and associated diseases in this chromosome 15q11.2 BP1-BP2 deletion did support a role in the neurodevelopmental-autism phenotype seen in this emerging syndrome. Interaction with genes found and their paralogs may have contributed, but our observations are preliminary on a small sample size requiring replication. The authors hope that our findings will stimulate more research and directions for study, shedding light on diagnosis, treatment, and prognosis for affected individuals with this emerging syndrome having the most frequent microarray defect seen in patients presenting with neurodevelopmental disorders.

Supplementary Materials: The following are available online at https://www.mdpi.com/1422-0067/22/4/1660/s1.

Author Contributions: Research design conceptualization, O.J.V., M.G.B.; methodology, validation, investigation, formal analysis, data curation, I.B., R.L.S., W.A.H., S.G., O.J.V.; the networks, functional analyses were generated through the use of Ingenuity Pathway Analysis by O.J.V.; writing—original draft preparation, I.B., R.L.S., W.A.H., S.G., O.J.V., M.G.B.; writing—review and editing, I.B., O.J.V., M.G.B.; supervision, M.W.M., M.G.B.; funding acquisition, O.J.V., M.W.M., M.G.B. All authors have read and agreed to the published version of the manuscript.

Funding: We acknowledge the National Institute of Child Health and Human Development (NICHD) grant number HD02528, KUMC Research Institute Clinical Pilot Research Grant Program, Kansas Intellectual and Developmental Disabilities Research Center (KIDDRC) grant number U54HD090216, the National Center for Advancing Translational Sciences (NCATS) Clinical and Translational Science Award (CTSA) awarded to the Frontiers: University of Kansas Clinical and Translational Science Institute (TL1TR002368), the National Institute of Mental Health (R01MH112734) and the National Library of Medicine (K01LM012870).

Institutional Review Board Statement: Participants were consented under an IRB-approved protocol (IRB#141167) that allows research. The University of Kansas Medical Center (KUMC) IRB-approved forms were signed by the participant and/or guardian prior to entry into the study.

Informed Consent Statement: All study participants or their legal guardian provided informed written consent prior to study enrollment.

Data Availability Statement: Genomic data that support the findings of this study are available in the Supplemental Table S1 and additional data are available from the authors upon reasonable request.

Conflicts of Interest: The authors declare no conflict of interest.

References

1. Nicholls, R.D.; Knoll, J.H.; Butler, M.G.; Karam, S.; Lalande, M. Genetic imprinting suggested by maternal heterodisomy in nondeletion Prader-Willi syndrome. *Nature* **1989**, *342*, 281–285. [CrossRef]
2. Butler, M.G.; Manzardo, A.M.; Forster, J.L. Prader-Willi Syndrome: Clinical Genetics and Diagnostic Aspects with Treatment Approaches. *Curr. Pediatr. Rev.* **2016**, *12*, 136–166. [CrossRef]
3. Butler, M.; Lee, P.D.K.; Whitman, B. Management of Prader-Willi syndrome. In *Management of Prader-Willi Syndrome*, 3rd ed.; Springer: Berlin/Heidelberg, Germany, 2006; pp. 1–550.
4. Williams, C.A.; Driscoll, D.J.; Dagli, A.I. Clinical and genetic aspects of Angelman syndrome. *Genet. Med.* **2010**, *12*, 385–395. [CrossRef]
5. Bittel, D.C.; Butler, M.G. Prader-Willi syndrome: Clinical genetics, cytogenetics and molecular biology. *Expert Rev. Mol. Med.* **2005**, *7*, 1–20. [CrossRef] [PubMed]
6. Zarcone, J.; Napolitano, D.; Peterson, C.; Breidbord, J.; Ferraioli, S.; Caruso-Anderson, M.; Holsen, L.; Butler, M.G.; Thompson, T. The relationship between compulsive behaviour and academic achievement across the three genetic subtypes of Prader-Willi syndrome. *J. Intellect. Disabil. Res.* **2007**, *51*, 478–487. [CrossRef] [PubMed]
7. Butler, M.G.; Bittel, D.C.; Kibiryeva, N.; Talebizadeh, Z.; Thompson, T. Behavioral differences among subjects with Prader-Willi syndrome and type I or type II deletion and maternal disomy. *Pediatrics* **2004**, *113*, 565–573. [CrossRef] [PubMed]
8. Hartley, S.L.; Maclean, W.E., Jr.; Butler, M.G.; Zarcone, J.; Thompson, T. Maladaptive behaviors and risk factors among the genetic subtypes of Prader-Willi syndrome. *Am. J. Med. Genet. A* **2005**, *136*, 140–145. [CrossRef] [PubMed]

9. Burnside, R.D.; Pasion, R.; Mikhail, F.M.; Carroll, A.J.; Robin, N.H.; Youngs, E.L.; Gadi, I.K.; Keitges, E.; Jaswaney, V.L.; Papenhausen, P.R.; et al. Microdeletion/microduplication of proximal 15q11.2 between BP1 and BP2: A susceptibility region for neurological dysfunction including developmental and language delay. *Hum. Genet.* **2011**, *130*, 517–528. [CrossRef]

10. Cox, D.M.; Butler, M.G. The 15q11.2 BP1-BP2 microdeletion syndrome: A review. *Int. J. Mol. Sci.* **2015**, *16*, 4068–4082. [CrossRef]

11. Butler, M.G. Clinical and genetic aspects of the 15q11.2 BP1-BP2 microdeletion disorder. *J. Intellect. Disabil. Res.* **2017**, *61*, 568–579. [CrossRef]

12. Ho, K.S.; Wassman, E.R.; Baxter, A.L.; Hensel, C.H.; Martin, M.M.; Prasad, A.; Twede, H.; Vanzo, R.J.; Butler, M.G. Chromosomal Microarray Analysis of Consecutive Individuals with Autism Spectrum Disorders Using an Ultra-High Resolution Chromosomal Microarray Optimized for Neurodevelopmental Disorders. *Int. J. Mol. Sci.* **2016**, *17*, 2070. [CrossRef]

13. Rafi, S.K.; Butler, M.G. The 15q11.2 BP1-BP2 Microdeletion (Burnside–Butler) Syndrome: In Silico Analyses of the Four Coding Genes Reveal Functional Associations with Neurodevelopmental Disorders. *Int. J. Mol. Sci.* **2020**, *21*, 3296. [CrossRef]

14. Delis, D.C.; Kramer, J.H.; Kaplan, E.; Ober, B.A. *California Verbal Learning Test*, 2nd ed.; Psychological Corporation: San Antonio, TX, USA, 2000.

15. Dunn, L.M.; Dunn, D.M. *Peabody Picture Vocabulary Test*, 4th ed.; Pearson Education: Minneapolis, MN, USA, 2007.

16. Reitan, R.M. Validity of the Trail Making Test as an Indicator of Organic Brain Damage. *Percept. Mot. Skills* **1958**, *8*, 271–276. [CrossRef]

17. Gotham, K.; Pickles, A.; Lord, C. Standardizing ADOS scores for a measure of severity in autism spectrum disorders. *J. Autism Dev. Disord.* **2009**, *39*, 693–705. [CrossRef]

18. Lord, C.; Luyster, R.; Guthrie, W.; Pickles, A. Patterns of developmental trajectories in toddlers with autism spectrum disorder. *J. Consult. Clin. Psychol.* **2012**, *80*, 477–489. [CrossRef]

19. Sparrow, S.S.; Ciccheti, D.V.; Saulnier, C.A. *Vineland Adaptive Behavior Scales*, 3rd ed.; Pearson Education: London, UK, 2016.

20. Esbensen, A.J.; Seltzer, M.M.; Lam, K.S.; Bodfish, J.W. Age-related differences in restricted repetitive behaviors in autism spectrum disorders. *J. Autism Dev. Disord.* **2009**, *39*, 57–66. [CrossRef]

21. Hurley, R.S.; Losh, M.; Parlier, M.; Reznick, J.S.; Piven, J. The broad autism phenotype questionnaire. *J. Autism Dev. Disord.* **2007**, *37*, 1679–1690. [CrossRef] [PubMed]

22. Sasson, N.J.; Lam, K.S.L.; Childress, D.; Parlier, M.; Daniels, J.L.; Piven, J. The broad autism phenotype questionnaire: Prevalence and diagnostic classification. *Autism Res.* **2013**, *6*, 134–143. [CrossRef] [PubMed]

23. Bodfish, J.W.; Symons, F.J.; Parker, D.E.; Lewis, M.H. Varieties of repetitive behavior in autism: Comparisons to mental retardation. *J. Autism Dev. Disord.* **2000**, *30*, 237–243. [CrossRef]

24. Quamme, G.A. Molecular identification of ancient and modern mammalian magnesium transporters. *Am. J. Physiol. Cell Physiol.* **2010**, *298*, C407–C429. [CrossRef]

25. Rainier, S.; Chai, J.-H.; Tokarz, D.; Nicholls, R.D.; Fink, J.K. NIPA1 Gene Mutations Cause Autosomal Dominant Hereditary Spastic Paraplegia (SPG6). *Am. J. Hum. Genet.* **2003**, *73*, 967–971. [CrossRef]

26. Maenner, M.J. Prevalence of Autism Spectrum Disorder Among Children Aged 8 Years—Autism and Developmental Disabilities Monitoring Network, 11 Sites, United States, 2016. *MMWR Surv. Summ.* **2020**, *69*, 1–12. [CrossRef] [PubMed]

27. Capodaglio, P.; Menegoni, F.; Vismara, L.; Cimolin, V.; Grugni, G.; Galli, M. Characterisation of balance capacity in Prader-Willi patients. *Res. Dev. Disabil.* **2011**, *32*, 81–86. [CrossRef] [PubMed]

28. Wang, Z.; Hallac, R.R.; Conroy, K.C.; White, S.P.; Kane, A.A.; Collinsworth, A.L.; Sweeney, J.A.; Mosconi, M.W. Postural orientation and equilibrium processes associated with increased postural sway in autism spectrum disorder (ASD). *J. Neurodev. Disord.* **2016**, *8*, 43. [CrossRef] [PubMed]

29. Lim, Y.H.; Partridge, K.; Girdler, S.; Morris, S.L. Standing Postural Control in Individuals with Autism Spectrum Disorder: Systematic Review and Meta-analysis. *J. Autism Dev. Disord* **2017**, *47*, 2238–2253. [CrossRef] [PubMed]

30. Wang, Z.; Khemani, P.; Schmitt, L.M.; Lui, S.; Mosconi, M.W. Static and dynamic postural control deficits in aging fragile X mental retardation 1 (FMR1) gene premutation carriers. *J. Neurodev. Disord.* **2019**, *11*, 2. [CrossRef]

31. Errico, A.; Ballabio, A.; Rugarli, E.I. Spastin, the protein mutated in autosomal dominant hereditary spastic paraplegia, is involved in microtubule dynamics. *Hum. Mol. Genet.* **2002**, *11*, 153–163. [CrossRef] [PubMed]

32. Evans, K.J.; Gomes, E.R.; Reisenweber, S.M.; Gundersen, G.G.; Lauring, B.P. Linking axonal degeneration to microtubule remodeling by Spastin-mediated microtubule severing. *J. Cell Biol.* **2005**, *168*, 599–606. [CrossRef] [PubMed]

33. Alber, B.; Pernauer, M.; Schwan, A.; Rothmund, G.; Hoffmann, K.T.; Brummer, D.; Sperfeld, A.D.; Uttner, I.; Binder, H.; Epplen, J.T.; et al. Spastin related hereditary spastic paraplegia with dysplastic corpus callosum. *J. Neurol. Sci.* **2005**, *236*, 9–12. [CrossRef]

34. Munhoz, R.P.; Kawarai, T.; Teive, H.A.; Raskin, S.; Sato, C.; Liang, Y.; St George-Hyslop, P.H.; Rogaeva, E. Clinical and genetic study of a Brazilian family with spastic paraplegia (SPG6 locus). *Mov. Disord.* **2006**, *21*, 279–281. [CrossRef]

35. Matthews, A.M.; Tarailo-Graovac, M.; Price, E.M.; Blydt-Hansen, I.; Ghani, A.; Drögemöller, B.I.; Robinson, W.P.; Ross, C.J.; Wasserman, W.W.; Siden, H.; et al. A de novo mosaic mutation in SPAST with two novel alternative alleles and chromosomal copy number variant in a boy with spastic paraplegia and autism spectrum disorder. *Eur. J. Med. Genet.* **2017**, *60*, 548–552. [CrossRef]

36. Henkhaus, R.S.; Kim, S.J.; Kimonis, V.E.; Gold, J.A.; Dykens, E.M.; Driscoll, D.J.; Butler, M.G. Methylation-specific multiplex ligation-dependent probe amplification and identification of deletion genetic subtypes in Prader-Willi syndrome. *Genet. Test Mol. Biomark.* **2012**, *16*, 178–186. [CrossRef]

37. Liu, C.; Mei, M.; Li, Q.; Roboti, P.; Pang, Q.; Ying, Z.; Gao, F.; Lowe, M.; Bao, S. Loss of the golgin GM130 causes Golgi disruption, Purkinje neuron loss, and ataxia in mice. *Proc. Natl. Acad. Sci. USA* **2017**, *114*, 346–351. [CrossRef]
38. Matsuki, T.; Matthews, R.T.; Cooper, J.A.; van der Brug, M.P.; Cookson, M.R.; Hardy, J.A.; Olson, E.C.; Howell, B.W. Reelin and stk25 have opposing roles in neuronal polarization and dendritic Golgi deployment. *Cell* **2010**, *143*, 826–836. [CrossRef]
39. Futreal, P.A.; Cochran, C.; Rosenthal, J.; Miki, Y.; Swenson, J.; Hobbs, M.; Bennett, L.M.; Haugen-Strano, A.; Marks, J.; Barrett, J.C.; et al. Isolation of a diverged homeobox gene, MOX1, from the BRCA1 region on 17q21 by solution hybrid capture. *Hum. Mol. Genet.* **1994**, *3*, 1359–1364. [CrossRef]
40. Mankoo, B.S.; Skuntz, S.; Harrigan, I.; Grigorieva, E.; Candia, A.; Wright, C.V.; Arnheiter, H.; Pachnis, V. The concerted action of Meox homeobox genes is required upstream of genetic pathways essential for the formation, patterning and differentiation of somites. *Development* **2003**, *130*, 4655–4664. [CrossRef] [PubMed]
41. Ricard-Blum, S. The collagen family. *Cold Spring Harb. Perspect. Biol.* **2011**, *3*, a004978. [CrossRef] [PubMed]
42. Fitzgerald, J.; Holden, P.; Hansen, U. The expanded collagen VI family: New chains and new questions. *Connect. Tissue Res.* **2013**, *54*, 345–350. [CrossRef] [PubMed]
43. Mukhopadhyay, A.; Kramer, J.M.; Merkx, G.; Lugtenberg, D.; Smeets, D.F.; Oortveld, M.A.; Blokland, E.A.; Agrawal, J.; Schenck, A.; van Bokhoven, H.; et al. CDK19 is disrupted in a female patient with bilateral congenital retinal folds, microcephaly and mild mental retardation. *Hum. Genet.* **2010**, *128*, 281–291. [CrossRef] [PubMed]
44. Wechsler, D.; Zhou, X. *WASI-II: Wechsler Abbreviated Scale of Intelligence*; The Pychological Corporation: San Antonio, TX, USA, 2011.
45. Wilkinson, G.S.; Robertson, G.J. *WRAT 4: Wide Range Achievement Test*; Psychological Assessment Resources: Lutz, FL, USA, 2006.
46. Cohen, J. *Statistical Power Analysis for the Behavioral Sciences*, 2nd ed.; L. Erlbaum Associates: Hillsdale, NJ, USA, 1988.
47. Andrews, S. FastQC: A Quality Control Tool for High Throughput Sequence Data. Available online: http://www.bioinformatics. babraham.ac.uk/projects/fastqc2010 (accessed on 10 June 2020).
48. Li, H.; Durbin, R. Fast and accurate short read alignment with Burrows-Wheeler transform. *Bioinformatics* **2009**, *25*, 1754–1760. [CrossRef]
49. Van der Auwera, G.A.; Carneiro, M.O.; Hartl, C.; Poplin, R.; Del Angel, G.; Levy-Moonshine, A.; Jordan, T.; Shakir, K.; Roazen, D.; Thibault, J.; et al. From FastQ data to high confidence variant calls: The Genome Analysis Toolkit best practices pipeline. *Curr. Protoc. Bioinform.* **2013**, *43*, 11.10.1–11.10.33. [CrossRef]
50. Cingolani, P.; Platts, A.; Wang, L.L.; Coon, M.; Nguyen, T.; Wang, L.; Land, S.J.; Lu, X.; Ruden, D.M. A program for annotating and predicting the effects of single nucleotide polymorphisms, SnpEff: SNPs in the genome of Drosophila melanogaster strain w1118; iso-2; iso-3. *Fly* **2012**, *6*, 80–92. [CrossRef]
51. McLaren, W.; Gil, L.; Hunt, S.E.; Riat, H.S.; Ritchie, G.R.; Thormann, A.; Flicek, P.; Cunningham, F. The Ensembl Variant Effect Predictor. *Genome Biol.* **2016**, *17*, 122. [CrossRef]
52. Ng, P.C.; Henikoff, S. SIFT: Predicting amino acid changes that affect protein function. *Nucleic Acids Res.* **2003**, *31*, 3812–3814. [CrossRef] [PubMed]
53. Adzhubei, I.; Jordan, D.M.; Sunyaev, S.R. Predicting functional effect of human missense mutations using PolyPhen-2. *Curr. Protoc. Hum. Genet.* **2013**, *76*, 7.20.1–7.20.41. [CrossRef]
54. Grantham, R. Amino acid difference formula to help explain protein evolution. *Science* **1974**, *185*, 862–864. [CrossRef] [PubMed]
55. Krämer, A.; Green, J.; Pollard, J., Jr.; Tugendreich, S. Causal analysis approaches in Ingenuity Pathway Analysis. *Bioinformatics* **2014**, *30*, 523–530. [CrossRef] [PubMed]
56. Wang, W.; Corominas, R.; Lin, G.N. De novo Mutations From Whole Exome Sequencing in Neurodevelopmental and Psychiatric Disorders: From Discovery to Application. *Front. Genet.* **2019**, *10*, 258. [CrossRef]
57. Davis, K.W.; Serrano, M.; Loddo, S.; Robinson, C.; Alesi, V.; Dallapiccola, B.; Novelli, A.; Butler, M.G. Parent-of-Origin Effects in 15q11.2 BP1-BP2 Microdeletion (Burnside-Butler) Syndrome. *Int. J. Mol. Sci.* **2019**, *20*, 1459. [CrossRef] [PubMed]

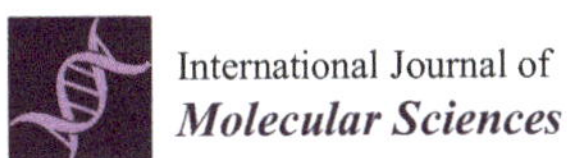

International Journal of
Molecular Sciences

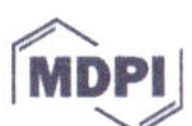

Case Report

40-Hz Auditory Steady-State Response (ASSR) as a Biomarker of Genetic Defects in the *SHANK3* Gene: A Case Report of 15-Year-Old Girl with a Rare Partial *SHANK3* Duplication

Anastasia K. Neklyudova [1], Galina V. Portnova [1], Anna B. Rebreikina [1], Victoria Yu Voinova [2,3], Svetlana G. Vorsanova [2,3], Ivan Y. Iourov [2,3] and Olga V. Sysoeva [1,*]

[1] Laboratory of Human Higher Nervous Activity, Institute of Higher Nervous Activity and Neurophysiology, Russian Academy of Science, 117485 Moscow, Russia; anastacia.neklyudova@gmail.com (A.K.N.); caviter@list.ru (G.V.P.); anna.rebreikina@gmail.com (A.B.R.)

[2] Veltischev Research and Clinical Institute for Pediatrics of the Pirogov, Russian National Research Medical University, Ministry of Health of Russian Federation, 125412 Moscow, Russia; vivoinova@yandex.ru (V.Y.V.); svorsanova@mail.ru (S.G.V.); ivan.iourov@gmail.com (I.Y.I.)

[3] Mental Health Research Center, 117152 Moscow, Russia

[*] Correspondence: olga.v.sysoeva@gmail.com

Citation: Neklyudova, A.K.; Portnova, G.V.; Rebreikina, A.B.; Voinova, V.Y.; Vorsanova, S.G.; Iourov, I.Y.; Sysoeva, O.V. 40-Hz Auditory Steady-State Response (ASSR) as a Biomarker of Genetic Defects in the *SHANK3* Dene: A Case Report of 15-Year-Old Girl with a Rare Partial *SHANK3* Duplication. *Int. J. Mol. Sci.* **2021**, 22, 1898. https://doi.org/ 10.3390/ijms22041898

Academic Editor: Merlin G. Butler

Received: 12 January 2021
Accepted: 9 February 2021
Published: 14 February 2021

Publisher's Note: MDPI stays neutral with regard to jurisdictional claims in published maps and institutional affil-iations.

Abstract: *SHANK3* encodes a scaffold protein involved in postsynaptic receptor density in gluta-matergic synapses, including those in the parvalbumin (PV)+ inhibitory neurons—the key players in the generation of sensory gamma oscillations, such as 40-Hz auditory steady-state response (ASSR). However, 40-Hz ASSR was not studied in relation to SHANK3 functioning. Here, we present a 15-year-old girl (SH01) with previously unreported duplication of the first seven exons of the *SHANK3* gene (22q13.33). SH01's electroencephalogram (EEG) during 40-Hz click trains of 500 ms duration binaurally presented with inter-trial intervals of 500–800 ms were compared with those from typically developing children ($n = 32$). SH01 was diagnosed with mild mental retardation and learning disabilities (F70.88), dysgraphia, dyslexia, and smaller vocabulary than typically developing (TD) peers. Her clinical phenotype resembled the phenotype of previously described patients with 22q13.33 microduplications (≈30 reported so far). SH01 had mild autistic symptoms but below the threshold for ASD diagnosis and microcephaly. No seizures or MRI abnormalities were reported. While SH01 had relatively preserved auditory event-related potential (ERP) with slightly attenuated P1, her 40-Hz ASSR was totally absent significantly deviating from TD's ASSR. The absence of 40-Hz ASSR in patients with microduplication, which affected the *SHANK3* gene, indicates deficient temporal resolution of the auditory system, which might underlie language problems and represent a neurophysiological biomarker of *SHANK3* abnormalities.

Keywords: 22q13.3 duplication; auditory steady-state response; ASSR; *SHANK3*; biomarker; auditory event-related potential; ERP; autism spectrum disorders; intellectual disabilities

1. Introduction

SH3 and multiple ankyrin repeat domain 3 (*SHANK3*), also known as proline-rich synapse-associated protein 2 (ProSAP2), is a gene that encodes scaffolding proteins that organize postsynaptic density in excitatory synapses [1,2]. This gene is in the 22nd chromo-some, 22q13.33 region. Deletion of this region as well as mutations lead to 22q13 Deletion Syndrome also known as Phelan–McDermid Syndrome (PMS) [3–8]. In most PMS cases, the *SHANK3* gene is affected that is believed to be the major cause of PMS.

Phelan–McDermid Syndrome (PMS) is a rare neurodevelopmental disorder with about 2000 cases identified so far [6]. However, many PMS cases can go unnoticed, as the diagno-sis of PMS is often difficult due to the subtle appearance of the deletion of chromosome 22 and relatively mild physical and nonspecific clinical manifestation of the syndrome.

171

Dysmorphic features in PMS include dysplastic nails, large or prominent ears, long eye-lashes, wide nasal bridge, bulbous nose, and sacral dimple [3]. Major dysfunctions in PMS are hypotonia [3], global developmental delay, and severely delayed or absent speech [4]. Autistic traits are also present in most patients with PMS, suggesting PMS as a syndromic form of autism spectrum disorder (ASD) [9,10]. According to a recent meta-analysis, 0.7% of patients with ASD have *SHANK3* mutations, and this number is even higher (2.1%) for ASD patients with moderate to profound intellectual disability [11]. Moreover, altered methylation patterns in *SHANK3* were detected in ≈15% of postmortem autistic brain tissue [12], suggesting even more widespread implication of altered *SHANK3* expression to ASD development through epigenetic influence. Copy-number of variance (CNV) and point mutations of *SHANK3* have been also associated with intellectual disability and schizophrenia [11,13–19].

Few cases (*n*≈30) of duplication involving the *SHANK3* gene has been described in the literature: among patients with Asperger's syndrome, attention-deficit hyperactivity disorder (ADHD), bipolar disorder [20], schizophrenia [21], intellectual disabilities, de-layed speech and language development [20–24]. While ASD is reported in patients with *SHANK3* duplication, ASD prevalence seems to be smaller than in *SHANK3* deletions or mutations (≈15% vs. >50%). Dysmorphic features of patients with duplications and mutations affected *SHANK3* gene included full lips, slightly upturned nose/anteverted nares, protruding ears, arch-shaped eyebrows. Microcephaly was reported in 15% of re-ported cases [23]. Resemblances between the cases with *SHANK3* duplication noticed by the researchers points to a distinct 22q13.33 duplication syndrome (for a recent update, see [23,24]). At the same time, the implication of both *SHANK3* deletion and duplication in neurodevelopmental and neuropsychiatric disorders suggests that *SHANK3* gene dosage is essential for correct brain function. However, one must be aware that microduplications does not always mean overexpression of the coded proteins, as an insertion of genetic material within the gene can alter nucleotide sequence and lead to abnormal protein code. Thus, detailed molecular genetic analysis is needed to infer whether the microduplication leads to gain or loss of *SHANK3* functioning.

Several animal models of ASD with deficient *Shank3* gene were developed. Mice with *Shank3* mutations/deletion exhibit ASD-like symptoms including social abnormalities and motor coordination problems [12,14,16,24–32]. The transgenic mice with mildly overex-press Shank3 proteins (≈50%) were also created [20,33,34]. These mice display manic-like hyperkinetic behaviors and decreased social interaction; however, unlike *Shank3* knockout mice (KO), *Shank3* transgenic mice did not exhibit repetitive behavior.

Shank3 determines the postsynaptic density of N-methyl-D-aspartate (NMDA) recep-tors. NMDAR is one of three ionotropic receptors to the main excitatory mediator in the brain: glutamate. Deviation in NMDAR function alters excitation/inhibition balance in neuronal circuitry and associates with autistic-like behavior in patients with ASD as well as in its animal models [26]. It is noteworthy that different *Shank3* mouse lines show similar NMDAR hypofunction [14,16,25–31].

Recent studies pointed to the abnormalities in inhibitory signaling in *Shank3*-mouse models of ASD. In particular, several studies [16,35] reported the reduced number of synaptic puncta containing parvalbumin (PV) as well as reduced PV expression of the PV-expressing gamma-aminobutyric acid (GABA) interneuron—the most abundant subtype of the inhibitory interneurons, which contribute to the perisomatic inhibition of glutamatergic principal cells. Supporting the implication of reduced inhibition to Shank3 deficits, an en-hancer of GABA-mediated inhibitory transmission, clonazepam, normalizes the abnormal network firing pattern in cultured cortical neurons of *Shank3* KO mice [36].

Cortical gamma oscillations (30–100 Hz) are generated in recurrent circuits of excita-tory and inhibitory neurons [37–39] and reflect the excitatory state of the neural network. While baseline, spontaneous gamma oscillations are studied in humans and animals, high-frequency oscillations are most reliably induced in response to sensory stimuli [40–43]. The evoked gamma-band activity can be studied with auditory steady-state response

(ASSR) [41–43]. ASSR refers to the ability of the neural populations to synchronize the timing of neural discharges with the frequency of external periodic auditory stimulation, e.g., click trains or amplitude modulated tone. ASSR is most pronounced in response to 40 Hz stimulation [44], coinciding with an intrinsic resonance frequency of cortical PV+ fast-spiking interneurons [45,46]. This 40-Hz ASSR was recently proposed as a non-invasive biomarker of NMDA receptor function [47–50]. In mice the pharmacological modulation of NMDAR function by NMDA antagonists such as MK-801 or ketamine suggested an inverse relationship between ASSR and NMDA occupancy [48,51]. Nakao and colleagues [47] demonstrated robust ASSR deficits in the mutant mice with selective elimination of NM-DARs from PV+ interneurons in neocortex (Ppp1r2-cre/fGluN1 KO mice), suggesting a causal role of the NMDA receptors on this PV+ interneurons for neural entrainment at 40 Hz. Modeling studies supported this finding, emphasizing the link between NMDAR on PV+ interneurons and 40-Hz ASSR [52,53].

ASSR is reduced in schizophrenia (for meta-analysis see [54]), bipolar disorders [55–58], and autism spectrum disorders (ASD) [59,60], which are the disorders with implicated GABAergic dysfunctions and altered NMDA signaling. The 40-Hz ASSR deficit occurs in non-psychotic first-degree relatives of patients with schizophrenia [61] and ASD [59], which is consistent with an effect of familial or genetic risk factors. However, recent larger sample studies in children with ASD did not confirm ASSR reduction [62,63]. Such discrepancy might be related to the well-known heterogeneity of the ASD population. Even remarkably similar behavioral manifestations can be caused by different biological underpinnings, e.g., genetic etiology. Thus, examination of ASSR for the patient with known genetic abnormalities, associated with ASD, might be the Rosetta stone for the identification of subgroups of ASD patients based on common molecular–genetic and neurophysiological causes.

Gamma oscillations have been associated with perceptual organization, attention, memory, consciousness, language processing, and motor coordination [64]. The 40-Hz ASSR has been suggested as a candidate mechanism underlying the fast temporal integration and resolution of auditory inputs [41,42,65,66]. In neurotypical controls and elderly population, ASSR was correlated with gap detection threshold [66] and attenuation of speech perception under the presence of noise [65], pointing to the relevance of ASSR to language processing. In patients with schizophrenia, the 40-Hz ASSR positively correlated with the working memory performance [67], attentional functioning [68], and predicted the future global symptomatic outcome (GAF-S2) [69]. Thus, ASSR is linked to the cognitive functioning, which is altered in patients with *SHANK3* abnormalities.

The promising approach in building the causal link between genes and behavior is relating the genetic pathways converging on candidate cellular/molecular processes to the target neurophysiological phenotype. In line with this approach, here, we present the clinical and neurophysiological description of a 15-year-old girl with rare microduplication in 22q13.33, which affects the *SHANK3* gene. The study focused on examination of the 40-Hz ASSR response, which is crucially dependent on PV+ interneurons activity, one of the key targets of the *SHANK3* gene. At the behavioral level, ASSR is thought to reflect temporal integration and resolution of the auditory system and is linked to memory and speech-in-noise processing. Based on this logic, we hypothesize that this girl will have altered ASSR.

2. Results

2.1. Genetic Information

The girl, further referred as SH01, has normal karyotype (46, XX). Molecular genetics analysis using an SNP array revealed a duplication (size: 16,389 bp) spanning partially *SHANK3*. The duplication affected the first seven exons of the gene (Figure 1).

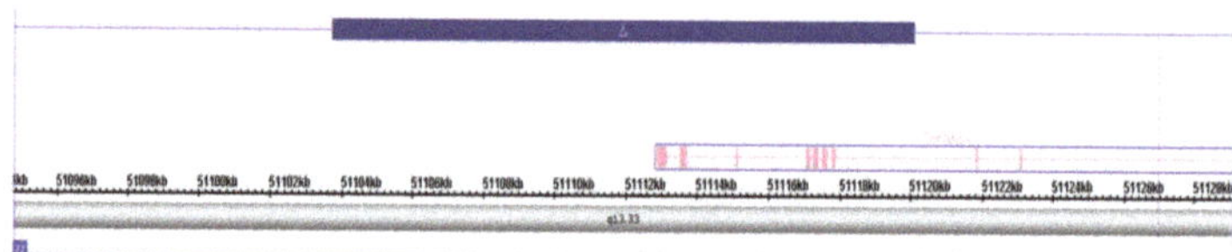

Figure 1. SNP array analysis demonstrating the duplication affecting the first seven exons of the *SHANK3* gene.

2.2. Phenotyping, Clinical Description

Anamnesis. SH01 was from full-term pregnancy from healthy parents, who were 39 years old at the time of the girl's birth. Her weight at birth was 3.040 g and length 52 cm, Apgar score was 7/8. Motor milestones were achieved within normal limits with holding her head at 2 months, sat down at 6 months, stood with the support at 10 months, began to walk alone at 11 months. However, language milestones were slightly delayed with the first syllables appeared at 12 months followed by a relatively long time of no phrases. Short sentences appeared at the age of 3. Cognitive development was also delayed, with a lack of interest in books and cartoons until age 3. At about this age, SH01 developed aggressiveness toward peers (e.g., biting) and protest behavior. At kindergarten, she referred her bad behavior to a fictional peer-boy. Aggressive behavior was resolved when she was about 10 years old. Currently, she might have some rare periods of self-aggression (biting) when too angry and unsatisfied. SH01 started normal school together with typically developing (TD) peers, but by the end of primary school, she was referred to specialists due to the problems with dealing with the school program (especially Math). However, she managed to continue the study in the school with TD peers with the support of the specialists and parents. Menstruation was regular and started at 10 years of age.

SH01 took part in our EEG/ERP experiment at age 15.06 years old. Her official diagnoses were mild mental retardation and other deficits of behavior due to other specified causes (F70.88), and organic emotionally labile [asthenic] disorder with unspecified cause (F06.69). Diagnoses were obtained from the recent clinical reports provided by experienced psychiatrists from the Moscow Research Institute of Psychiatry and Scientific and Practical Center for Mental Health of Children and Adolescents, which is a leading Moscow organization for the diagnosis of mental health problems. The report from a psychologist confirmed mild mental retardation by the Wechsler Intelligence Scale for Children (Russian adaptation based on original Wechsler Intelligence Scale for Children [70]): verbal IQ = 71; nonverbal/performance IQ = 64; full-scale IQ = 64. The psychologist also pointed to unstable attention, smaller memory span, a fluctuating but lower speed of performance, quicker tiredness and loss of work efficiency, as well as infantilism, protest behavior, irritability, emotional liability, problems with understanding the social context, lack of self-critique and motivation to overcome difficulties, and a preponderance of recreational entertaining interests over educational and cognitive ones. A speech therapist revealed mild forms of dysgraphia and dyslexia.

Parents' major concerns at age 15 were learning disabilities, behavioral disorders, and irritability. The girl was sociable, and her mild cognitive impairment was hardly noticeable in daily routines. Her mild speech underdevelopment manifested in rare problems to pronounce long and complex words and smaller vocabulary than typically developing (TD) peers. She attended the 9th grade of normal middle school that required great efforts from her parents. While she hardly managed to make any homework by herself, she was considering continuing her education in high school, pointing to the lack of adequate self-assessment. Among her interests was performing in a school theater. She used her right hand to write and to eat. At EEG/ERP examination, she showed infantile childish behavior, demanding attention of others and especially her mom, which was not typical for her age (e.g., she asked her mom to stay with her in the experimental room).

Physical parameters at the age of 15: 163 cm (50–75 percentile), 50 kg (50–75 percentile), head circumference of 51.5 cm (lower than 3rd percentile). Facial phenotype included elongated face, protruding auricles. There were short 5th fingers on the hands, a sandal gap. The girl had mild scoliosis, valgus deformity of the knee joints, and planovalgus feet.

Autistic characteristics as assessed at age 15. SH01's T-scores on social responsiveness scale (SRS) equals 63, which referred to mild autistic symptoms [71], while neither the Autism Diagnostic Interview-Revised [72] (ADI-R, with subscale social interaction A-4 scores, Communication and language B-2, repetitive and restricted behavior C-1, early developmental problems, 1-36 months, D-1) nor psychiatric assessment support the ASD diagnosis.

Magnetic resonance imaging (MRI) at age 15: The hemispheres of the brain were symmetrical. No focal changes in the intensity of the MR signal from the substance of the brain, cerebellum, or brain stem were found. Differentiation into cortical and medullary substances was expressed satisfactorily. The lateral ventricles were symmetrical, not dilated. The hind horns were deepened. The cerebellum was typically located. The pituitary gland was not changed with preserved structure. The adeno- and neurohypophysis was clearly differentiated. Chiasma did not change. The optic nerves were clearly visible. The median structures were not displaced. The craniovertebral junction was not changed.

Other laboratory examinations at age 15. Echocardiography revealed ectopic chords and trabeculae in the left ventricular cavity, mitral valve prolapse with 1+ regurgitation, tricuspid valve prolapse with 1.5+ regurgitation. Ultrasound examination showed bilateral nephroptosis. X-ray showed a short fifth finger metacarpal bone of the left hand. Pulmonary examination revealed moderate bronchial asthma, atopic, with polyvalent sensitization.

Medications at age 15: SH01 took phenibut, 250 mg three times a day to control behavior and levothyroxine (L-thyroxine) 50 mL to treat her asthma (diagnosis J45.0—Predominantly allergic asthma).

2.3. Clinical EEG

The voltage of EEG activity was in accordance with the healthy peers' EEG voltage; significant asymmetry of the background EEG was not detected. EEG recordings with eyes closed demonstrated normal background EEG with dominate alpha rhythm (Figure 2a). In 2018, it had an amplitude of 107 μV and 87 μV (maximal and mean, respectively) and a frequency of 9.1 Hz in the left hemisphere and amplitude of 104 μV and 69 μV (maximal and mean, respectively) and frequency 9.3 Hz in the right hemisphere. In 2020, the dominate alpha rhythm in the eyes closed condition had an amplitude of 93 μV and 67 μV (maximal and mean, respectively) and frequency of 9.5 Hz in the left hemisphere and amplitude of 94 μV and 63 μV (maximal and mean, respectively) and frequency of 9.7 Hz in the right hemisphere. The abnormalities of the background EEG (Figure 2b) could be described as intermittent theta, slowing (3.5–5.5 Hz and 80–140 μV) in the right hemisphere in 2018; in 2020, abnormalities of the background EEG could be described as sporadic spike and polyspike discharges (100–150 μV) arising from the right centrotemporal region.

2.4. ASSR/Auditory ERP

SH01's 40-Hz ASSR and auditory ERP were compared with two control groups of typically developing (TD) children: the first one ("old", n = 13, seven females, mean age 16.04 (SD = 1.9), ranged 12–18) was age-matched with our patient SH01 (age = 15.06). The second subgroup ("young") consisted of 19 participants (14 female, five male) with an average age of 7.8 (SD = 2.6), ranged 3–12. Comparison groups of different ages were selected to examine if the suggested alternation in SH01's neurophysiological responses to sounds might be linked to the developmental delay in brain maturation (as changes of auditory ERP and ASSR with age are known, see Section 3) or represent more general phenomena. Table 1 summarizes the results.

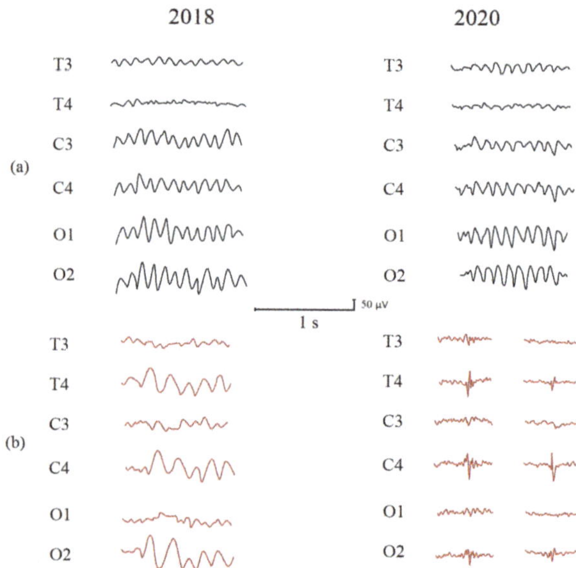

Figure 2. (**a**) Dominate alpha rhythm with eyes closed, (**b**) the abnormalities of the background EEG.

Table 1. Amplitudes of 40-Hz auditory steady-state response (ASSR) and event-related potential (ERP) components (mean ± STD) for two comparison groups of typically developing children and SH01 in Fz electrode.

	ASSR, µV	P1, µV	N1, µV	P2, µV
SH01 (15.1 y o)	−0.002	1.359	1.102	3.670
Old group (16.1 ± 1.9 y o)	0.274 ± 0.103	3.159 ± 2.017	1.829 ± 1.885	2.332 ± 2.241
Young group (7.8 ± 2.6 y o)	0.158 ± 0.155	4.267 ± 1.886	6.059 ± 3.801	6.455 ± 4.754

The 40-Hz ASSR was clearly identified in the TD groups and was dominant at frontal sites (Figures 3 and 4). Consistent with previous reports, 40-Hz ASSR peaked about 200 ms post-train onset and persisted over the whole period of stimuli presentation in all TD participants, which were significantly higher in the older control group than in the younger one (t (30) = 2.362, p = 0.025), as can be also seen in Figure 5, which represents the individual 40-Hz ASSR values averaged over the whole period of stimuli presentation. At the same time, 40-Hz ASSR were totally absent in SH01 (Figure 3), being significantly smaller compared to any of the TD groups (old vs. SH01: t (12) = 9.6602, p < 0.0001; young vs. SH01: t (18) = 5.684, p < 0.0001). Moreover, there were no TD participant in the old, age-matched group who had 40-Hz ASSR value below that of SH01 (minimum value in the TD old group being 0.053 µV, SH01's ASSR = −0.015 µV), suggesting a very robust effect (Figure 4, Figure A1 in Appendix A).

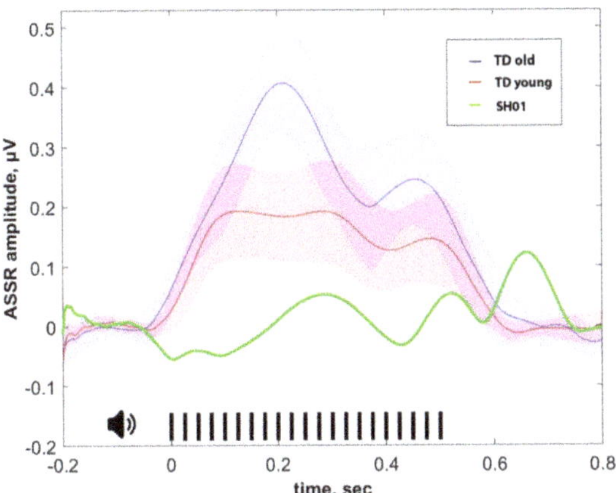

Figure 3. Envelope curve of 40-Hz ASSR obtained after Hilbert transform from electrode Fz. The ASSR of SH01 is shown in green, that of the young group of typically developing children (TD young) is in red, and that of the old, age-matched to SH01 group (TD old) is in blue. Opaque blue and red shading illustrate the 95% confidence interval. The time of stimulus presentation is 0.

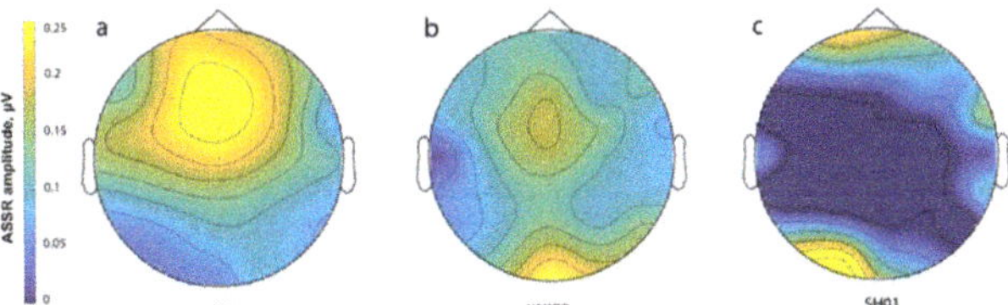

Figure 4. Topographic map of 40-Hz ASSR amplitude averaged over the period of 0–500 ms. The "old" group is represented in (**a**), the "young" group is represented in (**b**), and the values of SH01 are represented in (**c**).

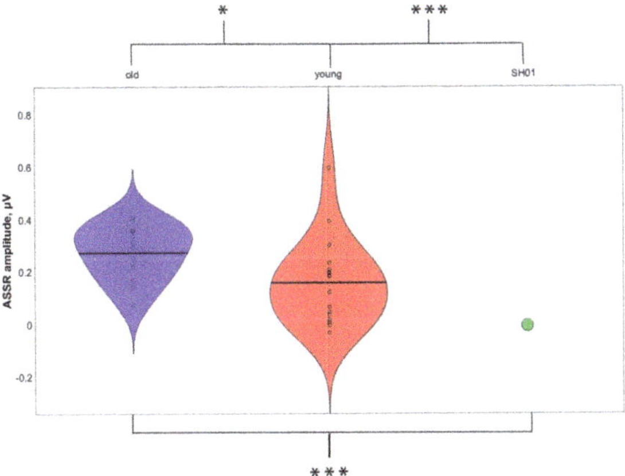

Figure 5. Individual values of 40-Hz ASSR across the groups (Fz electrode). The old TD group's values are shown in the first column, the young TD group's values are shown in the second, and SH01's values are shown in the third. (* shows significant differences $p < 0.05$, *** shows significant differences $p < 0.0001$).

Figure 6 represents the auditory event-related potentials to the same stimuli that fail to elicit 40-Hz ASSR in SH01. Despite such a drastic alteration in ASSR response, auditory ERP in SH01 were much more similar to that of TD groups (Figure 6, Figure A2 for individual ERPs). The old TD group was characterized by prominent P1, N1, and N2 components, which were registered after the 40-Hz train onset. SH01's ERP generally resembled that of the old TD ERPs, with only SH01's P1 components being significantly smaller than that in her age-matched group (t (12) = 3.484, p = 0.005), while N1 (t (12) = 1.864, p = 0.087) and P2 (t (12) = −2.099, p = 0.058) were unremarkable as represented in Figures 6 and 7. For the peak values of major ERP components, see Table 1. As for younger TD participants, their ERPs was characterized by the absence of a clear N1 response, corresponding with well-known developmental change in the ERPs structure (old TD vs. young TD: t (30) = −3.524, p = 0.0014). For all components, the SH01's ERPs differed from the young groups (P1: t (18) = 5.683, p < 0.0001; N1: t (18) = 5.863, p < 0.0001; P2: t (18) = 2.554, p = 0.02). Thus, the auditory ERP in SH01 was more similar to her peers than to the young control group, pointing to a generally preserved development of auditory ERP structure.

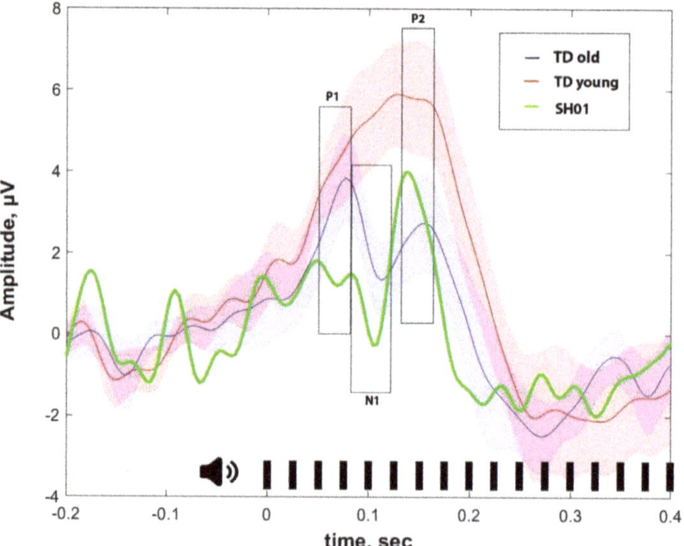

Figure 6. Auditory event-related potentials (ERPs), in Fz electrode with SH01 shown in green, the younger TD group (TD young) is shown in red, and the old, age-matched with SH01 control group (TD old) is shown in blue. Opaque blue and red shading illustrate 95% confidence interval. The time of stimulus presentation is 0. Time windows for P1 (50–80 ms), N1 (80–120 ms), and P2 (130–160 ms) are shown in rectangles.

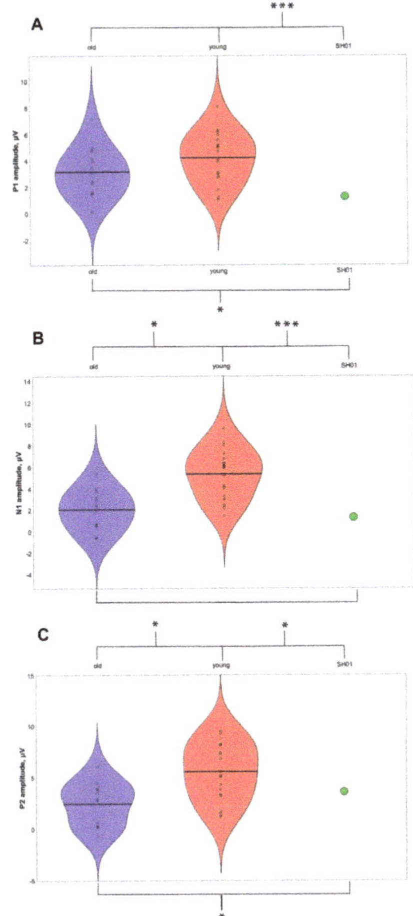

Figure 7. ERPs components across groups. P1 component is shown in (**a**), N1 is shown in (**b**), P2 is shown in (**c**). The old typically developing (TD) group's values are shown in the first column, the young TD's values are shown in a second, and SH01's value is shown in the third (* shows significant differences $p < 0.05$, *** shows significant differences $p < 0.0001$).

3. Discussion

Our report presents a new patient with unique duplication of the first seven exons of the *SHANK3* gene, adding one more case to the about 30 patients with 22q13.3 duplications described in previous studies [23]. For the first time, we describe the neurophysiological phenotype of a patient with 22q13.3 duplications. The major focus of our study was on the 40-Hz ASSR, a brain response to high-frequency auditory stimulation, which is thought to underlie temporal binding and speech-in-noise processing [65]. This choice was motivated by the studies that reported 40-Hz ASSR as a biomarker of NMDAR density and PV+ interneurons functioning, as they are dependent on *SHANK3* gene activity [48–51]. Here, we report a striking absence of 40-Hz ASSR in SH01, collaborating our initial hypothesis. Below, we discuss our findings in more detail.

The clinical phenotype of SH01 resembles that described for few patients with 22q13.3 microduplication ($n = 29$, [23], Table 2), although clinical features in the 22q13.3 duplication syndromes show great variability. Among common features are intellectual disabilities

(n = 15), attention deficits (n = 5), and language problems (n = 11). Physical dysmorphic features have been also reported in these patients previously, including sandal gap (n = 1) and protruding or low-set deformed ears (n = 3), microcephaly (n = 5). One previously described patient with 22q13.3 microduplication [21] shared with our patient irritability and scoliosis, as well as mild mental retardation and attention deficits. It is noteworthy that a girl showed normal development until 13 years old but later was diagnosed with borderline intellectual functioning and disorganized schizophrenia. At the same time, unlike few patients with 22q13.3 microduplication who were diagnosed with autism spectrum disorders (n = 5) and epilepsy (n = 4), our patient SH01 does not have epilepsy, only some minor epileptiform activity in EEG, and does not have enough symptoms to get a diagnosis of autism spectrum disorder, while her SRS score suggested some autistic features. SH01 phenotype was also compared to the more studied 22q13.3 deletion syndrome. SH01 shared with patients of this syndrome intellectual disabilities and language problems, as well as autistic features, although their manifestations are milder in SH01 [3,73–75]. Among the dysmorphic features reported in patients with PMS, SH01 also has an elongated skull. Thus, the clinical description of SH01 contains both common and distinct features with patients with different types of abnormalities affecting *SHANK3*, while it more resembles those with *SHANK3* microduplications, pointing to a partially distinct phenotype of 22q13.3 duplication and deletion. For convenience, Table 2 shows the prevalence of individual clinical features in patients with *SHANK3* duplication and deletion.

Table 2. Clinical phenotype of patients with 22q13.3 duplication and 22q13.3 deletion/mutations. In addition to individual cases of patients with 22q13.3 duplication (that include *SHANK3* gene), the last two lines show the overall occurrence (in percentage) of the symptoms in patients with 22q13.3 duplication (based on [21] and our own review of individual cases reported previously) and 22q13.3 deletion/mutations (taken from previous reviews). Our subject, SH01, is also included for comparison. As patients of different ages are described, both IQ and developmental quotient (DQ) are used to characterize mental retardation. +/− reflects the presence/absence of the symptom.

	Language Problem	Mental Retardation	Autism	Microcephaly	Seizures	Attention Deficit	Affective/ Psychiatric Symptoms	Physical Abnormalities/ Dysmorphism
SH01, our patient	mild dyslexia, dysgraphia	mild, IQ 64	SRS = 63, no diagnosis	+	−	+	irritability, aggressiveness	elongated skull, protruding auricles, sandal gap
Johannessen et al. (2019) [23]	n/a	mild	n/a	n/a	+	+	bipolar disease	Tourette syndrome (motor tics), mild dysmorphism
Han et al. (2013) [20] Patient 1	n/a	mild	n/a	n/a	+	+	destructive behavior	dysmorphism
Han et al. (2013) [20] Patient 2	n/a	mild	n/a	n/a	+	+	bipolar disorder	−
Chen et al. (2017) [76]	language delay, echolalia	mild, IQ 62	autistic traits, no diagnosis	n/a	n/a	+	irritability	−
Ujfalusi et al. (2020) [24] Patient 1	−	mild, IQ 72	n/a	−	−	n/a	−	dysmorphism
Ujfalusi et al. (2020) [24] Patient 2	dyslexia, dysgraphia	mild, IQ 79	n/a	−	+	−	bipolar disorder, temper tantrums	dysmorphism
Okamoto et al. (2007) [77] Patient 1	language delay	moderate, DQ 40	−	−	-	−	−	hypotonia, dysmorphism
Okamoto et al. (2007) [77] Patient 2	language delay	moderate, DQ 46	−	−	−	−	−	hypotonia, dysmorphism

Table 2. *Cont.*

	Language Problem	Mental Retardation	Autism	Microcephaly	Seizures	Attention Deficit	Affective/ Psychiatric Symptoms	Physical Abnormalities/ Dysmorphism
Failla et al. (2007) [21]	incoherent speech	mild, IQ 73	−	+	−	+	schizophrenia, irritability, aggressiveness	dysmorphism
Destrée et al. (2011) [78] Patient 1	language delay	mild	n/a	+	n/a	n/a	n/a	dysmorphism, growth retardation
Destrée et al. (2011) [78] Patient 2	language delay	mild	n/a	+	n/a	n/a	n/a	dysmorphism, growth retardation
Duplication ($n = 31$), %	35%	80% (from mild to severe)	19%	17%	17%	16%	bipolar disorder –4% psychosis–7%	Dysmorphism-54%
Deletion/PMS, %	100% (no speech in 50%) [79]	96% (with profound in 53%) [74]	31–84% [74,79]	6–14% [80]	63% [81]	11% [74]	bipolar disorder –54% psychosis–12% irritability– 36% [82]	68–93% dysmorphism [74]

Our study indicates a general preservation of auditory ERP in SH01 with the pronounced N1-P2 response, which is typical for TD teens. At the same time, the P1 component that usually decreases with age [83,84] is not evident in SH01, with amplitude within P1 latency being significantly smaller in SH01 not only as compared to the younger cohort but also as compared to the age-matched control group. Unfortunately, we are not aware of any ERP study conducted in patients with the 22q13.3 microduplication. Thus, we compare our results with those obtained in patients with point mutations or deletion in 22q13.3 (PMS). Consistent with our finding of reduced P1 response to auditory stimuli, Reese and colleagues [85] found a reduction of P50 in response to the repeated tone in patients with PMS. It is noteworthy that the reduction was significant only for the female participants. Thus, there might be some common deficits in the early stage of auditory processing in the auditory cortex in patients with abnormalities related to the *SHANK3* gene. The decrease in the early component of visual ERP to checkerboard stimuli, which was registered within the same latency range, 50-75 ms post-stimulus, was also reported in PMS [86,87], pointing to the fact that neurophysiological abnormalities occur in PMS at the early stages of sensory processing regardless of the modality of stimulation. Whether such deficits also spread to the visual system in our patient was not studied. It is noteworthy that the attenuation of P1 in response to auditory stimuli was also reported in patients with idiopathic autism [88–90], linking these behavioral and neurophysiological abnormalities.

As for the later components, patients with PMS showed a reduction of P2 component in response to the repeated tones [85,91] as well as a decrease in the latency of N250 in response to oddball stimuli [92]. In our study, neither P2 nor N250 were affected, and P2 even tended to be larger in SH01 than in the age-matched controls. Such discrepancy might indicate different neurophysiological phenotypes for 22q13.3 duplication/deletion or just be related to a methodological difference between the studies.

The focus of our study was 40-Hz ASSR, as we hypothesize its abnormality in our patient based on previous literature. Indeed, we found a striking absence of 40-Hz ASSR in SH01. Considering relatively normal auditory ERP in SH01, such finding points to specific deficits in following high-frequency auditory signals. An absence of 40-Hz ASSR might underlie a disruption of temporal integration and binding mechanism in audition that is linked with PV+ interneurons functioning [41,42]. As 40-Hz ASSR was correlated with speech-in-noise perception [65], an absence of ASSR might be related to speech decoding. At the same time, 40-Hz ASSR seems to reflect not a primary mechanism for speech comprehension, as the total absence of 40-Hz ASSR does not prevent SH01 from learning language and being fluent in everyday life. Rather, 40-Hz ASSR reflects some modulatory mechanism that helps to differentiate speech sounds, making it easier to learn and communicate. Abnormalities in such modulatory mechanism can cause low vocabulary and some complex words' pronunciation problems, as well as mild dysgraphia and dyslexia, as observed in SH01. Further studies are needed to fully examine SH01's phonematic abilities, which are related to speech perception, to shed light on the particular process disrupted with the absence of 40-Hz ASSR related to *SHANK3* abnormality.

While ASSR is modulated by age [44,93,94], our 15-year-old patient's 40-Hz ASSR was significantly smaller not only as compared to age-matched control group but also in relation to data obtained in children aged 3–12 years old. Thus, her 40-Hz ASSR deficiency is hard to explain by the developmental delay, or such a delay should be very profound with SH01's ASSR corresponding to that from TD children under 5–8 years old [95,96].

While 40-Hz ASSR was previously studied neither in patients with 22q13.3 deletion/duplication nor their animal models, Engineer and colleagues [97] observed a drastic attenuation of neuronal firing rate in response to rapidly presented sounds in the *Shank3*-deficient rat model. These authors showed that the number of driven spikes evoked by noise bursts and speech sounds as well as the spontaneous firing rate were significantly weaker in *Shank3*-deficient rats compared to control rats. In relation to our results, the effect was most pronounced when the stimuli were presented with short inter-stimulus intervals below 100 ms, especially in the primary auditory cortex and anterior auditory field. Taken together, the results point to the problems of following the rapidly presented auditory signal as general phenomena, which is related to *SHANK3* abnormalities. This might indicate that the gain and loss of *SHANK3* function share a common neurophysiological phenotype. It might also point to the potential loss-of-function effect of microduplication within the *SHANK3* gene. More detailed molecular genetic analysis and modeling might help resolve these alternatives.

Our study has implications to the heterogeneous population of idiopathic ASD with a significant percentage of its cases related to *SHANK3* abnormalities and having language problems. ASSR being easy to assess as a non-invasive index of functioning of PV+ neurons and NMDAR signaling, stemming from *SHANK3* abnormalities, can help segregate the ASD population based on neurophysiological and molecular genetic underpinnings.

Our study is not without limitations. First, it is just a case report of one patient's data. While SH01 is an incredibly unique patient, more studies are needed to confirm our observations. As there have been about 30 patients described so far, our study aims to promote the ASSR paradigm among other researchers and clinicians, inviting them to run 40-Hz ASSR in other patients with the 22q13.3 duplication identified world-wide. These studies are an important step toward the validation of this neurophysiological biomarker.

SH01 also took phenibut as regular medicine. As this drug is a GABA-receptor agonist, it might potentially influence ASSR. To rule out such an explanation, we compared SH01 with a kid without known genetic abnormalities, who also took Phenibut for migraine treatment. Such control kid exhibits typically pronounced 40-Hz ASSR (Appendix B, Figure A3). At the same time, more research on a larger sample is needed to examine the effects of phenibut on ASSR.

One may also relate absent 40-Hz ASSR to the hearing problems, arousal level, or attention deficits, as some researchers found ASSR modulation by these factors [44,98,99]. However, normal auditory ERP in response to the same stimuli rule out these explanations, as e.g., an N1 component was also shown to be modulated by attention and stimuli-subjective intensity [100]. Moreover, the P2 component, that was reported to be attenuated in participants with moderate to severe sensorineural hearing loss [101] even tended to be larger in SH01, pointing to an increased rather than decreased auditory sensitivity in SH01.

4. Materials and Methods

4.1. Participants

Thirty-two typically developing (TD) children were recruited from the local community to take part in a study as a comparison group. According to their parents or guardians, they did not have a history of neuropsychiatric conditions and had normal or corrected to normal vision and hearing. Except for one participant (this case is described in Appendix B), none of the participants reported to be taking any medicines. TD participants were divided into two subgroups by age (Appendix C, Table A1). The first one ("old") was age-matched with the participant SH01 (age = 15.06). It consisted of 13 people (7 female, 6 male) with an average age of 16.04 (SD = 1.9). The second subgroup "young") consisted of 19 participants (14 female, 5 male) with an average age of 7.8 (SD = 2.6).

Almost all participants' guardians filled in the Russian translation of the Social Responsiveness Scale, second edition (SRS-2) [71], the school age version for the "young" group and the school age or adult version for the "old" group. Threshold values for any social behavior deficiencies are 58 T-scores for males and 63 T-scores for females. None of the participants from the "old" group exceeded the threshold value (range 16–56, mean = 37, SD = 13), and only one participant from the "young" group had a greater value (range 11–62, mean = 27, SD = 14). Six participants did not have SRS values. More detailed characteristics of comparison samples are presented in Table A1.

The SH01 patient underwent a full clinical assessment at the Research Clinical Institute of Pediatrics by experienced clinicians. In addition, Autism Diagnostic Interview–Revised [72], an investigator-based semi-structured instrument, was administered by a trained interviewer to SH01's mom. It was used to assess autistic traits in SH01.

The study was approved by the local ethics committee of the Institute of Higher Nervous Activity and Neurophysiology, Russian Academy of Sciences, protocol number 3, date of approval July, 10th, 2020, and was conducted following the ethical principles regarding human experimentation (Helsinki Declaration). All children provided their verbal consent to participate in the study and were informed about their right to withdraw from the study at any time during the testing. Written informed consent was also obtained from a parent/guardian of each child.

4.2. EEG Recording

Electroencephalographic data were recorded using the NeuroTravel system with 32-scalp electrodes arranged according to the international 10–10 system. Ear lobe electrodes were used as reference, and the grounding electrode was placed centrally. For clinical EEG, periods of resting activity were recorded as well as a test on closing and opening the eyes.

4.3. Stimuli and Paradigm

The ASSR paradigm consisted of 40-Hz click train stimuli, which were presented binaurally through foam insert earphones for 500 ms at 80 dB sound pressure level. Inter-trial intervals varied from 500 to 800 ms. The total number of trials was 150, and the duration of the whole paradigm was around three minutes. Stimuli were presented via Presentation software (NeuroBehavioral Systems, Albany, CA, USA). During the experiment, participants were sitting in a dimmed room and watching a silent video of their choice.

4.4. Data Analysis

EEG analysis was performed using MATLAB (Version—b, The MathWorks, Natick, MA, USA), Fieldtrip software (https://www.fieldtriptoolbox.org/, [102]), as well as customized scripts. Peak values were compared using two-tailed Student's t-test for independent groups.

4.4.1. ASSR Analysis

First, the raw data were segmented into epochs with an interval of 200 ms before the stimulus and 800 ms after it. Then, the signal was filtered at a frequency of 35–45 Hz, and trials with amplitude within 3 STD of the mean were averaged. The mean number of selected trials was 97 ± 34 for the "old" group and 80 ± 17 for the "young" group. There were 182 good trials for SH01. To better characterize 40-Hz ASSR, we extracted the envelope of the signal using the Hilbert transform. The absolute value of this linear integral transformation reflects the envelope of the grand-average waveform (see Figure A4). Baseline correction for the 200–0 ms was applied. These steps were conducted for all participants, including the patient with microduplication affecting *Shank3*, SH01. For further analysis, we chose the Fz electrode, since according to topographic data (see Figure 3), ASSR has a maximum response near Fz. It is also consistent with the literature, which reports that ASSR is most pronounced in this site [103,104]. Then, we averaged the values of the envelope curve after Hilbert transform in the Fz electrode over the whole period of stimuli presentation (0–500 ms) and compared the results of SH01 with the average values of each comparison group.

4.4.2. ERP Analysis

ERP for auditory stimuli were created with filtering band-pass 1–30 Hz using the Fieldtrip function for all participants. The averaging epoch was the same as in ASSR analysis: 200 ms before the stimulus and 800 ms after it, but for later analysis, we focused on the period of –200–400 ms. Only trials with an amplitude within 3 STD of the mean were averaged. The mean number of good trials was 99 ± 43 for the old group, 96 ± 18 for the young group, and 69 for SH01. Then, we calculated ERPs peak values for all participants. The timeframes for each component were chosen based on grand-averaged peak latencies (P1: 50–80 ms; N1: 80–120 ms; P2: 130–160 ms).

4.5. Molecular Genetic Analysis

Molecular genetic analysis of SH01 was performed by CytoScan HD Arrays (Affymetrix, Santa Clara, CA, USA), which consists of about 2.7 million markers (resolution: >1 kbp). The results were visualized by the Affymetrix ChAS (Chromosome Analysis Suite) CytoScan® HD Array software (reference sequence GRCh37/hg19). The procedures were earlier described in detail [105,106]. All the genomic variations uncovered by the molecular genetic analysis were analyzed using a panel of bioinformatic techniques targeting the phenotypic outcome of each variation. The procedure was described previously in a step-by-step manner [107,108].

5. Conclusions

Our study demonstrates a link between duplication of the first seven exons of the *SHANK3* gene and alteration of brain response to high-frequency auditory input, 40-Hz ASSR: a neurophysiological phenotype believed to be mediated by hypofunctional NMDA receptor signaling on the parvalbumin (PV)+ inhibitory neurons, which depends on SHANK3 abnormality. As reported in our manuscript, the absence of 40-Hz ASSR in the patient with microduplication that affected *SHANK3* gene points to a deficient temporal resolution of this patient's auditory system, which might underlie the language problems observed in our patient as well as in many patients with abnormal functioning of the *SHANK3* gene.

Author Contributions: Conceptualization, O.V.S.; methodology, O.V.S. and V.Y.V.; data collection, A.K.N., A.B.R., O.V.S. and V.Y.V.; data analysis, A.K.N., G.V.P. and O.V.S.; resources and data curation, O.V.S. and V.Y.V.; genetic analysis, I.Y.I. and S.G.V.; writing—original draft preparation, O.V.S. and A.K.N.; writing—review and editing—all authors; visualization, A.K.N. All authors have read and agreed to the published version of the manuscript.

Funding: This research was funded by the Russian Science Foundation (RSF), grant #20-68-46042.

Institutional Review Board Statement: The study was conducted according to the guidelines of the Declaration of Helsinki, and approved by the Ethics Committee of the Institute of Higher Nervous Activity and Neurophysiology (protocol code 3, date of approval 10 July 2020).

Informed Consent Statement: All children provided their verbal consent to participate in the study and were informed about their right to withdraw from the study at any time during the testing. Written informed consent was also obtained from a parent/guardian of each child to publish this paper.

Data Availability Statement: Data available on request due to restrictions.

Acknowledgments: We thank all the participants of our study and their parents for their support and dedication to science. This work would not be possible without them.

Conflicts of Interest: The authors declare no conflict of interest. The funders had no role in the design of the study; in the collection, analyses, or interpretation of data; in the writing of the manuscript, or in the decision to publish the results.

Abbreviations

ASD	Autism Spectrum Disorders
ASSR	Auditory Steady State Response
EEG	Electroencephalogram
ERP	Event-related potential
GABA	Gamma-aminobutyric acid
TD	Typically developing children
PMS	Phelan-McDermid Syndrome
SRS	Social Responsiveness Scale

Appendix A

Individual ASSRs and ERPs

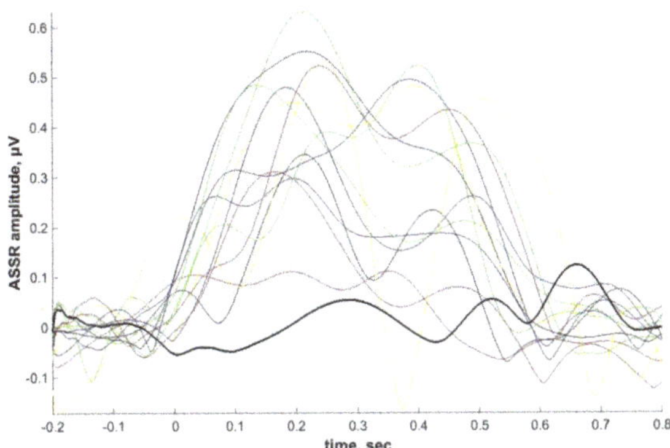

Figure A1. Individual values (µV) of 40-Hz ASSR obtained after Hilbert transform for age-matched comparison group ('old') and values of SH01 (presented in bold black). The time of stimulus presentation is 0.

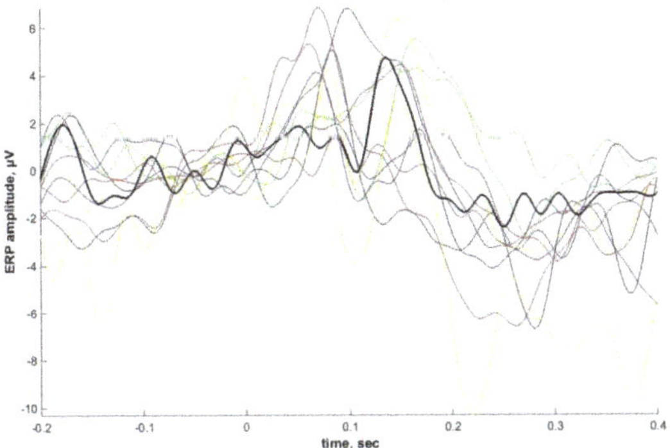

Figure A2. Individual ERPs (µV) for age-matched comparison group ('old') and SH01's ERP (presented in bold black).

Appendix B

Phenibut effect on ASSR

As mentioned above, one of the participants from the young group reported to be taking Phenibut. He was 8.41 years old and had normal SRS T-scores (19). He was taking half a tablet (250 mg) twice a day and was prescribed phenibut for a migraine attack. As it can be seen in Figure A3, D038 has ASSR within the range of other TD children from the young group (t (17) = −0.333, p = 0.743) and clearly above that of SH01. Thus, we can conclude that phenibut does not cause abnormally low ASSR in SH01.

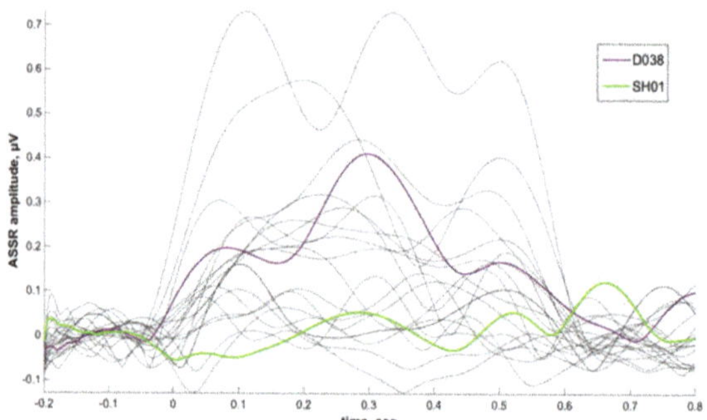

Figure A3. Comparison of ASSR values (µV) for the participant D038 who took phenibut (violet) and the participant SH01 (green). Individual amplitudes of 'young' group are shown in grey. The time of stimulus presentation is 0.

Appendix C

Table A1. Description of comparison groups including age, sex and SRS T-scores.

'Old' Group				'Young' Group			
Participant	Age	Sex	SRS, T-Scores	Participant	Age	Sex	SRS, T-Scores
D015	12.65	f	16	D043	2.58	f	26
D020	12.68	f	39	D033	3.04	m	
D021	13.45	f		D007	5.04	f	
D041	13.94	m	56	D009	5.86	f	22
D002	14.10	f	42	D022	6.01	m	23
D025	14.47	m	24	D012	6.42	f	21
D027	14.76	m	22	D004	7.93	f	15
D047	15.18	m	35	D001	8.18	f	28
D046	15.4	m	52	D006	8.24	f	41
D048	15.74	m	49	D013	8.4	f	22
D049	17, 98	f	38	D038	8.41	m	19
D050	17.98	f	37	D011	9.04	f	47
D030	17.99	f		D035	9.13	m	62
				D016	9.43	f	11
				D045	9.6	m	12
				D017	9.83	f	
				D014	10.69	f	
				D003	11.98	f	37
				D023	12.04	f	24

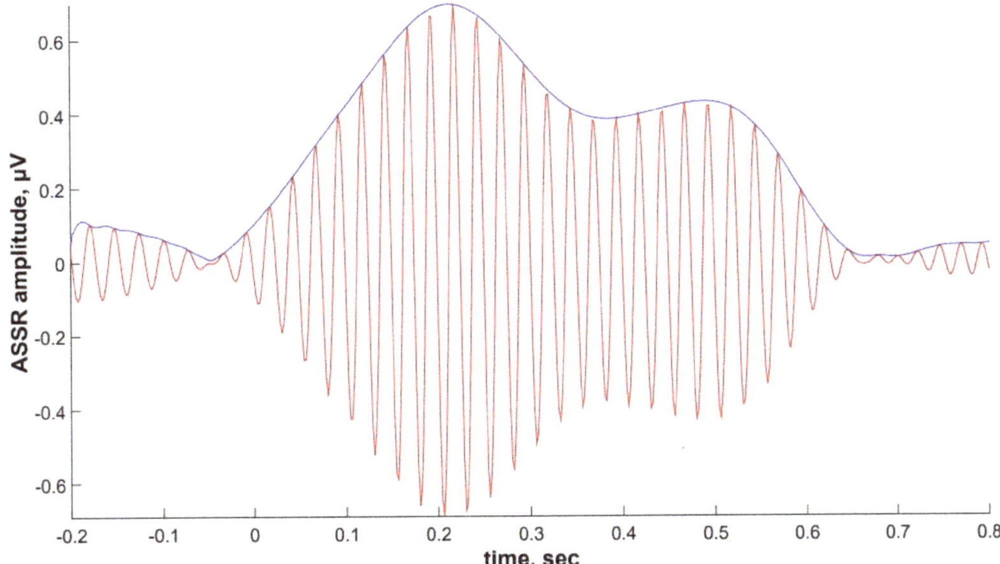

Figure A4. Illustration of Hilbert transformation performed for the analysis of ASSR. Red line corresponds with the signal obtained after filtering the data (35–45 Hz) and averaging all good trials. Blue line indicates Hilbert transformation of 35–45 Hz filtered ERPs.

References

1. Naisbitt, S.; Kim, E.; Tu, J.C.; Xiao, B.; Sala, C.; Valtschanoff, J.; Weinberg, R.J.; Worley, P.F.; Sheng, M. Shank, a Novel Family of Postsynaptic Density Proteins that Binds to the NMDA Receptor/PSD-95/GKAP Complex and Cortactin. *Neuron* **1999**, *23*, 569–582. [CrossRef]
2. Sheng, M.; Kim, E. The Shank Family of Scaffold Proteins. *J. Cell Sci.* **2000**, *113*, 1851–1856. [PubMed]
3. Phelan, K.; McDermid, H. The 22q13.3 Deletion Syndrome (Phelan-McDermid Syndrome). *Mol. Syndr.* **2011**, *2*, 186–201. [CrossRef]
4. Sarasua, S.M.; Dwivedi, A.; Boccuto, L.; Chen, C.-F.; Sharp, J.L.; Rollins, J.D.; Collins, J.S.; Rogers, R.C.; Phelan, K.; Dupont, B.R. 22q13.2q13.32 Genomic Regions Associated with Severity of Speech Delay, Developmental Delay, and Physical Features in Phelan–McDermid Syndrome. *Genet. Med.* **2013**, *16*, 318–328. [CrossRef] [PubMed]
5. Wilson, H.L.; Wong, A.C.C.; Shaw, S.R.; Tse, W.-Y.; Stapleton, A.G.; Phelan, M.C.; Hu, S.; Marshall, J.; McDermid, H.E. Molecular Characterisation of the 22q13 Deletion Syndrome Supports the Role of Haploinsufficiency of SHANK3/PROSAP2 in the Major Neurological Symptoms. *J. Med. Genet.* **2003**, *40*, 575–584. [CrossRef] [PubMed]
6. Bassell, J.; Srivastava, S.; Prohl, A.K.; Scherrer, B.; Kapur, K.; Filip-Dhima, R.; Berry-Kravis, E.; Soorya, L.; Thurm, A.; Powell, C.M.; et al. Diffusion Tensor Imaging Abnormalities in the Uncinate Fasciculus and Inferior Longitudinal Fasciculus in Phelan-McDermid Syndrome. *Pediatr. Neurol.* **2020**, *106*, 24–31. [CrossRef]
7. Costales, J.L.; Kolevzon, A. Phelan–McDermid Syndrome and SHANK3: Implications for Treatment. *Neurotherapeutics* **2015**, *12*, 620–630. [CrossRef]
8. Harony-Nicolas, H.; De Rubeis, S.; Kolevzon, A.; Buxbaum, J.D. Phelan McDermid Syndrome. *J. Child Neurol.* **2015**, *30*, 1861–1870. [CrossRef] [PubMed]
9. Betancur, C.; Buxbaum, J.D. SHANK3 Haploinsufficiency: A "Common" but Underdiagnosed Highly Penetrant Monogenic Cause of Autism Spectrum Disorders. *Mol. Autism* **2013**, *4*, 17. [CrossRef]
10. Oberman, L.M.; Rotenberg, A.; Pascual-Leone, A. Use of Transcranial Magnetic Stimulation in Autism Spectrum Disorders. *J. Autism Dev. Disord.* **2013**, *45*, 524–536. [CrossRef]
11. Leblond, C.S.; Nava, C.; Polge, A.; Gauthier, J.; Huguet, G.; Lumbroso, S.; Giuliano, F.; Stordeur, C.; Depienne, C.; Mouzat, K.; et al. Meta-Analysis of SHANK Mutations in Autism Spectrum Disorders: A Gradient of Severity in Cognitive Impairments. *PLoS Genet.* **2014**, *10*, e1004580. [CrossRef]

12. Zhu, L.; Wang, X.; Li, X.-L.; Towers, A.; Cao, X.; Wang, P.; Bowman, R.; Yang, H.; Goldstein, J.; Li, Y.-J.; et al. Epigenetic Dysregulation of SHANK3 in Brain Tissues from Individuals with Autism Spectrum Disorders. *Hum. Mol. Genet.* **2014**, *23*, 1563–1578. [CrossRef] [PubMed]

13. Grabrucker, A.M.; Schmeisser, M.J.; Schoen, M.; Boeckers, T.M. Postsynaptic ProSAP/Shank Scaffolds in the Cross-Hair of Synaptopathies. *Trends Cell Biol.* **2011**, *21*, 594–603. [CrossRef] [PubMed]

14. Duffney, L.J.; Zhong, P.; Wei, J.; Matas, E.; Cheng, J.; Qin, L.; Ma, K.; Dietz, D.M.; Kajiwara, Y.; Buxbaum, J.D.; et al. Autism-Like Deficits in Shank3-Deficient Mice Are Rescued by Targeting Actin Regulators. *Cell Rep.* **2015**, *11*, 1400–1413. [CrossRef] [PubMed]

15. Alexandrov, P.N.; Zhao, Y.; Jaber, V.; Cong, L.; Lukiw, W.J. Deficits in the Proline-Rich Synapse-Associated Shank3 Protein in Multiple Neuropsychiatric Disorders. *Front. Neurol.* **2017**, *8*, 670. [CrossRef] [PubMed]

16. Monteiro, P.; Feng, P.M.G. SHANK Proteins: Roles at the Synapse and in Autism Spectrum Disorder. *Nat. Rev. Neurosci.* **2017**, *18*, 147–157. [CrossRef] [PubMed]

17. Mei, Y.; Monteiro, P.; Zhou, Y.; Kim, J.-A.; Gao, X.; Fu, Z.; Feng, Y.M.P.M.Y.Z.J.-A.K.X.G.Z.F.G. Adult Restoration of Shank3 Expression Rescues Selective Autistic-like Phenotypes. *Nat. Cell Biol.* **2016**, *530*, 481–484. [CrossRef] [PubMed]

18. Sala, C.; Vicidomini, C.; Bigi, I.; Mossa, A.; Verpelli, C. Shank Synaptic Scaffold Proteins: Keys to Understanding the Pathogenesis of Autism and Other Synaptic Disorders. *J. Neurochem.* **2015**, *135*, 849–858. [CrossRef] [PubMed]

19. Moessner, R.; Marshall, C.R.; Sutcliffe, J.S.; Skaug, J.; Pinto, D.; Vincent, J.; Zwaigenbaum, L.; Fernandez, B.; Roberts, W.; Szatmari, P.; et al. Contribution of SHANK3 Mutations to Autism Spectrum Disorder. *Am. J. Hum. Genet.* **2007**, *81*, 1289–1297. [CrossRef]

20. Han, K.; Jr, J.L.H.; Schaaf, C.P.; Lu, H.-C.; Chen, H.; Kang, H.; Tang, J.; Wu, Z.; Hao, S.; Cheung, S.W.; et al. SHANK3 Overexpression Causes Manic-Like Behaviour with Unique Pharmacogenetic Properties. *Nat. Cell Biol.* **2013**, *503*, 72–77. [CrossRef]

21. Failla, P.; Romano, C.; Alberti, A.; Vasta, A.; Buono, S.; Castiglia, L.; Luciano, D.; Di Benedetto, D.; Fichera, M.; Galesi, O. Schizophrenia in a Patient with Subtelomeric Duplication of Chromosome 22q. *Clin. Genet.* **2007**, *71*, 599–601. [CrossRef]

22. Durand, C.M.; Betancur, C.; Boeckers, T.M.; Bockmann, J.; Chaste, P.; Fauchereau, F.; Nygren, G.; Rastam, M.; Gillberg, I.C.; Anckarsäter, H.; et al. Mutations in the Gene Encoding the Synaptic Scaffolding Protein shank3 Are Associated with Autism Spectrum Disorders. *Nat. Genet.* **2006**, *39*, 25–27. [CrossRef] [PubMed]

23. Johannessen, M.; Haugen, I.B.; Bakken, T.L.; Braaten, Ø. A 22q13.33 Duplication Harbouring the SHANK3 Gene: Does It Cause Neuropsychiatric Disorders? *BMJ Case Rep.* **2019**, *12*, e228258. [CrossRef] [PubMed]

24. Ujfalusi, A.; Nagy, O.; Bessenyei, B.; Lente, G.; Kántor, I.; Borbély, Á.J.; Szakszon, K. 22q13 Microduplication Syndrome in Siblings with Mild Clinical Phenotype: Broadening the Clinical and Behavioral Spectrum. *Mol. Syndr.* **2020**, *11*, 146–152. [CrossRef]

25. Kouser, M.; Speed, H.E.; Dewey, C.M.; Reimers, J.M.; Widman, A.J.; Gupta, N.; Liu, S.; Jaramillo, T.C.; Bangash, M.; Xiao, B.; et al. Loss of Predominant Shank3 Isoforms Results in Hippocampus-Dependent Impairments in Behavior and Synaptic Transmission. *J. Neurosci.* **2013**, *33*, 18448–18468. [CrossRef] [PubMed]

26. Lee, J.; Chung, C.; Ha, S.; Lee, D.; Kim, D.-Y.; Kim, H.; Kim, E. Shank3-Mutant Mice Lacking Exon 9 Show Altered Excitation/Inhibition Balance, Enhanced Rearing, and Spatial Memory Deficit. *Front. Cell. Neurosci.* **2015**, *9*, 94. [CrossRef] [PubMed]

27. Speed, H.E.; Kouser, M.; Xuan, Z.; Reimers, J.M.; Ochoa, C.F.; Gupta, N.; Liu, S.; Powell, C.M. Autism-Associated Insertion Mutation (InsG) of Shank3 Exon 21 Causes Impaired Synaptic Transmission and Behavioral Deficits. *J. Neurosci.* **2015**, *35*, 9648–9665. [CrossRef] [PubMed]

28. Jaramillo, T.C.; Speed, H.E.; Xuan, Z.; Reimers, J.M.; Liu, S.; Powell, C.M. Altered Striatal Synaptic Function and Abnormal Behaviour inShank3Exon4-9 Deletion Mouse Model of Autism. *Autism Res.* **2016**, *9*, 350–375. [CrossRef] [PubMed]

29. Jiang, Y.-H.; Ehlers, M.D. Modeling Autism by SHANK Gene Mutations in Mice. *Neuron* **2013**, *78*, 8–27. [CrossRef] [PubMed]

30. Yoo, J.; Bakes, J.; Bradley, C.; Collingridge, G.L.; Kaang, B.-K. Shank Mutant Mice as an Animal Model of Autism. *Philos. Trans. R. Soc. B Biol. Sci.* **2014**, *369*, 20130143. [CrossRef]

31. Schmeisser, M.J. Translational Neurobiology in Shank Mutant Mice—Model Systems for Neuropsychiatric Disorders. *Ann. Anat. Anat. Anz.* **2015**, *200*, 115–117. [CrossRef]

32. Dhamne, S.C.; Silverman, J.L.; Super, C.E.; Lammers, S.H.T.; Hameed, M.Q.; Modi, M.E.; Copping, N.A.; Pride, M.C.; Smith, D.G.; Rotenberg, A.; et al. Replicable in Vivo Physiological and Behavioral Phenotypes of the Shank3B Null Mutant Mouse Model of Autism. *Mol. Autism* **2017**, *8*, 1–19. [CrossRef] [PubMed]

33. Choi, S.-Y.; Pang, K.; Kim, J.Y.; Ryu, J.R.; Kang, H.; Liu, Z.; Kim, W.-K.; Sun, W.; Kim, H.; Han, K. Post-transcriptional Regulation of SHANK3 Expression by MicroRNAs Related to Multiple Neuropsychiatric Disorders. *Mol. Brain* **2015**, *8*, 74. [CrossRef] [PubMed]

34. Lee, S.; Lee, E.; Kim, R.; Kim, J.; Lee, S.; Park, H.; Yang, E.; Kim, H.; Kim, E. Shank2 Deletion in Parvalbumin Neurons Leads to Moderate Hyperactivity, Enhanced Self-Grooming and Suppressed Seizure Susceptibility in Mice. *Front. Mol. Neurosci.* **2018**, *11*, 209. [CrossRef] [PubMed]

35. Filice, F.; Vörckel, K.J.; Sungur, A.Ö.; Wöhr, M.; Schwaller, B. Reduction in Parvalbumin Expression Not Loss of the Parvalbumin-Expressing GABA Interneuron Subpopulation in Genetic Parvalbumin and Shank Mouse Models of Autism. *Mol. Brain* **2016**, *9*, 1–17. [CrossRef] [PubMed]

36. Lu, C.; Chen, Q.; Zhou, T.; Bozic, D.; Fu, Z.; Pan, J.Q.; Feng, G. Micro-Electrode Array Recordings Reveal Reductions in Both Excitation and Inhibition in Cultured Cortical Neuron Networks Lacking Shank3. *Mol. Psychiatry* **2015**, *21*, 159–168. [CrossRef]

37. Bartos, M.; Vida, I.; Jonas, P. Synaptic Mechanisms of Synchronized Gamma Oscillations in Inhibitory Interneuron Networks. *Nat. Rev. Neurosci.* **2007**, *8*, 45–56. [CrossRef]
38. Vinck, M.; Womelsdorf, T.; Buffalo, E.A.; DeSimone, R.; Fries, P. Attentional Modulation of Cell-Class-Specific Gamma-Band Synchronization in Awake Monkey Area V4. *Neuron* **2013**, *80*, 1077–1089. [CrossRef]
39. Carlen, M.; Meletis, K.; Siegle, J.; Cardin, J.; Futai, K.; Vierling-Claassen, D.; Rühlmann, C.; Jones, S.R.; Deisseroth, K.; Sheng, M.; et al. A Critical Role for NMDA Receptors in Parvalbumin Interneurons for Gamma Rhythm Induction and Behavior. *Mol. Psychiatry* **2011**, *17*, 537–548. [CrossRef] [PubMed]
40. Hoogenboom, N.; Schoffelen, J.-M.; Oostenveld, R.; Parkes, L.M.; Fries, P. Localizing Human Visual Gamma-Band Activity in Frequency, Time and Space. *NeuroImage* **2006**, *29*, 764–773. [CrossRef] [PubMed]
41. Ross, B.; Picton, T.W.; Pantev, C. Temporal Integration in the Human Auditory Cortex as Represented by the Development of the Steady-State Magnetic Field. *Hear. Res.* **2002**, *165*, 68–84. [CrossRef]
42. Ross, B.; Pantev, C. Auditory Steady-State Responses Reveal Amplitude Modulation Gap Detection Thresholds. *J. Acoust. Soc. Am.* **2004**, *115*, 2193–2206. [CrossRef] [PubMed]
43. Onitsuka, T.; Oribe, N.; Nakamura, I.; Kanba, S. Review of Neurophysiological Findings in Patients with Schizophrenia. *Psychiatry Clin. Neurosci.* **2013**, *67*, 461–470. [CrossRef]
44. Picton, T.W.; John, M.S.; Dimitrijevic, A.; Purcell, D. Human Auditory Steady-State Responses: Respuestas Auditivas de Estado Estable en Humanos. *Int. J. Audiol.* **2003**, *42*, 177–219. [CrossRef] [PubMed]
45. Tateno, T.; Harsch, A.; Robinson, H.P.C. Threshold Firing Frequency–Current Relationships of Neurons in Rat Somatosensory Cortex: Type 1 and Type 2 Dynamics. *J. Neurophysiol.* **2004**, *92*, 2283–2294. [CrossRef]
46. Golomb, D.; Donner, K.; Shacham, L.; Shlosberg, D.; Amitai, Y.; Hansel, D. Mechanisms of Firing Patterns in Fast-Spiking Cortical Interneurons. *PLoS Comput. Biol.* **2007**, *3*, e156. [CrossRef] [PubMed]
47. Enakao, K.; Enakazawa, K. Brain State-Dependent Abnormal LFP Activity in the Auditory Cortex of a Schizophrenia Mouse Model. *Front. Neurosci.* **2014**, *8*, 168. [CrossRef]
48. Sivarao, D.V.; Chen, P.; Senapati, A.; Yang, Y.; Fernandes, A.; Benitex, Y.; Whiterock, V.; Li, Y.-W.; Ahlijanian, M.K. 40 Hz Auditory Steady-State Response Is a Pharmacodynamic Biomarker for Cortical NMDA Receptors. *Neuropsychopharmacology* **2016**, *41*, 2232–2240. [CrossRef] [PubMed]
49. Sullivan, E.M.; Timi, M.P.; Hong, L.E.; O'Donnell, P. Effects of NMDA and GABA-A Receptor Antagonism on Auditory Steady-State Synchronization in Awake Behaving Rats. *Int. J. Neuropsychopharmacol.* **2015**, *18*, pyu118. [CrossRef] [PubMed]
50. Leishman, E.; O'Donnell, B.F.; Millward, J.B.; Vohs, J.L.; Rass, O.; Krishnan, G.P.; Bolbecker, A.R.; Morzorati, S.L. Phencyclidine Disrupts the Auditory Steady State Response in Rats. *PLoS ONE* **2015**, *10*, e0134979. [CrossRef]
51. Sivarao, D.V.; Frenkel, M.; Chen, P.; Healy, F.L.; Lodge, N.J.; Zaczek, R. MK-801 Disrupts and Nicotine Augments 40 Hz Auditory Steady State Responses in the Auditory Cortex of the Urethane-Anesthetized Rat. *Neuropharmacology* **2013**, *73*, 1–9. [CrossRef] [PubMed]
52. Kirli, K.K.; Ermentrout, G.B.; Cho, R.Y.; Kirli, K.K. Computational Study of NMDA Conductance and Cortical Oscillations in Schizophrenia. *Front. Comput. Neurosci.* **2014**, *8*, 8. [CrossRef] [PubMed]
53. Spencer, K.M. The Functional Consequences of Cortical Circuit Abnormalities on Gamma Oscillations in Schizophrenia: Insights from Computational Modeling. *Front. Hum. Neurosci.* **2009**, *3*, 33. [CrossRef] [PubMed]
54. Thuné, H.; Recasens, M.; Uhlhaas, P.J. The 40-Hz Auditory Steady-State Response in Patients with Schizophrenia. *JAMA Psychiatry* **2016**, *73*, 1145–1153. [CrossRef]
55. Parker, D.A.; Hamm, J.P.; McDowell, J.E.; Keedy, S.K.; Gershon, E.S.; Ivleva, E.I.; Pearlson, G.D.; Keshavan, M.S.; Tamminga, C.A.; Sweeney, J.A.; et al. Auditory Steady-State EEG Response Across the Schizo-Bipolar Spectrum. *Schizophr. Res.* **2019**, *209*, 218–226. [CrossRef] [PubMed]
56. Isomura, S.; Onitsuka, T.; Tsuchimoto, R.; Nakamura, I.; Hirano, S.; Oda, Y.; Oribe, N.; Hirano, Y.; Ueno, T.; Kanba, S. Differentiation between Major Depressive Disorder and Bipolar Disorder by Auditory Steady-State Responses. *J. Affect. Disord.* **2016**, *190*, 800–806. [CrossRef] [PubMed]
57. Rass, O.; Krishnan, G.; Brenner, A.C.; Hetrick, W.P.; Merrill, C.C.; Shekhar, A.; O'Donnell, B.F. Auditory Steady State Response in Bipolar Disorder: Relation to Clinical State, Cognitive Performance, Medication Status, and Substance Disorders. *Bipolar Disord.* **2010**, *12*, 793–803. [CrossRef] [PubMed]
58. Oda, Y.; Onitsuka, T.; Tsuchimoto, R.; Hirano, S.; Oribe, N.; Ueno, T.; Hirano, Y.; Nakamura, I.; Miura, T.; Kanba, S. Gamma Band Neural Synchronization Deficits for Auditory Steady State Responses in Bipolar Disorder Patients. *PLoS ONE* **2012**, *7*, e39955. [CrossRef]
59. Rojas, D.C.; Teale, P.D.; Maharajh, K.; Kronberg, E.; Youngpeter, K.; Wilson, L.B.; Wallace, A.; Hepburn, S. Transient and Steady-State Auditory Gamma-Band Responses in First-Degree Relatives of People with Autism Spectrum Disorder. *Mol. Autism* **2011**, *2*, 11. [CrossRef]
60. Seymour, R.A.; Rippon, G.; Gooding-Williams, G.; Sowman, P.F.; Kessler, K. Reduced Auditory Steady State Responses in Autism Spectrum Disorder. *Mol. Autism* **2020**, *11*, 1–13. [CrossRef]
61. Hong, L.E. Evoked Gamma Band Synchronization and the Liability for Schizophrenia*1. *Schizophr. Res.* **2004**, *70*, 293–302. [CrossRef]

62. Ono, Y.; Kudoh, K.; Ikeda, T.; Takahashi, T.; Yoshimura, Y.; Minabe, Y.; Kikuchi, M. Auditory Steady-State Response at 20 Hz and 40 Hz in Young Typically Developing Children and Children with Autism Spectrum Disorder. *Psychiatry Clin. Neurosci.* **2020**, *74*, 354–361. [CrossRef]

63. Stroganova, T.A.; Komarov, K.S.; Sysoeva, O.V.; Goiaeva, D.E.; Obukhova, T.S.; Ovsiannikova, T.M.; Prokofyev, A.O.; Orekhova, E.V. Left Hemispheric Deficit in the Sustained Neuromagnetic Response to Periodic Click Trains in Children with ASD. *Mol. Autism* **2020**, *11*, 1–22. [CrossRef] [PubMed]

64. Uhlhaas, P.J.; Haenschel, C.; Nikolić, D.; Singer, W. The Role of Oscillations and Synchrony in Cortical Networks and Their Putative Relevance for the Pathophysiology of Schizophrenia. *Schizophr. Bull.* **2008**, *34*, 927–943. [CrossRef] [PubMed]

65. Ross, B.; Fujioka, T. 40-Hz Oscillations Underlying Perceptual Binding in Young and Older Adults. *Psychophysiology* **2016**, *53*, 974–990. [CrossRef] [PubMed]

66. Baltus, A.; Herrmann, C.S. Auditory Temporal Resolution Is Linked to Resonance Frequency of the Auditory Cortex. *Int. J. Psychophysiol.* **2015**, *98*, 1–7. [CrossRef] [PubMed]

67. Light, G.A.; Hsu, J.L.; Hsieh, M.H.; Meyer-Gomes, K.; Sprock, J.; Swerdlow, N.R.; Braff, D.L. Gamma Band Oscillations Reveal Neural Network Cortical Coherence Dysfunction in Schizophrenia Patients. *Biol. Psychiatry* **2006**, *60*, 1231–1240. [CrossRef]

68. Tada, M.; Nagai, T.; Kirihara, K.; Koike, S.; Suga, M.; Araki, T.; Kobayashi, T.; Kasai, K. Differential Alterations of Auditory Gamma Oscillatory Responses Between Pre-Onset High-Risk Individuals and First-Episode Schizophrenia. *Cereb. Cortex* **2016**, *26*, 1027–1035. [CrossRef]

69. Koshiyama, D.; Kirihara, K.; Tada, M.; Nagai, T.; Fujioka, M.; Ichikawa, E.; Ohta, K.; Tani, M.; Tsuchiya, M.; Kanehara, A.; et al. Electrophysiological Evidence for Abnormal Glutamate-GABA Association Following Psychosis Onset. *Transl. Psychiatry* **2018**, *8*, 1–10. [CrossRef]

70. Filimonenko, Y.I.; Timofeev, V.I. *Wechsler Intelligence Scale for Children. Methodological Manual*; Imaton: Saint Petersburg, Russia, 2006; p. 112. (In Russian)

71. Constantino, J.N.; Davis, S.A.; Todd, R.D.; Schindler, M.K.; Gross, M.M.; Brophy, S.L.; Metzger, L.M.; Shoushtari, C.S.; Splinter, R.; Reich, W. Validation of a Brief Quantitative Measure of Autistic Traits: Comparison of the Social Responsiveness Scale with the Autism Diagnostic Interview-Revised. *J. Autism Dev. Disord.* **2003**, *33*, 427–433. [CrossRef] [PubMed]

72. Lord, C.; Rutter, M.; Le Couteur, A. Autism Diagnostic Interview-Revised: A Revised Version of a Diagnostic Interview for Caregivers of Individuals with Possible Pervasive Developmental Disorders. *J. Autism Dev. Disord.* **1994**, *24*, 659–685. [CrossRef]

73. Philippe, A.; Boddaert, N.; Vaivre-Douret, L.; Robel, L.; Danon-Boileau, L.; Malan, V.; De Blois, M.-C.; Heron, D.; Colleaux, L.; Golse, B.; et al. Neurobehavioral Profile and Brain Imaging Study of the 22q13.3 Deletion Syndrome in Childhood. *Pediatrics* **2008**, *122*, 376–382. [CrossRef] [PubMed]

74. Soorya, L.; Kolevzon, A.; Zweifach, J.; Lim, T.; Dobry, Y.; Schwartz, L.; Frank, Y.; Wang, A.T.; Cai, G.; Parkhomenko, E.; et al. Prospective Investigation of Autism and Genotype-Phenotype Correlations in 22q13 Deletion Syndrome and SHANK3 Deficiency. *Mol. Autism* **2013**, *4*, 18. [CrossRef] [PubMed]

75. Zwanenburg, R.J.; Ruiter, S.A.; Heuvel, E.R.V.D.; Flapper, B.C.; Van Ravenswaaij-Arts, C.M. Developmental Phenotype in Phelan-McDermid (22q13.3 Deletion) Syndrome: A Systematic and Prospective Study in 34 Children. *J. Neurodev. Disord.* **2016**, *8*, 16. [CrossRef] [PubMed]

76. Chen, C.-H.; Chen, H.-I.; Liao, H.-M.; Chen, Y.-J.; Fang, J.-S.; Lee, K.-F.; Gau, S.S.-F. Clinical and Molecular Characterization of Three Genomic Rearrangements at Chromosome 22q13.3 Associated with Autism Spectrum Disorder. *Psychiatr. Genet.* **2017**, *27*, 23–33. [CrossRef]

77. Okamoto, N.; Kubota, T.; Nakamura, Y.; Murakami, R.; Nishikubo, T.; Tanaka, I.; Takahashi, Y.; Hayashi, S.; Imoto, I.; Inazawa, J.; et al. 22q13 Microduplication in Two Patients with Common Clinical Manifestations: A Recognizable Syndrome? *Am. J. Med Genet. Part A* **2007**, *143*, 2804–2809. [CrossRef]

78. Destrée, A.; Hilbert, P.; Boulanger, S. A 273-kb Duplication at 22q13.33 Encompassing the Shank3 Gene in 2 Sibs with Microcephaly, Behavioral Disorder and Learning Disabilities. In Proceedings of European Society of Human Genetics Conference, Amsterdam, The Netherlands, 28–31 May 2011, P02.034. *Eur. J. Hum. Genet.* **2011**, *19*, 76.

79. Sarasua, S.M.; Boccuto, L.; Sharp, J.L.; Dwivedi, A.; Chen, C.-F.; Rollins, J.D.; Rogers, R.C.; Phelan, K.; Dupont, B.R. Clinical and Genomic Evaluation of 201 Patients with Phelan–McDermid Syndrome. *Qual. Life Res.* **2014**, *133*, 847–859. [CrossRef] [PubMed]

80. Kolevzon, A.; Angarita, B.; Bush, L.; Wang, A.T.; Frank, Y.; Yang, A.; Rapaport, R.; Saland, J.; Srivastava, S.; Farrell, C.; et al. Phelan-McDermid Syndrome: A Review of the Literature and Practice Parameters for Medical Assessment and Monitoring. *J. Neurodev. Disord.* **2014**, *6*, 39. [CrossRef] [PubMed]

81. Reierson, G.; Bernstein, J.; Froehlich-Santino, W.; Urban, A.; Purmann, C.; Berquist, S.; Jordan, J.; O'Hara, R.; Hallmayer, J. Characterizing Regression in Phelan McDermid Syndrome (22q13 Deletion Syndrome). *J. Psychiatr. Res.* **2017**, *91*, 139–144. [CrossRef] [PubMed]

82. Kolevzon, A.; Delaby, E.; Berry-Kravis, E.; Buxbaum, J.D.; Betancur, C. Neuropsychiatric Decompensation in Adolescents and Adults with Phelan-McDermid Syndrome: A Systematic Review of the Literature. *Mol. Autism* **2019**, *10*, 1–22. [CrossRef]

83. Hileman, C.M.; Henderson, H.A.; Mundy, P.; Newell, L.C.; Jaime, M. Developmental and Individual Differences on the P1 and N170 ERP Components in Children with and without Autism. *Dev. Neuropsychol.* **2011**, *36*, 214–236. [CrossRef] [PubMed]

84. Itier, R.J.; Taylor, M.J. Effects of Repetition and Configural Changes on the Development of Face Recognition Processes. *Dev. Sci.* **2004**, *7*, 469–487. [CrossRef] [PubMed]

85. Reese, M. Effects of Age, Gender, and Genotype on Auditory Processing in Phelan-McDermid Syndrome. Master's Thesis, University of Oklahoma, Norman, OK, USA, 2019.

86. Brittenham, C. Objective Measures of Electrophysiological Responses of Children with Idiopathic Autism Spectrum Disorder and Phelan-McDermid Syndrome to a Contrast-Reversing Checkerboard. Master's Thesis, Hunter College, University of New York, New York, NY, USA, 18 December 2017.

87. Siper, P.; George-Jones, J.; Lurie, S.; Rowe, M.; Durkin, A.; Weissman, J.; Meyering, K.; Rouhandeh, A.; Buxbaum, J.; Kolevzon, A. 23. Biomarker Discovery in ASD: Visual Evoked Potentials as a Biomarker of Phelan-McDermid Syndrome. *Biol. Psychiatry* **2018**, *83*, S9. [CrossRef]

88. Whitehouse, A.J.; Bishop, D.V. Do Children with Autism 'Switch off' to Speech Sounds? An Investigation Using Event-Related Potentials. *Dev. Sci.* **2008**, *11*, 516–524. [CrossRef] [PubMed]

89. Stroganova, T.A.; Kozunov, V.V.; Posikera, I.N.; Galuta, I.A.; Gratchev, V.V.; Orekhova, E.V. Abnormal Pre-Attentive Arousal in Young Children with Autism Spectrum Disorder Contributes to Their Atypical Auditory Behavior: An ERP Study. *PLoS ONE* **2013**, *8*, e69100. [CrossRef] [PubMed]

90. Madsen, G.F.; Bilenberg, N.; Jepsen, J.R.; Glenthøj, B.; Cantio, C.; Oranje, B. Normal P50 Gating in Children with Autism, Yet Attenuated P50 Amplitude in the Asperger Subcategory. *Autism Res.* **2015**, *8*, 371–378. [CrossRef] [PubMed]

91. Isenstein, E.; Durkin, A.; Zhang, Y.; Feldman, E.; Servedio, N.; Harony-Nicolas, H.; Buxbaum, J.; Kolevzon, A.; Siper, P.; Foss-Feig, J. T185. Electrophysiological Evidence of Auditory Habituation Abnormalities in Young Adults with Phelan-McDermid Syndrome. *Biol. Psychiatry* **2018**, *83*, S200. [CrossRef]

92. Ponson, L.; Gomot, M.; Blanc, R.; Barthelemy, C.; Roux, S.; Munnich, A.; Romana, S.; Aguillon-Hernandez, N.; Malan, V.; Bonnet-Brilhault, F. 22q13 Deletion Syndrome: Communication Disorder or Autism? Evidence from a Specific Clinical and Neurophysiological Phenotype. *Transl. Psychiatry* **2018**, *8*, 146. [CrossRef]

93. Griskova-Bulanova, I.; Dapsys, K.; Maciulis, V. Does Brain Ability to Synchronize with 40 Hz Auditory Stimulation Change with Age? *Acta Neurobiol. Exp.* **2013**, *73*, 564–570.

94. Poulsen, C.; Picton, T.W.; Paus, T. Age-Related Changes in Transient and Oscillatory Brain Responses to Auditory Stimulation during Early Adolescence. *Dev. Sci.* **2009**, *12*, 220–235. [CrossRef]

95. Maurizi, M.; Almadori, G.; Paludetti, G.; Ottaviani, F.; Rosignoli, M.; Lucianob, R. 40-Hz Steady-State Responses in Newborns and in Children. *Int. J. Audiol.* **1990**, *29*, 322–328. [CrossRef] [PubMed]

96. Stapells, D.; Herdman, A.; Small, S.; Dimitrijevic, A.; Hatton, J. *Current Status of the Auditory Steady-State Responses for Estimating an Infant's Audiogram*; Phonak: Zurich, Sweden, 2005; pp. 43–59.

97. Engineer, C.T.; Rahebi, K.C.; Borland, M.S.; Buell, E.P.; Im, K.W.; Wilson, L.G.; Sharma, P.; Vanneste, S.; Harony-Nicolas, H.; Buxbaum, J.D.; et al. Shank3-Deficient Rats Exhibit Degraded Cortical Responses to Sound. *Autism Res.* **2017**, *11*, 59–68. [CrossRef] [PubMed]

98. Griškova-Bulanova, I.; Rukšėnas, O.; Dapšys, K.; Mačiulis, V.; Arnfred, S.M. Distraction Task Rather Than Focal Attention Modulates Gamma Activity Associated with Auditory Steady-State Responses (ASSRs). *Clin. Neurophysiol.* **2011**, *122*, 1541–1548. [CrossRef] [PubMed]

99. Griskova, I.; Morup, M.; Parnas, J.; Ruksenas, O.; Arnfred, S.M. The Amplitude and Phase Precision of 40 Hz Auditory Steady-State Response Depend on the Level of Arousal. *Exp. Brain Res.* **2007**, *183*, 133–138. [CrossRef] [PubMed]

100. Bensmann, W.; Vahid, A.; Beste, C.; Stock, A.-K. The Intensity of Early Attentional Processing, but Not Conflict Monitoring, Determines the Size of Subliminal Response Conflicts. *Front. Hum. Neurosci.* **2019**, *13*, 13. [CrossRef]

101. Martin, B.A.; Tremblay, K.L.; Korczak, P. Speech Evoked Potentials: From the Laboratory to the Clinic. *Ear Hear.* **2008**, *29*, 285–313. [CrossRef]

102. Oostenveld, R.; Fries, P.; Maris, E.; Schoffelen, J.-M. FieldTrip: Open Source Software for Advanced Analysis of MEG, EEG, and Invasive Electrophysiological Data. *Comput. Intell. Neurosci.* **2010**, *2011*, 1–9. [CrossRef]

103. Griskova, I.; Morup, M.; Parnas, J.; Rukšėnas, O.; Arnfred, S.M.; Griškova-Bulanova, I. Two Discrete Components of the 20 Hz Steady-State Response Are Distinguished through the Modulation of Activation Level. *Clin. Neurophysiol.* **2009**, *120*, 904–909. [CrossRef]

104. Hirano, Y.; Nakamura, I.; Tamura, S.; Onitsuka, T. Long-Term Test-Retest Reliability of Auditory Gamma Oscillations Between Different Clinical EEG Systems. *Front. Psychiatry* **2020**, *11*, 11. [CrossRef]

105. Iourov, I.Y.; Vorsanova, S.G.; Korostelev, S.A.; Zelenova, M.A.; Yurov, Y.B. Long Contiguous Stretches of Homozygosity Spanning Shortly the Imprinted Loci Are Associated with Intellectual Disability, Autism and/or Epilepsy. *Mol. Cytogenet.* **2015**, *8*, 77. [CrossRef]

106. Iourov, I.Y.; Vorsanova, S.G.; Yurov, Y.B.; Zelenova, M.A.; Kurinnaia, O.S.; Vasin, K.S.; Kutsev, S.I. The Cytogenomic "Theory of Everything": Chromohelkosis May Underlie Chromosomal Instability and Mosaicism in Disease and Aging. *Int. J. Mol. Sci.* **2020**, *21*, 8328. [CrossRef] [PubMed]

107. Iourov, I.Y.; Vorsanova, S.G.; Voinova, V.Y.; Yurov, Y.B. 3p22.1p21.31 Microdeletion Identifies CCK as Asperger Syndrome Candidate Gene and Shows the Way for Therapeutic Strategies in Chromosome Imbalances. *Mol. Cytogenet.* **2015**, *8*, 82. [CrossRef] [PubMed]

108. Iourov, I.Y.; Vorsanova, S.G.; Yurov, Y.B. In Silico Molecular Cytogenetics: A Bioinformatic Approach to Prioritization of Candidate Genes and Copy Number Variations for Basic and Clinical Genome Research. *Mol. Cytogenet.* **2014**, *7*, 98. [CrossRef] [PubMed]

MDPI

St. Alban-Anlage 66

4052 Basel

Switzerland

Tel. +41 61 683 77 34

Fax +41 61 302 89 18

www.mdpi.com

International Journal of Molecular Sciences Editorial Office

E-mail: ijms@mdpi.com

www.mdpi.com/journal/ijms

9 783036 536118